T0220704

My Search

Susaik Chu

Order this book online at www.trafford.com
or email orders@trafford.com

Most Trafford titles are also available at major online book retailers.

Print information available on the last page.

ISBN: 978-1-4907-5584-7 (sc)
ISBN: 978-1-4907-5583-0 (hc)
ISBN: 978-1-4907-5585-4 (e)

Library of Congress Control Number: 2015902706

Trafford rev. 03/30/2016

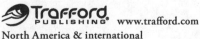

North America & international
toll-free: 1 888 232 4444 (USA & Canada)
fax: 812 355 4082

In God We Trust

To my children, Sirena and Shaun

Contents

Contents

Acknowledgments

All these years while I was searching to prove that allergies and sickness are from the white birch trees in our neighborhood and was serving the country from home, it was not easy for my two children, Sirena and Shaun, to support me physically and financially; they had to work hard to get themselves through higher education to get good jobs for their future. I am very pleased and grateful for their love and their strength in supporting me and helping me physically and financially all these years. I am very thankful to my two children, Sirena and Shaun; all my sisters and brothers; my godmother Ada Lundgren; and Dr. Thomas Tan for helping me when I needed them.

I would like to thank Renee Perko, the city attorney of the city of Pleasanton, Marlene Peterson, Charlene Swierkowski, and Cara Houck from Pleasanton Senior Supporting Group, who visited me all these years and saw the whole situation I had been through and how I suffered badly because of the allergies and sickness caused by my neighbor's white birch tree. I would like to thank and remember the elderly Catherine Nugent from Pleasanton, who gave her time to listen to my complaints about my allergies and sickness due to the birch trees. I would like to thank Dr. Ma Aye Myint and Dr. Teddy Young from Kaiser Permanente Medical group, who helped me identify the allergies and sickness that I got from the white birch trees. I would like to thank all the doctors, the nurses, the medical assistants, and the friends who helped me and protected me within their capacities.

Finally, I would like to thank all the readers who will read this book and will participate to pass the news to all their relatives, their friends, and their neighbors to persuade them to cut down the bad allergic birch family trees in their neighborhoods if they want to clean up the communities to provide a healthy environment for all the people who live in the communities. Only when we are healthy can we live happily.

Chapter One

Moving In

My family and I moved into a brand-new house in Pleasanton, California, in November 1984, after we moved out from King of Prussia, Pennsylvania, in early May 1984. My family was originally from California. My grandfather was an American, adopted by Chinese railroad workers. He worked with his adopted father in the railroad after he grew up. I discovered all the relatives from my grandfather side in California after we moved into this house. Senator George Hearst and Phoebe Apperson Hearst were my great-great-grandparents. William R. Hearst was my great-grandfather. Elaine Cohen was my great-grandmother, and Howard Hughes was my grand-uncle. My parents were Hee Chu and Kitty Chu. My parents went to Burma after they got married and lived in a small town called Mergui, situated in the southern part of Burma. They gave birth to nine children in Mergui. I was the youngest child in the family. My father was a mine owner. My mother was a housewife. My father did very well in his mining business. He brought home many hundred tons of wolfram from his mines each time he came back home. He invested all the money that he got from the mining business into the rubber plantation business. He also owned a pawn shop in Mergui. My father and his friends together started an elementary school in Mergui. They hired the best teachers to provide the best education to all the children. He hired an English teacher who came to our home to teach English to all the children. My father would dress me up like a boy. After I was born, each year, when he bought the materials to make shirts and pants for himself, he bought extra materials to make shirts and pants for me just like him. I did not go to school until

1

I was seven years old. I went to elementary school in Mergui. My parents moved all their children to Rangoon to attend a Catholic school. I grew up in the Catholic school. I graduated from elementary school in St. Emily Convent High School and graduated from middle and high school in St. Philomena Convent High School. I received my bachelor's degree, majoring in chemistry, from Rangoon Arts and Science University in 1970. After I graduated from the university, my mom insisted all of us to apply for immigration visas to go back to America. So we all applied for visa and came back to America in 1971. I lived in Philadelphia, Pennsylvania, with my sisters and my brother Edward Chu and his family. After one year, my sister Daisy Khaw and her family bought a house in King of Prussia. We all moved to King of Prussia in 1972.

I was working for J. C. Penney departmental store as an accountant clerk in audit department. Siok was working as a machinist in Philadelphia Gear Corporation after he moved to King of Prussia from California in 1972. I knew Siok since I was in university. We got married in 1973, and we lived in DeKalb Pike apartment. We bought a brand-new two-story house in General Scott Road, King of Prussia, after our first daughter Sirena was born. Sirena was born in Lankernau Hospital, Upper Merion County, Pennsylvania, in 1974. After we moved into our new house in King of Prussia, Siok designed and laid out the yard himself, planting a lot of floral trees. We took turns to take care of our daughter Sirena as we both were working. Siok took care of Sirena during the day while I went to work in J. C. Penney. After I came back from work at 5:00 p.m., I babysat Sirena, while Siok went to work until next morning. I miscarried a baby in 1976 after I lifted heavy boxes in the office. I felt very upset on losing my baby, so I quit my job and became a housewife. I took care of my daughter Sirena until my son Shaun was born. He was born in Sacred Heart Hospital, Norristown, Pennsylvania, in 1978. When I was five months' pregnant with Shaun, every day, amazingly, on and off, my room smelled of good perfume. I did not use any perfume at home. I did not know where the perfume smell came from, but it made me feel very comfortable. When I delivered Shaun, I did not feel any pain like I had done when I delivered Sirena. I took care of my two beautiful children, Sirena and Shaun that God gave me until they were quite a bit older. Then I went back to school to study my master's degree, majoring in computer science, in 1981 at Villanova University. I was lucky to have my two lovely children who understood that they had to take care of themselves when I went to school. Sirena took the responsibility of taking care of her brother while I was in school at night. They both watched television until 8:00 p.m. Then Sirena would turn off the light, and they both would sleep in my room. When I came back home from school at 9:00 p.m., both my children would be already asleep. I had to work hard to study. Finally, I received my master's degree diploma from Villanova University in December 1983. After I graduated from Villanova University, Siok and I decided to move our family to California. Siok contacted his longtime friend, Jim, who owned a moving and storage company in Oakland, for a job in his company. When Jim agreed to offer him a job in his company and move us out to California in his truck, we were very excited that we had got the chance to move ourselves to California. I informed all my sisters and brothers about my family moving to California real soon. Then I started to pack all our stuff that we needed to take to California and waited for Jim to call us to confirm the date for moving our household goods to California.

At the time when we decided to move to California, Sirena was in third grade, and Shaun was in kindergarten at Caley Road Elementary School in King of Prussia. Every day, I sent my children to school in the morning, and I picked Shaun in the afternoon. Sirena came home by herself after school. They took violin lessons at school and piano lessons at home with the piano teacher once a week. They practiced their piano and violin lessons at home after school. They both joined the scouts and attended the scout meeting once a week. I packed all our belongings all by myself at home when my children were at school. Siok did not have time to help me to pack because he had to work twelve hours a day, seven days a week. I just kept pulling out all the stuff that we needed to take to California from the cabinet shelves and packed in packing boxes every day. It took three months to get all the things to get ready to move. Finally, Jim called us to confirm the date in April when his truck driver would come and load all our household goods and belongings to move to California. We set a date to move to California in early May 1984. My children were excited that we were ready to move to California. They informed all their teachers and friends about our move to California. Jim's truck driver came in the end of April and loaded all our household goods on the truck and took them to California. We flew to California from Philadelphia in early May 1984. We lived in a Fremont apartment until we bought a house in Pleasanton.

When we moved into this new house in late 1984, Siok carefully designed our yard to plant the bushes and the trees to match the structure of our house. Siok planted the slow-growing trees and bushes such as cherry trees, tropical trees, Japanese maples, cypress trees, evergreen trees, carnations, camellias, azaleas, lily, iris, and other green bushes. They all were very healthy, beautiful flowering plants. After six months, Mr. Ackerman and his family moved into the house on the right side of our house. He planted three white birch trees in his left-side yard close to our garage. When he met Siok after he planted the white birch trees, he told Siok that the birch trees were medicinal trees and that Native American people used the birch leaves as tea and medicines. After Siok heard this news, he believed Mr. Ackerman and brought home two small paper birch trees and planted in our backyard. They were fast-growing trees and very messy. Years went by and our paper birch trees grew very big. I also saw a lot of birch trees were planted in our community. All these trees were getting so big, just like our paper birch trees. Siok would take care of the outside lawn and yard. After he was done working in the lawn, he would complain his face and body were itching. Sometimes, lots of rashes formed on his both hands, sometimes on his whole face and body. When Siok was not at home, my son Shaun took care of the lawn for me. Shaun complained that he got a bad itch and allergy rashes on his face after working in the outside yard. Siok and Shaun kept on complaining about the bad itch and the allergy rashes forming on their faces and bodies after they worked outside in the yard. They both told me that something, about which they did not know, was in the outside air that caused a bad itch and allergy rashes on their faces and bodies. After I heard the complaints from Siok and Shaun, I talked to the people in my neighborhood about the bad itch and allergies. They told me they also got bad itch and allergies on their bodies when they worked outside in their yards, and they also did not know what was in the air that was causing them the bad itch and allergies.

Siok and I bought a moving and storage company in Benicia after we moved out to Pleasanton. After our moving and storage company picked up the businesses from the corporations and was growing, we moved our company to Livermore. I worked with Siok in Best-way International Moving and Storage Company in Livermore. We met a lot of good people in Tri Valley. In particular, I was very lucky to meet my godmother Ada Lundgren and elderly Catherine Nugent in Pleasanton. My godmother

Ada was a navy captain's wife. Catherine was an elderly who was a retired school teacher from Amador High School. They had both lived in Pleasanton almost all their lives. I got to know elderly Catherine in Pleasanton Women Club when my godmother Ada took me to join the club. I met her in Ada's house several times when they both were working on a project for their Baptist Church. I got to know her so well, and I liked her a lot. I would talk to her on the phone almost every week. Catherine was different from Ada; she had a lot of knowledge in different fields. She would listen to me patiently whenever I called her and talked to her. She would always guide me to do what was best for me. She would explain to me a lot of things that I did not know; she would advise me on solving the problems that I faced. She was the person that I could rely on very much.

My godmother Ada was a very energetic and outgoing lady. She joined all kind of churches and went out to meet and made friends with a lot of people. She always liked to take me to visit her aunt Bertha in Pleasanton Convalescent Home. When we visited her aunt, she would always go to the nearby garden to pick flowers from the floral tree without asking for permission from the owner. Then she would take the flowers inside the convalescent home to give her aunt and other elderlies. The way she did that really scared me. I told her she should not do this. She laughed and said there was nothing to be afraid of. She said that she had been living in Pleasanton so long that almost all people from her church and her neighbors knew her quite well and was very friendly with her and that no one complained and said anything to her. I remember that I carried my two cockatiel birds, Sunny and Shadow, while visiting Aunt Bertha to show her. Shadow flew away in front of the convalescent home when I took Sunny and Shadow out from my car. Ada and I looked for Shadow in front of the convalescent home and nearby areas and could not find him, but we heard his weeping voice on the tree in front of the convalescent home. So I just took Sunny inside the convalescent home to show Aunt Bertha. Aunt Bertha loved Sunny so much. She played with Sunny after I put the bird on her arm. Ada went over to the nurses of the convalescent home to let them know we had lost a cockatiel bird in front of the convalescent home. She gave them her telephone number and requested them to call her if they saw the cockatiel bird in the outside yard of the convalescent home or anywhere nearby. The nurses agreed to call her and then we left.

After we came out from the convalescent home, we looked for Shadow again. One of the nurses came out and told us that she had just seen Shadow on the tree branches crying out loudly and then flying away toward the back of the convalescent home. I told Ada that I would bring Shaun to the convalescent home after he came back from school to look for Shadow. She told me she would inform all her neighbors and friends about Shadow being lost and would request them to inform her if they saw Shadow in the surrounding areas. I dropped Ada in her house and went home with Sunny, without Shadow. When Shaun came back from school, I told him that Shadow was lost in the convalescent home when we had been visiting Ada's aunt. He cried bitterly and asked me to take him to the convalescent home to look for Shadow. I took him to the convalescent home. When we reached there, we heard Shadow weeping somewhere near the convalescent home. Shaun kept on calling loudly, "Shadow! Shadow! Shadow!" When Shadow heard Shaun's voice, he cried out loudly, responding to him. We followed the direction of Shadow's weeping voice and walked to the backyard of the convalescent home. But we could not find him. There was a small hill behind the convalescent home. As it was dark, we decided against climbing the hill and returned home. When I took Sirena and Shaun to Ada's house during the weekend, Shaun kept on crying in front of Ada when he saw her and told her that I had lost his cockatiel bird Shadow and that he wanted his Shadow back. When Ada saw him crying, she promised him that she would get another cockatiel bird to replace Shadow. But Shaun told her he did not want any replacement bird and just wanted Shadow back, and he kept on crying. She could not console him and stop his crying. Then she promised that she would find Shadow for him. After we left Ada's house, Ada drove around her neighborhood, looking for Shadow. She kept telling all her friends to call her if they saw the cockatiel bird. I took Shaun to the convalescent home almost every day after he would come back home from school. We kept looking at the places where we heard Shadow's weeping voice. We went to the convalescent home again during the weekend at noon time. We climbed up the small hill behind the convalescent home. Shaun kept on calling, "Shadow! Shadow! Shadow!" When Shadow heard Shaun's voice, he responded back in his weeping voice from a tree on the top of the hill behind the convalescent home. We climbed up all the way to the top of the hill, following the direction of Shadow's weeping voice. Shadow's weeping voice was getting closer and closer when we were on top of the hill. Then when we stopped under a big tree, Shadow's weeping voice got louder and louder. From Shadow's voice, we knew that he was somewhere very close-by. Shaun kept calling him, and we kept looking around the surroundings. Suddenly, Shadow jumped down from the tree and landed on Shaun's shoulder. When Shaun turned around and saw Shadow on his shoulder, he was so happy. He gripped Shadow in his hands and kissed Shadow. Then we went down the hill behind the convalescent home and went home. Shaun was very grateful and happy to get Shadow back from the wild environment near the place where we had lost him. After we were home, he settled Shadow with Sunny in the cage. Then he called Ada to inform her he had got Shadow back. Ada was very happy to hear that. She told Shaun and me that she had been driving around in her neighborhood almost every day looking for Shadow. She was very grateful and relieved to hear we got Shadow back from the wild environment. She told all her friends that we had got Shadow back from the wild. She had so many friends to keep her busy in this city and nearby cities. She did not have much time to listen to my problems and my complaints, but she loved me and my family dearly and supported me whatever I did. Whenever I needed her help, she was always there for me. After my car accident, she took me to the farm when Sirena was busy and could not take me to the farm. Catherine and Ada both were very conservative, sincere, and kind persons. I have so many things to talk about both of them. I did not have anything to complain about them. I loved both of them so much. They were my family members in Pleasanton.

I stopped commuting to Livermore office and worked at home in early 1993, after an employee Randy J. from our company forced me to issue him a check to pay him. Randy had his own moving and storage company in southern California. I did not understand why Siok hired him and Phil S. to work for our company. I did not know how Siok set up their contracts to deal with the company. I heard from Siok that he had hired Randy J. as salesman and Phil S. as traffic manager to work for our company. After they worked in the office, they took over all the accounts of the company. When Randy came to me and asked me to issue a check for him, I suggested that he should talk to Siok first to get the approval before asking me to cut a check for him. He refused to talk to Siok and kept insisting me to cut the check for him. I told him I would not cut any check without Siok's approval. Then he left. Phil S. also came to me and asked me to issue the checks for him again without the approval from Siok. I was getting upset and frustrated every time they came to me, asking me to issue the checks for them without getting approval from Siok. I felt this was not a good idea to let the employee keep asking me to cut the checks for them without any approval from their boss in the office. Hence, I decided to move back home, and I started working from home. After I moved back home, I worked in my study room. I worked hard to manage the company to let it grow big. We kept the company so busy under our management. The truck drivers brought in a lot of household goods to our Livermore warehouse every day. I asked Siok to bring home all the paperwork from the office when he came home. I designed the computer programming for my company and took care of all the company accounts and payroll.

My right-side neighbor planted three big birch trees next to my garage and my study room. I used to open the window when I was working in my study room. My seat faced the opposite side of the garage. The study room window was on my left side and my left ear toward the study room window. After I worked a period of time in my study room, my left ear started to itch and got infected badly. A lot of fluid started flowing out of my infectious ear. I called my brother, Dr. Harvey Chu, to tell him that my ear had got infected badly. He sent out allergy and antibiotic medicines to me by mail. After I received the medicines, I took them as instructed by Harvey, but it did not stop my ear infection. I called him again to let him know that my allergy and left ear infection were getting worse. I told him the medicines that he had mailed to me did not help my ear infection get better. The black liquid kept flowing out of my left infectious ear.

My sister Rosie Yip and my brother Dr. Harvey Chu came to California and took me to New York on September 14, 1994, to stay with Harvey in New York. I did not have any say regarding my trip to New York to live with Harvey. I just went with my sister and brother to New York. After I arrived in New York, I stayed with Harvey. The first thing Harvey did was ask all his sons to find the best ear surgeon in New York to take care of my infectious ear. After one week, one of his sons, Dr. Mark Chu, got the information about Dr. Lins, C. J. (MD, CM, FRCS, FACS), from his friends and informed his father, Harvey, that Dr. Lins of New York Eye and Ear Infirmary National Care Medical Center (NYEAEINCMC) on East Fourteenth Street, New York, was one of the best doctors in New York to take care of patients with ear infections. Harvey asked Mark to set up an appointment for me to see Dr. Lins. After Mark set up the appointment with Dr. Lins, Harvey, Rosie, and Harvey's wife, Margaret Chu, took me to see Dr. Lins to check on my left ear. After Dr. Lins checked my left ear, he told Harvey that he needed to do the surgery in my left ear because of the bad infection. My brother Harvey agreed to let Dr. Lins operate my ear. Before my ear surgery, I had to take CAT scan X-ray of my ears. Harvey, Margaret, and Rosie took me to the hospital radiology department to take CAT scan X-ray first. After I was done taking CAT scan X-ray, they took me to see Dr. Noel E. T. (Psychiatry and Psychopharmacology) in Beth Medical Center (BMC), Tenth Avenue and Fourteenth Street, New York. When I was in Dr. Noel's clinic, she asked me to tell her anything I wanted to tell her.

I told her that I did not have anything to tell her, because I did not do anything wrong while I was working in my company in California. I explained to her that on the day the police officer pulled me into the psychiatric hospital I just went in to my company to get the truck driver John's time card that I had not got it from Siok when he came home. I kept calling the office, asking the clerk for John's time card for almost three months. I was getting upset that I had not got the time card from the office. I drove my car to the office. When I arrived at the office, Siok blocked me in front of the company door and did not let me go inside the company. I was upset, and I pushed him away and just went into my office, looking for John's time card. But I could not find it. All the paperwork and time cards were piled up in one corner of the office. No one was taking care of them. Hence, I asked Siok in the office where the driver John's time card was. He did not give me any answer. Then I went back home without getting the time card, which I needed to check and adjust the payroll for John, so I called the office again to ask the clerk for John's time card. I asked her whether she understood my language or not. She did not say anything. I told her that I had been asking her a couple of months to get John's time card for me and I still had not got the right time card from her. So I told her to leave the company if she could not understand what I was asking her to do, and then I hung up the phone. After a while, I called the office again because I needed John's time card. The office clerk picked up the phone again. After I heard her voice, I told her to leave the company. Then I drove in my car to the office to find John's time card. I saw John was working on his truck outside the company. I called him to talk to him. He came to my car and talked to me. I asked him how he liked his job and how he was doing in the company. He started telling me he was doing fine and was very happy to work for our company. While I was talking to John, I saw two police cars pull up and park behind my car. One of the police officers got down from his car. He came to me and asked me to give him my driving license. I did not know what was happening. I gave him my driving license. He took my driving license and left. I called him and asked him what was happening. He turned around his head and looked at me. Then he ignored me and walked to his car. I opened my car door and asked him again, "Sir, what happened?" He came to me and accused me he did not like the way I used my finger to point at him. He caught my right hand and pulled me out of my car. He pushed my body so that I faced my car and used the criminal chain to lock both my hands and then locked me inside the police car. I asked him loudly to let me out of the police car. Lots of people from other companies came out and stood near the police car, watching me. No one came to help me. I just had to stay inside the police car. The police officer must have called the ambulance. After half an hour, the ambulance arrived. An employee from the ambulance opened its back door and took out the bed from it. Then they pulled me out from the police car and forced me to lie down on the ambulance bed. I tried to get up from the ambulance bed and suggested that he let me go. But they tied my hands and body with the ambulance bed's belts. Then they pushed the ambulance bed inside the ambulance van and took me to Alameda County Psychiatric Hospital. After I arrived in the Alameda County Psychiatric Hospital, they treated me like a criminal. They locked both my hands and legs on the criminal beds. They kept asking me the reason that the police officer brought me into the psychiatric hospital. I kept telling them the same answer that I did not know and I did not understand the reason the police officer got so upset with me after I asked him what was happening. I also told them how he had accused me of pointing my finger at him and taken me to the psychiatric hospital. I told them that I did not point my finger at the police officer. No one would point their fingers at somebody when they are asking a question. They would just flip their hands to ask the questions. Then I showed them in action how I flipped over my both hands and repeatedly explained to them I had never pointed my finger at him. Then I realized the police officer must have got a call from somebody accusing me of something that I did not know about.

Then they asked me to stay in my room until the next day when Ada and Siok came to visit me in the psychiatric hospital. After three days, Rosie and Harvey came to California and visited me. They told me they would pick me up from the psychiatric hospital and take me to New York the next day. As said, they came and took me to New York. I explained to Dr. Noel about the police officer in California and how I ended in jail. After I talked to Dr. Noel about the police officer, she did not say anything and released me. I went back to Harvey's clinic with Harvey, Margaret, and Rosie. Then Rosie and I went back to Harvey's home by bus.

Dr. Lins called Harvey after he received and reviewed my ears' CAT scan X-rays. He was amazed and informed Harvey about what he had found from the CAT scan X-rays. He told Harvey that I did not have an eardrum in my left ear and it was infected badly. He also added that he would have to operate my left ear to clean up the infection right away and to replace a new skin eardrum in my left ear. Harvey agreed to let him perform the ear surgery. He set the surgery date for me. After Harvey heard from Dr. Lins that I did not have an eardrum in my left ear, he got very upset. He pointed his finger at me and yelled at me as to why I had pointed my finger at the police officer. He said to me in a very upset tone that it was so bad that I let the police officer hurt me and lose my ear drum. I looked at him and the way he was getting so upset. I reminded him to look at his own finger himself, just to let him know what was called pointing the finger at somebody. Harvey looked at his own finger and realized that he was pointing his finger at me. Then I explained to him that I did not point my finger at the police officer when I called him and asked him about the situation in front of our company, and then I used my hands to show Harvey how I had flipped over my hands when I asked the question to the police officer. Then he asked me what had happened on that day before the police officer took me to the psychiatric hospital. I explained to him all that had happened on that day. Then Harvey asked me whether I knew I had lost my eardrum. I told him I did not know about that and also informed him that my left ear had been itching badly all the time and was infected quite bad with black and yellow fluid flowing out, after I started to work from home in my study room. Then Harvey told me I had to perform ear surgery on my left ear. I looked at him and said OK.

Harvey, Margaret, and Rosie took me to NYEAEINCMC early in the morning for my ear surgery on the day that they had set up for me.

Harvey helped me to check in at the hospital front desk and took care of all the paperwork. They took me upstairs to the third floor to check in with the administration nurse. Then the nurse took me to the surgery room. Harvey went back to his office to take care of his patients in his clinic. Rosie and Margaret stayed in the hospital's waiting room for the whole day until I was done with my surgery. Dr. Lins took more than six hours to clean and fix my eardrum during my ear surgery. After my surgery, the nurses pushed my bed out of the surgery room to the hallway and tried to wake me up. I woke up a little bit, looked at the nurse, and went back to sleep. Then the nurse tried to wake me up again after half an hour. I woke up and looked at her again. I was just about to go back to sleep when I saw Harvey come in from the hallway. Then I told the nurse to help me get dressed right away to go home. The nurse told me to wait for a while. She said I did not look good, but I insisted her to help me get dressed. So she helped me to change my clothing and get dressed. After I was done, she said to me I had looked terrible a moment ago after the surgery. She prepared all the release paperwork to get ready and gave them to me. She released me to go home. Harvey, Margaret, and Rosie took me home. Harvey settled me inside the room to let me get more privacy and rest. Every morning, Harvey checked on my left ear to change the Band-Aid for me before he went to his clinic with Margaret. Rosie stayed home with me and took care of me.

On my next checkup date with Dr. Lins, Harvey, Margaret, and Rosie took me to see Dr. Lins. Dr. Lins checked my left ear and said to Harvey that while he was operating my left ear, the fluid kept flowing out badly even after he had prescribed me a strong antibiotic medicine before the surgery. He said my ear was really infected so bad that it took him quite a bit of time to clean up all the infectious area in my ear. Then he mentioned about his regular patients from Southern America, who got ear infections and kept coming back to him for their ear surgeries. He said he believed most of these people's ear infections were caused by plants, but he did not know the patients' activities and how their ears got infected all the time. Dr. Lins knew the plants were the main source, which caused his patients' ears to get infected, but he did not mention the type of plants that caused those ear infections.

While I was in New York, Rosie stayed with me in Harvey's house and took care of me. We did not have anything to do every day, so being restless, we walked to the Queen mall near Harvey's house to spend our time inside the mall and ate all kind of foods from different restaurants. Every week, Harvey, Margaret, and Rosie took me to see Dr. Noel in her clinic. Every time I was in Dr. Noel's clinic, I repeatedly told her I did not have anything to tell her, because I was a quiet person, and I did not do anything wrong to harm anybody. I told her that I was just worried and tried to get things done for the company. I tried very hard to help and manage the company, guided our employees to do the right things, and helped them to solve their problems when they were in need. The truck drivers who worked with us were very happy to come to our company and were very friendly to us. They tried to deliver their household goods to our warehouse as much as they could to fill up our warehouse. I kept telling her about the incident with the police officer in front of our company in Livermore. I explained to her that I did not dare to point my finger at any person to demand them to do anything for me. I had never hurt any person. I did not have any intention to hurt anybody. She told me not to worry about anything after I kept on explaining to her about the incident with the police officer in front of my company in California. She said she wanted me to fix my ear to get well. I thanked her. Then I mentioned to her about the purple color chicken wire shape that I saw every time when I looked at the sky. She told me not to say any nonsense thing, but I told her it was a true fact and that I did see a purple color chicken wire shape above the sky. Dr. Noel told me not to say anything. Then she released me. Rosie and Harvey asked me whether I got relief from the stress or not after I talked to Dr. Noel. I said I felt much better after I talked to Dr. Noel. They both looked at me and were very pleased to see me feeling better.

Every day, I called my son Shaun in California between three and four o'clock to make sure he was home after school and studied his homework. Shaun told me he went to Pleasanton Library to study after his dinner every day. Every weekend, all my sisters, brothers, and their families came to visit me at Harvey's house. When they heard that I had lost my eardrum, they were all very upset. They gave me money and asked me to buy things that I needed for myself while I was in New York. I stayed in New York until my ear was in good condition. After both my doctors, Dr. Noel and Dr. Lins, released me to go back to California, Rosie took me to King of Prussia, Pennsylvania, to stay with her for three weeks, waiting for Sirena to pick me up in King of Prussia during her winter break in December. Then Sirena came during her winter break and stayed at Rosie's house with me for one week. Sirena and I went home to California in early January 1995.

I stayed in New York for three months. After I came back home from Pennsylvania, Siok refused to let me work in the company again. I stopped going to office and stayed at home. I had very little conversation with him after I came back from New York. I did not know the reason he did not want me to go to the company again. While I was in New York, Shaun had started raising fighting fishes and a lot of other big fishes in a hundred-gallon water fish tank at home. After I came back from New York, I bought some more gold fishes to put in his tank. I watched and studied them every day and played with them. I went to Eddie's fish shop in Pleasanton to buy small gold fishes and worms for the big fishes at home. One day, when I was in the fish shop, I talked to Eddie about my study regarding allergies and sickness. There was a very sick fish in the tank. Eddie told me that fish was very sick. He was just about to take it out from the fish tank to throw it away. I told him I would like to keep that sick fish. He said OK and let me have it. I took that fish home and kept it in a small plastic bowl. Then I hung the sick fish bowl in the big fish tank. Next day, I cleaned the fish tank and pumped out all the water from the fish tank. When I used the pipe from my backyard to refill the new water in the tank, accidentally, the plastic bowl with the sick fish in it dropped into the big tank. I picked up the sick fish from the big tank and put it back in the plastic bowl, hanging the plastic bowl back in the big fish tank. Next day, I saw the water in the plastic bowl and the fish tank had turned to a milky white color, and the sick fish in the plastic bowl had died. I did not know the reason the water in the fish tank had changed into a milky white color. I just kept the milky water in the tank. After a few days, a white, cloudy, silky fungus grew inside the tank so fast that they filled up the whole hundred-gallon fish tank. All of Shaun's valuable big fishes died inside the tank. I took all the dead fishes out from the tank and threw them away. Then I used a cloth to clean the four sides of the tank, and I filled up the fish tank with clean water. After a few days, the white, cloudy fungus grew again inside the tank. I cleaned up the fish tank and filled up with clean water. I bought some more gold fishes and put them inside the same fish tank. The cloudy fungus grew again inside the fish tank. All my gold fishes inside the fish tank died within two days. Then I cleaned the fish tank again and again until I felt it was really clean. Then I put in new water and new fishes again. But the white fungus grew again, and all my fishes died. I realized I could not use this fish tank to raise the fishes again, so I dumped out all the water from the tank and left it to dry. Every time I cleaned the fish tank with my hands, I washed my hands with soap and warm water. The white fungus from the fish tank did not cause any allergy to me.

We had eight cockatiel birds at home before I went to New York. After I came back from New York, there were only seven cockatiels left in the cage in our backyard. Sirena and Shaun told me about the female cockatiel Stacey that flew away when they took her out from the cage. They looked for her in our backyard. They had also heard her weeping voice in our backyard, but they could not locate where she was. They lost her. Then when I went outside my backyard to check on these birds, I found another male cockatiel Sebastian shaking badly inside the cage. He seemed like he was very scared, and his whole body was shaking. I took him out of the cage and brought him inside the house. I fed him one small piece of Advil pain reliever. Then I kept him inside a basket and covered him with a small blanket inside my house, but he was still shaking badly. I kept him in my room at night with me, but I still could not comfort him. He was getting really sick. Next day, I put some pieces of rice in front of him to eat, but he did not eat. I pushed a small piece of rice in his food pouch, but he threw out the rice. When Siok found out Sebastian was very sick, he took him to the vet. The vet kept him in the clinic overnight and called us to let us know he would not eat or drink anything and his body was still shaking no matter how she tried to cover him with a blanket. The following day, the vet called again to let us know Sebastian had died. I was very upset after hearing that Sebastian had died. I went to the bookstore and bought some books about cockatiel birds to study. I read and studied the book carefully to find the source of sickness that had caused Sebastian to die. Then I remembered a few days ago I had seen a big hawk landing on top of the bird's cage in our backyard. All the birds saw the big hawk, but they all stayed inside the cage quiet as usual except Sebastian. He was shaking badly when I went outside to check on them. Sebastian must have got hurt during the hawk's attack. I did not check his body to find out if he was hurt by the hawk or not after I found him shaking. I believed Sebastian was scared and choked to dead after he saw the big hawk in our backyard. I still remember how my two adult male cockatiels, Shadow and Sky, fought for three eggs to hatch. These two male cockatiels took turns to hatch the three eggs. Three baby cockatiels came out from the eggs after fifteen days. Sebastian was one of the babies from the three eggs. All male and female cockatiels took turns to feed the three baby birds. Every day, I spent time to play with those three baby cockatiels. They were very tame and cute. I fed them with my hands when they cried for food. Sometimes they fell asleep in my hands. They helped me to get rid of my stress and worry after I was home all these years.

After Shaun graduated from Amador High School and went to Davis University in Davis city, I was at home alone with Siok. I felt that I was wasting my time not doing anything at home. While I was playing with my baby birds, I got an idea to build an incubator myself to raise different kind of birds. I designed the bird incubator in early 1997. I tried to organize all the materials I needed for my incubator, using my own imagination. Then I went to Home Depot store and Orchard Supply Hardware store to buy the materials that I needed to build my incubator. After I got all the materials, I assembled my first glass incubator at home with my son Shaun. It took me three months to assemble and build the glass incubator. I bought the eggs from the supermarket and put them in my first incubator to test if they would hatch eggs. I did not get any baby chick. I asked Shaun to buy more chicken eggs from the supermarket to hatch in my incubator. He bought the eggs for me to hatch in my glass incubator. I still did not get any baby chick from those eggs bought from the supermarket. When I talked to a friend from New York about my incubator, my friend reminded me not to use the eggs from the supermarket to hatch in the incubator. He said those eggs from the supermarket were already hatched in the incubator. After I hung up the phone with my friend, I went to Pleasanton farmers' market to look for fresh eggs to hatch. I found the eggs of quails and ducks in the farmers' market. I bought two packs of quail eggs and two duck eggs home to test them in my glass incubator. When I was testing my glass incubator with the chicken eggs from the farmers' market, I knew my incubator would work and I would get a lot of baby chicks later. So I built another incubator of wood while I was testing my glass incubator. After I finished assembling my wooden incubator, I went to Pleasanton farmers' market almost every week to buy more quail eggs to hatch in my wooden incubator. I bought duck eggs to hatch in my glass incubator. I kept adding new quail eggs each week in my wooden incubator and duck eggs in my glass incubator. After one month, on May 30, 1997, I saw a shadow run to the back of the shelf and disappear behind the quail eggs in the wooden incubator. I opened the door and looked inside the incubator. I did not see anything. I closed the incubator door and went to the farmers' market to get more quail eggs. After I came back from the farmers' market, I opened my wooden incubator to find out what the shadow was. I saw a baby quail with a tall and skinny body, hiding among the quail eggs in the inner shelf of the wooden incubator. I was so happy to see my first incubated baby quail. I took him out from the wooden incubator in the garage and brought him to my kitchen to feed him. Then I named him Su-Nee right away, after I took him out from the wooden incubator in my garage. I picked "Su" word from my first name and "Nee" word from Angel's songs that I heard every day. Once in the kitchen, I took one small piece of cooked rice from the rice cooker to feed him. He did not eat the rice. I was worried because he was my first incubated baby bird, and I valued him and wanted him to eat. After I found out he would not eat the food himself, I went to Long Drug store to buy two small tubes right away. I came home, cooked rice soup, and tried to feed him with the tube. But unfortunately, he died in my hands while I was feeding him. I was very upset to see my first baby bird die. I preserved his body in vodka alcohol in a glass bottle and kept it in my garage shelf. Since I did not know how many days the eggs needed to hatch in the incubator to get the baby, I realized I should check my incubator every day to make sure there were babies inside the incubator. After two weeks, two more baby quails came out from their eggs in my wooden incubator. I named them Su-Na and Su-Nee. I called my children to let them know my wooden incubator worked well. I got the first alive two baby quails from my wooden incubator. I fed them cooked rice every day. They were getting big. Sue-Nee was a male quail and was very naughty. He liked to use his claws to attack me when I played with him. But Su-Na was very quiet; she liked to stay on my hands when I held her up.

When my niece Nolana Yip from Pennsylvania visited me on July 4, 1997, I took her to Alameda county fair with Shaun to look for the baby chicks in the agriculture section of Alameda county fair. They had all kinds of baby birds in the agriculture show room. I bought two male and female baby chicks. Nolana insisted on paying for the chicks, so I let her pay for these two chicks. After I was home, I thought about how to name them. I had to use the first letter of Nolana to name the chicks since she had paid for the chicks. I named the male chick as Nicky and the female chick as Necky. I raised them in my family room inside the bird cage. Then I got my first two baby ducklings Su-Yee and Su-Mi from the glass incubator after twenty-one days of hatching. When I found them inside the incubator, their whole bodies were still wet, and they tried to push themselves out from their eggshells. I took them out from the incubator, washed them with clean water, dried them with my dryer, fed them the cooked rice, and kept them inside the plastic box in my room. Next day, I saw them walking around inside the plastic box. They were very healthy ducklings and were growing fast. They kept making the "quack, quack" sound inside the box. After a couple of months, I had to keep them in the crib outside my backyard. But I found my duckling Su-Mi was missing the next morning. I looked around in my backyard to search for the baby duckling but could not find her. I only found the feathers and some small portions of my duckling's body left in the right side of my yard. I believed my neighbor's cat must have grabbed her out from the crib at night and eaten her. I was so upset. I went over to the cat's owner's house to complain to them about how their cat had killed my baby duckling and eaten it.

When I went to Alameda County Fair to look for the baby chicks in the agriculture section, I got the information about Mr. Larmar Stephenson from Tracy, California. I decided to call Mr. Stephenson to buy fresh chicken eggs from him if he had any in their farm. I called him in late July 1997. Mrs. Joyce Stephenson picked up the phone. I introduced myself to her and told her about my incubator that I had built and that I would like to buy some fresh eggs from her to hatch in my incubator. She said she had chicken eggs in their farms and promised me to provide eggs for free right away to help me to test my incubator. She told me to go to her farm to get the eggs right away and gave me the directions to go to their farm in Tracy. I drove myself to their farmhouse. When I reached Tracy, I saw all different kinds of big birds running around in the nearby farms even before I reached their house.

I parked my car in front of Mr. Stephenson's house. I saw Joyce was busy in the farm, feeding the birds. I got down from my car to go to her and introduced myself to her. She was a very nice and sincere lady. She welcomed me with a warm heart. She took me inside her house, asked me to sit down on the kitchen chair, and offered me a cup of hot tea. She told me that Mr. Stephenson was taking care of their farm. She asked me to wait for Mr. Stephenson to come inside the house so that he could talk to me. As soon as Mr. Stephenson came in from outside, Joyce introduced me to Mr. Stephenson. He was a very nice and sincere man, just like his wife. They both were very friendly to me and told me they would help me by providing fresh bird's eggs. They took me to their farm and showed me all their different kinds of birds. Their farmland was really big. Some of their big birds took over their neighboring farms and were running freely. Mr. Stephenson told me that after he had retired from the United States military he moved to Tracy with his wife. They had spent their time in the farmland raising different kinds of birds. They had so many different kinds of chickens, ducks, cockatiels, peacocks, and many other kinds of big birds whose names I did not know. They told me there was a lot of work involved in maintaining the farm and it was not an easy job to do the cleaning. I told them I knew this would not be easy and that I would like to get some eggs from them to try and hatch them in my glass incubator. Mr. Stephenson told me not to worry about the chicken eggs and that he would provide me as many eggs as I wanted from their farm. Then he took me to their big chicken farm buildings and showed me all their different kinds of chickens, explaining to me how they had raised the birds in their farm. I had never seen some of the chickens inside the farm in my life before. Mr. Stephenson took all the eggs from that they had collected in the morning the farm building and then took me to the garage to show me his small incubator in the garage. He said he had to use his hands to flick the eggs every day after he put all the fresh eggs in the incubator to hatch the eggs. Then he opened his incubator cover and showed me how he had to use his hands to flick the chicken eggs in the small incubator, and he then asked me how my incubators were built and worked. I told him I had built two big incubators and I did not need to flick or turn my eggs in the incubator just like him. I just distributed the heat to all the eggs inside the incubator to hatch the eggs. He asked me why I did not flick my eggs. He said he had seen all the female chickens using their legs to turn the eggs once in a while to hatch the eggs. I said that may be the chickens were using their legs to move the eggs to the comfortable places, which made them easy to hatch in the real world. But there were white and yellow gels inside the eggs. It did not make any difference whether the eggs were flicked or turned or not. After he heard what I said, he laughed, feeling stupid on flicking or turning the eggs. He put all the chicken eggs that he had collected in the morning inside the paper bag and gave it to me. I took the paper bag from him and thanked them. Then he asked me to come to their farm if I needed more eggs. I told them I would come to get more eggs until I got some baby chicks from my incubator. I thanked them and came home.

I put all their chicken eggs in my glass incubator to incubate them right away. I went to visit Mr. and Mrs. Stephenson every week to get more chicken eggs from them until baby chicks came out from the glass incubator. After seventeen days, I got my first baby hen, Sue-Me. Then a lot of other different kinds of chicks came out of their shells inside the glass incubator after her. I was very pleased to see all the baby chicks looking very healthy and running around inside the incubator. I was very thankful to Mr. and Mrs. Stephenson for providing me fresh chicken eggs from their farm to test my incubator. I was very pleased to see all the beautiful chicks successfully hatched and come out of their shells inside my incubator. I took all the baby chicks out of the incubator and kept them inside the plastic boxes in my room. I fed them with chicken food that I had bought from Livermore pet shop. All the chicks were getting big after a few months. They were very tame and friendly. They needed a bigger place to stay. I decided to build coops for them in my garage.

After one month, I built two big three-level coops for them in my garage. They loved to stay inside their coops. When I took them out in my backyard, they did not enjoy staying outside. They would all be waiting in front of my patio sliding door to go back into their coops in my garage. I turned on the music for them in my garage while I was building another coop. They stayed quiet and enjoyed the music very much. Once the music stopped, they would start crowing and make a lot of noises to remind me the music had stopped. When I turned on the music for them again, they stayed quiet. They would upset my neighbor across the street when they crowed early in the morning, making a lot of noises when they heard the sounds of the cars from the street passing by our house. They would also make a lot of noises when people passed by my front yard. My neighbor across the street called the city of Pleasanton to complain about my birds. He did not know before that I had raised the birds in this house. I went to my neighbors' houses to request them to allow me to raise the birds temporarily in my house for my research on the birds and their environments. I ordered different kinds of baby quails, chicks, and eggs from another state. The farmers from other states sent out all these chicks, baby quails, and eggs through the United States Postal Services and had them delivered at my house. My godmother,

Ada Lundgren, knew I was raising the birds, and she was happy to see me doing something for myself again. After she heard my neighbor was complaining about my birds, she was upset and went over to my neighbor's house across the street to tell him to stop the complaints to the city of Pleasanton, but he did not listen to Ada and kept complaining to the city of Pleasanton. So the city of Pleasanton created a small court inside the city of Pleasanton building, setting up a court date for the people who lived in our community to come to the court to listen and debate whether they should allow the people to raise chickens in our residential community or not.

The people from my neighborhood created a lot of arguments in the city of Pleasanton Courthouse about raising chickens in our residential community because the bird flu sickness was spreading in California. The people from California believed that the birds were the cause of the bird flu sickness. They complained that chickens, ducks, and other birds were responsible for spreading bird flu disease in the community. The people from our community were afraid that my chickens would spread bird flu sickness to them. They tried to stop me from raising the chickens. The people who were raising the chickens in their own homes in Pleasanton and Tri Valley said that there was no such law set before to prohibit the people from raising chickens in their homes. It was legal for me to raise birds in my house. The other side gave out excuses for the people that raising chickens would create bird flu sickness in the community. *The Valley Time* newspaper reporter came to my house to interview me and write an article about me and my chickens that I raised at home. The reporters from different television channels were looking for me to interview me, but I was tired. I did not like to show my face on television. I did not go out to meet them. Then the court of the city of Pleasanton ordered me to find a place to keep my birds. They wanted me to move my birds from my house as soon as I found a place to keep them safely. I told Sirena about the court order. She advised me to talk to Century 21 real estate agent. I called Century 21 to find a place to move all my chickens out of my house. Mrs. Lynn Phillips, a real estate agent from Century 21, took me to Livermore agriculture areas to look for a place to raise my chickens. She showed me ten acres of land up in the mountain in Livermore to raise my chickens, but Mrs. Phillips did not allow me to buy the mountain land to raise chickens alone in the mountain side. She advised me to rent a place in the agriculture area in

Livermore to raise my chickens to get more experience on how to raise and maintain the chicken farm. Then she helped me to find an old farm in front of Lawrence Livermore National Laboratory, and she gave me the farm owner Mr. Howard Liskin's telephone number to call. She asked me to talk to Howard about renting his farm building.

I called Howard the next day and talked to him about renting his farm buildings to raise chickens. He suggested going and looking at his farm first, to make sure I liked the place. I said OK. Then I set up a date with him to see his old farm buildings. When I was in Howard's farm, I looked around the environment on his farm. The surrounding environment was very quiet and peaceful. I saw lambs, goats, sheep, and cows were scattered all over his neighbors' farmlands. Some of these animals were eating grasses, some were resting under the shady trees, some were inside the huts, and some small animals were playing in their own farmlands. I decided to rent one old building in the farm from Howard. I talked it over with Howard about the rent. I rented one of the old farm buildings to keep all my birds. Howard offered me the use of his truck to help move all the bird coops from my house to the farm building. My neighbor Mr. Bob Novel came to my house and helped Howard load all the coops into the truck. After they were done loading the coops, Howard drove his truck to his farm, unloaded the coops, and carried them inside the farm building for me. My children helped me to move all my birds to the farm building and settled them inside the farm. Then I ordered different types of quail eggs, two hundred different types of baby quails, and four hundred different kinds of baby chicks from out-of-state farmers through mails. After a month, I got all the baby birds from the mail. They all were very healthy and grew very fast. They became hens and roosters in a few months. They were very tame and friendly. I took rice and cabbages to the farm every day to feed them. Sometimes I cooked noodles for them. Every morning when I drove my car to the farm and stopped in front of the farm building, all my chickens, quails, and ducks would make a lot of noises as soon as they heard my car's noise. When they saw me coming inside the building, they would run to me and some even would jump up on to my shoulders. I would take the cabbages from my basket and throw it to them. They would chase after the cabbages just like football players would chase the player who had the football and try to get the football from him. My hens and female quails laid a lot of eggs each day. In particular, my female quails laid more than forty eggs a day; my hens laid over twenty colored eggs each day. The colors of the eggs were pink, light red, purple, yellow, brown, different shades of blue, and green. I had never seen so many different kinds of colored chicken eggs in my life. I told my children and friends that I did not know before there were so many different kinds of chickens that would lay so many kinds of colored eggs in this world. They did not believe me at first when I told them about so many kinds of colored eggs being laid in my farm, and they were very amazed. They said they had never heard of chicken eggs in different colors other than the white and brown chicken eggs that were sold in the markets. I put all the fresh eggs from my farm in the incubator each day after I came back home from there. After six months, I had over one thousand chickens, one thousand quails, and two ducks in my Livermore farm. I decided to sell the chickens from my farm to the restaurants, so I registered my bird farm as Peak Farm in Alameda County in early 1998. All my birds were very healthy. I did not have any allergy when I was inside the farm. I did not hear any people from Livermore complaining about the allergy, except they complained about Hong Kong chicken flu sickness and that they had a lot of flies in Livermore. I did not see a lot of flies in my farm in Livermore, but a few flies flew in sometimes.

Three months after I had rented this farm, a group of people came in and rented the farm building and built coop rooms in the other section of my farm building. After they finished building the coop rooms, they moved in a lot of roosters and some hens to the farm. I was busy in the farm during the day preparing food and water for the birds. I built more coops for the birds in my garage at night. One Saturday, after I had finished building one of the coops in my garage, I could not lift it up because it was very heavy. I opened my garage door and went out to my driveway, looking for somebody from my neighbors to help me lift up the heavy coop. I saw my left-side neighbor Drew's son, Brent, standing outside in his driveway with his friends. I called him for help to lift up the finished coop in my garage. He came with his friends to help me lift up the heavy coop. After they lifted up the coop for me, I thanked him and his friends, and they went back to his house. I remember when Drew's family had moved into my neighbor's house, Brent was only a young boy. He always helped his father to cut the lawn. He grew up there and graduated from Amador High School. Then he went to Chico University. He came home to stay with his father in summer break. I noted that his face had a lot of red rashes when he lived here. I did not see any rash on his face after he moved out of his house to live at school, but I saw a lot of scars remained on both sides of his chins. I knew all those scars were left from the rashes that he had got before when he lived in my neighbor's house. When I saw so many scars on his young face, I felt very upset. I tried to compare his complexion with other teenagers who did not have to help at home to cut the lawn. He must have got the redness and blister rashes that ruined his complexion because of the allergic materials in our neighborhood. I talked to the people that I met in our neighborhood about the allergies, the blister rashes, and the scars left on this young teenager's face.

I built four more new coops. I moved them to the farm building with the help of my two children. Since I had not assembled the automatic water system and automatic feeding system in my farm yet, I had to go in my farm to feed my birds every day. I got so many baby chickens from my incubator. They were growing and getting big. When Shaun saw they were squeezed inside the coops, he advised me they would live better if we built big coop rooms for them. He kept on pushing me to build the coop rooms inside the farm for the birds every time he went to the farm with me. Hence, I started to lay out the structure on how to build the coop rooms in the farm building. Then I went to the Home Depot store to buy wood, wires, and all the accessories that I needed to build coop rooms inside the farm building. Sirena and Shaun helped me to take them to the farm building. I started to build coop rooms inside my farm building according to my own layout. While I was building the coop rooms, I saw a lot of people were visiting Howard. They came in and out of the farm. Sometimes I saw a few trucks would go in and out, loading a lot of shoeboxes from their truck in the old building next to my farm building. Sometimes the truck drivers brought their children with them to come into my farm building and talk to me. They told me they were Howard's longtime friends, their children are enjoying to see all kind of birds here. Every day, I saw the employees of Lawrence Livermore National Laboratory walk on the road in front of the farm. All my birds crowed when they heard the noises from outside. After I moved my chicken to Livermore farm building, the roads in front of my farm building became very busy because of the employees from Lawrence Livermore National Laboratory. They would move in and out, walking on the main road of Howard's farm during the day time.

One Saturday, Shaun went to my bird farm with me to help me unload the chicken food at the farm. I told Shaun I had seen wild animals in the surrounding neighborhoods of Livermore. Sometimes I saw a couple of foxes running around on the nearby roads in Livermore. He advised me to be careful of all these wild animals when I was working in the farm. When we arrived in front of my farm, I got down from my car and opened the farm building's sliding door. Shaun unloaded the chicken food from my car and took them inside the farm. Then he called me to look up at the roof. When I looked up at the roof, I saw there was a raccoon on top of the wooden roof bar of the farm building. The farm building had doors that would be closed when we were not inside the building. I told Shaun I did not know how the raccoon came inside the building and how to chase the raccoon out of the farm building. He asked me to stay outside. Then he went to get Howard in his house. Howard came with him and tried to chase the raccoon out of the building, but the raccoon was running back and forth on the roof wooden bar. I suggested that he climb up to the bar to chase the raccoon down. He said it was not a good idea to climb up to the bar. Then he told me he would go home to get his rifle gun to scare the raccoon down from the bar. He went back to his house and brought his rifle gun to the building. He shot many times, trying to scare the raccoon to make it come down from the roof wooden bar, but the raccoon did not come down and kept running back and forth from one end of the roof wooden bar to the other end on the roof of the building. Finally, Howard lost his patience and shot down the raccoon from the roof wooden bar with his gun. The raccoon fell onto the ground and was dead. Howard took the raccoon's dead body outside the building and then put it inside a plastic bag, leaving the plastic bag outside the building that was near his house. Shaun and I went back inside the building and prepared all food and water for the birds. After we were done, we went home.

On December 20, 1998, when I was coming back from the Livermore farm, I met with a bad car accident on Pimlico Drive, Pleasanton. On that day, we had cloudy weather, and it seemed like it was going to rain. I was driving my car carefully on the 580 freeway at less than 50 mph. When I took the Santa Rita Road exit and went on to Pimlico Drive at a speed of less than 25 mph, I saw a car suddenly pull out from Pimlico Drive shopping center at high speed. As soon as I saw the car, I hit my brakes quickly to stop my car. Then I turned my car wheel to the left to avoid the other car hitting my car. But the driver did not stop her car and just kept pushing her car forward, hitting my car with great force, damaging the front of my Cadillac car badly. Luckily, I saw her fast enough to turn my car wheel to the left to save both our lives; otherwise, we both would have died if my car had hit her car directly. She got down from her car and came to me. She told me that the sun had been blocking her eyes, that she did not see my car coming, and that she had just pulled out the car at high speed. I was very upset with her. I felt the reason that she gave out to me was an unacceptable excuse because it was a cloudy day and there was no sun on that day. I felt pain in my chest. I did not come down from my car. But I looked at her in anger, advising her in my very upset voice to call the police department to report the accident right away. She said she did not have a cellular phone to call the police department. I advised her to go to the nearby store to call the police department. She left and went to the nearby store to find a telephone to call the police department and report the accident.

After a few minutes, two police officers arrived in Pimlico Drive. One of the police officers came to my car and asked me to give him my driving license. I took out my driving license from my purse and handed it out to him. Then he asked me how the accident had happened. I described to the police officer how the car accident had happened. The police officer said to me, "This is what we call a car accident." I did not understand what he meant by that. I was just looking at him in surprise. He took my driving license and went to his police motorcycle. After half an hour, he came back and gave me back my driving license. Then he told me this car accident was because of the mistake of the lady driver Debbie Driscoll in the other car. He went back to his police motorcycle and called the ambulance. While we were waiting for the ambulance, I felt that I needed to go to the restroom. I got down from my car to request the police officer to give me permission to go to the restroom. The police officer said OK. I walked to the Chinese restaurant in the small shopping center to ask permission to use their restroom. One of the waiters came to me and guided me the way to go to the restroom. I went in the restroom and came back out after I had used it. I met the owner, Mrs. Lee, of Gold Chopstick restaurant on my way out of the restaurant. She asked me what had happened to me. I told her I had met with a car accident on the street in front of their restaurant. Then I left and went back to the street to report to the police officer that I was back.

After a while, the ambulance arrived. The ambulance driver came down from the ambulance van and opened the back door; the police officer asked us to get inside the ambulance van to go to the hospital emergency room for checkup. The woman driver of the other car went inside the ambulance van, but I did not go in. Then the police officer asked me to get into the ambulance van again. I told him I did not want to go to the hospital and that I would like to go home because I still had a lot of baby quails at home, which needed me to feed them. But the good-hearted police officer persuaded me again to go to the emergency hospital for a checkup to make sure I was OK. I told him I had much pain in my chest, but I would not go to the hospital and wanted to go home to my baby birds. They needed me to feed them at home. I had a lot of stuff also that I had brought back from the farm in my car trunk to take home. The police officer asked me how I would take my stuff home. He said he did not have a car to take me home. I told him I did not know how to go home. Then I saw the lady owner of Gold Chopstick restaurant, Mrs. Lee, who had come to check on me. Then she looked at my car and said, 'Terrible!' She offered to help me drive home. I said OK and thanked her. I accepted her offer to take me home. She went back to her restaurant to get her van from the parking lot. After a while, she came back in her big van. The two police officers pushed my car to the sidewalk to let me open my car trunk. I opened my car trunk and was just about to take the heavy bags out of the car when one of the police officers saw the way I tried to carry the heavy bags out from the trunk in great pain. He called to offer to help me. I responded to him, "OK, sir, thank you!" He got down from his police motorcycle to unload all the heavy bags from my car and loaded them into my friend's van. After he had loaded all the heavy bags for me in my friend's van, I said thanks to him with deep appreciation. The police officer went back to his police motorcycle and left. My friend took me home. When I opened the garage door after we arrived at my house, she saw I had over five hundred quails inside the coop in my garage. She said she did not believe that I was raising so many quails inside my garage. I told her I also had a lot of chickens inside my farm. Then she said she did not have to worry about the chickens for her restaurant anymore. She said that if she needed any chicken, she would get them from me. I told her to just let me know and I would let her have as many chickens she wanted from my farm. She said OK. She helped me unload all my heavy bags from her van into my garage, and she left. I filled in all the bowls of food and water for the quails in my garage before I went inside my house. After I settled the food and water for the quails, I went inside my house to take Advil pain-reliever pills. Then I called Sirena to inform her about the car accident in front of the Pimlico Drive shopping mall. I told her I needed her to take me to the farm tomorrow because I did not have a car to go to the farm. All the birds would die if they did not get food and water inside the farm. She said she would come home early to take me to the farm. I could not sleep the whole night because the pain in my chest increased greatly. I did not know my chest bone had dislocated. I took some more pain-reliever pills to overcome my pain the whole night.

Next day, Sirena came in the morning to take me to the farm. After she dropped me at the farm, she left for her office. As usual, I filled up the food and water bowls for all my birds. I was continuously building the coop rooms until I had finished all the coop rooms inside my farm building. Sirena came back to the farm in the evening to take me home. After she picked me up at the farm and dropped me home, she went back to her office again. On the third day after my car accident, I felt a bad pain in my right chest. I could not do anything inside the farm except fill up food and water bowls for the birds. When Sirena came home to take me to the farm the next day, I told her I had a bad pain in my chest. She suggested taking me to emergency hospital right away. But I insisted her to take me to the farm before she took me to the emergency hospital, because I had not assembled the automatic food and water system in the farm yet and the birds needed food and water for the day to eat and drink. She said OK. She took me to the farm and helped me fill up all the food and water bowls for the birds. After she was done, she took me to the emergency clinic in Valley Care Medical Center (VCMC) on Santa Rita Road. When we reached the VCMC emergency clinic, I registered myself with the front desk medical clerk first. The front desk clerk asked me the reason I had come there. I told her I had a bad pain in my right chest after I was in the bad car accident three days ago. The front desk clerk asked me to take an X-ray first before the doctor saw me. She asked me to wait in the waiting room for the technician to take me to the X-ray room. I waited in the front waiting room with Sirena. After a while, the technician came out and asked me to sit on the wheelchair and took me to the X-ray room. Once I was in the X-ray room, the technician asked me to remove all my jewelries from my body. I took all the jewelries from my body and changed to the patient outfit. After I was done, he asked me to stand in front of the X-ray machine. He took X-ray of my chest. After he was done taking X-ray, he asked me to sit on the wheelchair and took me back out to the hallway. Then the nurse came and took me to the emergency room. She told me to lie down on the patient's bed. She asked me where I felt the pain in my chest. I showed her my right chest and told her I did not know why I had so much pain in my chest. She checked my right chest and exclaimed that I had a big bruise on my right chest. The big bruise on my chest was because of the car accident when the two cars collided badly with each other due to strong force. I told her I had a lot of pain in my right chest and I could not even touch it. Then she covered my chest with a blanket and asked me to stay on the bed and wait for the doctor to look at my bruise on my right chest. She said the doctor would come and see me after she reviewed the X-ray films. She told me to let her know if I needed anything from her. I shook my head at her, and she left. Sirena was with me in the hospital emergency room to wait for the doctor to come and check on me.

After a few hours, the lady doctor came in and told me that my X-ray did not show any broken bone on my chest and body. She wanted me to let her look at the bruise on my right chest that caused me so much pain. After she looked at the big bruise on my chest, she checked my stomach by pressing it and asked me if I had any pain in my stomach. I shook my head to indicate that I did not have pain inside my stomach. Then she asked me to turn on my stomach to let her check my back. I turned my back to her. She pressed my spinal cord and asked me whether I had any pain. I shook my head and said no. After she was done checking my back, I told her again that I had a big pain in my right chest. She prescribed me Tylenol pain-reliever pills. Then she referred me to see Dr. David Chee as an outpatient and discharged me from the emergency clinic. I changed back to my normal clothing and left the emergency clinic. I met Dr. Chee in the hallway, and he told me to follow him. I went to his office with him. The nurse measured my blood pressure. After she finished measuring my blood pressure, she told me my blood pressure was in the normal data range and left. Then Dr. Chee came in and talked to me. He told me he had got all my information from the emergency clinic and wanted me to contact him right away if I had more pain in my chest. I told him I would call his office to set up an appointment for my next checkup with him. Before I left, he told me to contact him right away if I had great pain in my chest again. I said OK to him. He discharged me. Then Sirena took me home. When we arrived home, Sirena told me one of her friends had suggested that I needed a lawyer to solve this car accident problem. She said she would hire a lawyer for me. She was waiting for her friend to get the lawyer's name, address, and telephone number. Next day, after Sirena picked me up from the farm and dropped me home, she told me her friend had referred her to lawyer Randy Choy from San Francisco to take care of my car accident case. She said she had already talked to the lawyer Randy about my car accident and the lawyer Randy had referred her to contact Dr. Pono V. A., Advanced Sports Therapy Chiropractic Center (ASTCC) in Milpitas, to take me in for checkup. Sirena told me she had already contacted Dr. Pono to set up an appointment on December 30, 1998, for me to go in for a checkup with him, and then she left.

Sirena picked me up at home and took me to see Dr. Pono on Wednesday, December 30, 1998, in ASTCC in Milpitas. Sirena checked in with the front desk clerk for me. Then I had to wait for a while in the waiting room. The clerk came out and took me into one of the patient rooms. Then she asked me to change into the patient outfit. After I changed, I sat on the chair waiting for the doctor to come in. Dr. Pono came in the room after five minutes and introduced himself to me. Then he asked me about my car accident. I told him I had a lot of pain in my right chest after my car accident. I also told him that X-ray had been taken in the VCMC emergency clinic and that the doctor from the VCMC emergency clinic had told me I did not have any broken bone on my body after she reviewed my X-ray, but I had a big bruise on my right chest, which was causing me great pain. Then I showed him my big bruise. After he looked at my big bruise, he asked me to stand straight in front of him to check my body. I stood straight in front of him. When I bent my head down to look at my chest, I saw one of my right chest bones was sticking out distinctly through my patient outfit. I was surprised and did not know what to do. I just looked at Dr. Pono and then at my chest bone sticking out. Dr. Pono also saw my chest bone sticking out from my chest. He came to me and pressed softly on my right chest bone sticking out. Then he told me I had a dislocated chest bone on my right chest and that he could help me push my chest bone back into the right position without going through any surgery. I asked him how he was going to do it. He said he would show me when I came back to his clinic after five days. He did not explain to me how he was going to do it. He did not ask me whether I would like to accept his technique to take care of my dislocated bone. Since I did not have any idea how he was going to push the dislocated chest bone in for me, I did not know what to ask him at that moment. All I knew was I had to listen to the doctor, waiting for him to tell me how he was going to do it. I was afraid that if anything happened to me, people would blame me for not listening to the doctor. I did not dare to say one word back to the doctor other than to let him take care of me. After he discharged me, I went to the front desk clerk to set up an appointment on Monday, January 4, 1999, to come back to see him. Then Sirena took me back home. On our way back home, I told Sirena that I was scared, that I did not know how Dr. Pono was going to push my dislocated right chest bone back in for me, and that he had not told me anything. Sirena told me not to worry and just to let the doctor take care of me. Then she dropped me home and went back to her office. After I reached home, I was a bit of afraid of letting the doctor push my chest bone in. I took Advil pain-reliever pills to overcome my pain every night. Sirena picked me up in the morning and dropped me in the farm; then she came back to the farm and picked me up in the evening and dropped me at home and then she went back to her office.

On Monday morning, January 4, 1999, Sirena picked me up at home and took me to Dr. Pono's clinic. Once we were in front of Dr. Pono's clinic, Sirena wanted me to go in myself to checkup with Dr. Pono because she had a few important works to take care of in her office. I got down from her car and she left. I checked in the clinic with the front desk clerk. The clerk took me in one of the patient rooms. She gave me a patient outfit to change. I changed into the patient outfit and waited for Dr. Pono to come in. After a while, Dr. Pono came inside the room with two other people wearing white outfits. After these two people sat in the corner near the patient bed, he asked me to stand in front of him, facing inside the room. He turned his face to the two people and said that my chest bone number 4 had dislocated. He was explaining to them how he was going to push my chest bone back in for me. Then he held my chest with his right arm from around my back and pushed my chest bone in hard. After he was done, he asked me to lie down and turned my body down on the patient bed to give me massage machine treatment on my back. After fifteen to thirty minutes, he came in and told me he was done with me for the day and asked me to change back into my clothing. He did not prescribe any medicine to me. He did not tell me what I should do after I was home and how to take care of myself. He told me to come back and see him after a week and then discharged me. After I came out from the patient room, I asked the front desk clerk who were those two people that had come into my room with Dr. Pono. She told me that Dr. Pono was teaching in the chiropractic school, and they were the students from the chiropractic school. Then I asked the front desk clerk whether I could use their phone to call Sirena to pick me up at the clinic to take me home. The clerk said yes. She gave me the phone to call Sirena. I called Sirena to let her know I was done. After fifteen minutes, Sirena was in the clinic and took me home. After I was home, I took pain-reliever pills myself. I did not know what to ask and what to say after Dr. Pono had pushed my chest bone in for me. I did not know what would happen to my chest bone in the future.

When the car accident happened, I was in the middle of building the coop rooms inside my farm building. I did not have automatic food and water systems in my farm yet. I needed to go to the farm to feed my birds every day. I did not have a car, so I had to depend on Sirena to take me to the doctor for my treatment and to drop me at the farm every morning and then pick me up from the farm after four o'clock and take me home. After she dropped me home, she would go back to her office. I could only stay half an hour to fill up the food and water bowls inside the farm and then I had to go to checkup with my doctor. The rest of the week, I had to stay inside the farm to build the coop rooms until they were done. This was the way Sirena was taking me back and forth to the farm and then to the doctor, and after I was done with the doctor, she dropped me home and went back to office.

We had heavy rains in Livermore, California, in January and February, 1999. The old farm building was leaking badly and it was very muddy inside and outside the farm building. I tried to save the birds from dying by fixing the leaking building as much as I could, but the farm building was too old and it had so many leaking areas that I could not fix all of them. All the birds were forced to live in a very muddy and very cold building. A lot of mice and rats were migrating inside the farm building from the nearby areas in Livermore. Every day when I went into the farm, I would see all the birds looking like they were very tired and had not got enough sleep at night, feeling sick. I saw some of the birds had died inside the farm building. I searched for the reasons the birds were dying inside the farm building by moving the water and food bowls around to check what was underneath. I found there were so many small and big mice and rats underneath the bowls. I complained to Howard about the mice and the rats inside the building, which were making my birds so sick and dying. I called the city of Livermore to complain about the mice and the rats of which I had found a lot of them inside the farm building in Livermore. After I complained to the city of Livermore, Lawrence Livermore National Laboratory hired people to clean up all the bushes in their company compounds. Howard also cleaned all his other old farm buildings. A lot of mice and rats from his old building migrated into my building after he cleaned up his old farm building. I saw my chickens chasing the mice and the rats inside the farm and eating them. Every day, I found a lot of my chickens had died, their bodies black. A few dead bodies of mice were found outside my farm building. I predicted that the people of Livermore must be poisoning the mice and the rats in their farmhouses and their buildings after I called the city of Livermore to complain about the mice and the rats. When I talked to Howard, he told me they were using poisoned food inside and outside their houses and buildings to kill the mice and the rats to get rid of them. Some of those mice and rats must have run into my farm building after they ate the poisoned food and must have died inside my farm building. My chicken and quails that ate the dead mice died, their bodies turning black. Some of them died with their bodies flipped up. I tried my best to clean and maintain my farm building. Unfortunately, there was so much rain in the winter that the whole farm was filled with rainwater and it became very muddy. So many rats and mice migrated in daily from the nearby areas of Livermore. My birds did not have enough rest at night. They became very sick and many birds died every day. When Howard saw me take the dead chickens out from my farm, he came to me and complained about my dead chickens. I was very unhappy to hear him complaining about the dead chickens to me. I told him I had done my best to save the chickens inside the farm by fixing the farm building. I wanted him to take responsibility for fixing his building. After I complained to him many times, instead of fixing his building, he hired people to bring in barks in trucks to fix the muddy road in his farmland. I saw a lot of trucks were in and out the whole day in the farmland, fixing the muddy farm roads for almost a couple months.

I called the city of Livermore many times to inform them about the situation of chickens dying in my farm in Livermore because too many mice and rats in Livermore kept migrating into my farm building. I observed the way the birds died. Mostly, they died with their bodies turning fat and black. I saw in some of the chickens white thick layered pieces formed near their eyes' lacrimal gland. I tried to feed the sick chicken with antibiotic medicines. Some of them got better, but some died. When I went to the pet shop in Livermore to buy food for my birds, I talked to the people inside the pet shop. They told me they had a lot of flies, mosquitoes, mice, and rats in their farmland. Their chickens were also dying in their farms just like my chickens. I called some of my friends in different cities to find out whether they had allergies and sickness in their environments. They said they had a lot of big flies in their areas, and some said they had a lot of ants, but they did not have any allergic reactions. My sister Holly told me that one of the Burmese doctors was bitten by a poisonous spider from the evergreen tree at his house in Los Angeles and died. She said some of the spiders had very strong poisons and reminded me to stay away from the spiders.

While I was visiting the doctor, I was continuously building my coop rooms until all of them were done. Except my two children, I did not have anyone to help me in building the farm. Shaun would help me when he came home on weekends. Sirena was the only person who took the responsibility of providing me transportation to help me run around doing errands. My chest bone seemed like it had got twisted again and again, and it created a lot of pain. Dr. Pono leveled my chest bones and my spinal cord again and again, giving me the massage treatments continuously. I had a lot of pain in my body. It was getting harder and harder for me to maintain my farm. Finally, I gave up my farm in July 1999. Sirena talked to Howard about shutting down my farm and stop renting his building. Then she shut down the farm, brought home six small hens and two small roosters, and kept them in the garage. I stayed home to take care of the birds. At night, I trained my male chicken Nicky to make different kind of sounds at home. He could crow and make sounds like or-or-ah-ah-ah-ah-ah-ah-ah-ah-or. Every time he could not get my attention, he tried to crow the way I had taught him to do. My hen Kai-La could crow like a rooster. She crowed like a rooster in my garage when she heard the noises from outside my house. They were my strange and priceless chicken.

During this time, I was still going to Dr. Pono's clinic for treatments. The students always came in with Dr. Pono and gave massage treatment for me. Finally, in September 1999, Dr. Pono told me that my chest bone was healed and that I no longer needed any treatment. I was happy and relieved to know my chest bone was healed. Then Sirena told me that I was allowed to drive my car after my treatment with Dr. Pono was done. She rented a car for me. After this car accident, I had not gone anywhere. I felt like getting out of my house and visiting my cousin in Daly City. I called my cousin to let him know I would visit him on Saturday. Then I drove in my car to his house on Saturday. They were very happy to see me get well again. When I saw my cousin's grandson Brain, I called to him and lifted him up. Brain's weight was about thirty-five pounds. As soon as I lifted him up, I felt a bad pain in my chest. It seemed like I had twisted my chest bones, and my whole body was very uncomfortable. So I put him down on the ground. I told my niece that I did not feel good, that I had pain in my chest and had to go home. My niece insisted me to stay for lunch before I went home, and then my cousin also asked me to have lunch with them. After I ate lunch, I stayed for a while and went home. Next day, I called Dr. Pono in ASTCC to tell him I had bad pain in my chest again. He told me to set up an appointment to see him. I set up an appointment to checkup with Dr. Pono again.

On the appointment day, before I went to Dr. Pono's clinic, I went to the city of Pleasanton first to see the city attorney, Renee Perko, to turn in my letter that I had prepared for her in the night, informing her about the results of my study on the comparison of the environments of the two cities Pleasanton and Livermore, which I had carried out to find the causes of allergies and sickness. I met her in her office and gave her my letter and left. Then I went to see Dr. Pono in Milpitas. After Dr. Pono checked my chest and body, he told me that my healed dislocated chest bone had twisted. He helped me to level in my twisted chest bone again right away. Probably my dislocated bone was healed, but my chest bones with the connected vertebrae bones of my back were twisted at the same time when I lifted up Brain, which led to a lot of pain in my right chest and my back near the twisted vertebrae bones, making me very uncomfortable. I told Dr. Pono that I did not feel good at all even after he had leveled the twisted bones for me. Then he gave massage machine treatment on my back. Dr. S. C. Wong who had graduated from the Chinese chiropractic school was working with Dr. Pono in ASTCC. She came into the patient's room to help me massage my back and put lotion for me every time I was in the clinic.

After I told her that my chest bones and body had a lot of pain and that I did not feel good, Dr. Wong said that she would help me level the chest bones and vertebrae bones of my back to get rid of the pain. She asked me to lie down on the patient bed and turned my body so that my back faced the ceiling. Then she held up my right arm and pressed a bit harder on my right back. I yelled, 'Ah!' I was so scared and felt something was wrong in my neck and my back. I refused to let her continue pressing my left back again, and I said to her, 'No more.' She insisted on letting her finish on the left side of my back to level out the bones of my body, so I let her press the left side of my back. I told her something was still not right in my neck. I did not know how to describe to her the feeling that I had in the nerves of my neck at that time. She pressed and massaged my neck with her hands. Then she mentioned to me how she had tried to help Dr. Pono massage his back when he asked her to massage his back to fix the arthritis in his body. She said that sometimes she had to climb up on his back and use her legs to press harder on his back with her body weight. I reminded Dr. Wong that Dr. Pono did not have any dislocated bone on his chest; he was a big guy just like a big cow, and he could stand her body weight, but not me. I was only a small little lady. My body was unable to accept her pushing on my back. After she gave me the massage machine treatment, Dr. Pono came in the clinic room and discharged me. I went home. I did not feel good after I reached home. I went to bed early. I usually had a habit to check both my legs every day before I went to bed at night, and after I woke up in the morning, I usually looked at my legs and compared the sizes of my legs. Most of the times, both my legs would be swollen. I would put both my legs up on the big pillow to make the swelling from my legs go down when I slept. In the morning, there wouldn't be any swelling in my legs and it would be of normal size. Both my legs would always be of the same size whether there was swelling or not. After Dr. Wong pushed the right side of my back hard with her hands, my right leg swelled, and the swelling did not go down to its normal size as usual. However, the swelling on my left leg went down to normal size in the morning. I felt the nerves on my neck were not right, and it seemed like my nerves were twisting to the left side of my body. I told Dr. Pono about my twisted neck and the swelling in my right leg when I went back to see him on my next visit. He and Dr. Wong tried to give me both hand massages and machine treatments on my body, but I still did not feel good. The swelling on my right leg was getting worse and did not go down to the regular size in the morning. My twisted neck and chest bone were not getting better, and it caused a lot of pain, so I called Dr. David Chee in VCMC in Pleasanton to tell him about my twisted neck, chest bone, and swollen right leg. I requested him to come to my house to check on me to see whether he could help me to get better or not. He came to my house and examined my neck, chest bone, and legs. He suggested I should not let Dr. Pono push and level my chest bone again. He advised me to checkup with an orthopedic surgeon. He said he would call me after he found the orthopedic surgeon in Pleasanton, and then he left. After a couple of days, he called me back and gave me the telephone number of Dr. Robert D. S.'s clinic in Pleasanton for me to call to set up an appointment to checkup with him. I called Dr. Robert's clinic and set up the appointment on November 30, 1999.

I went to see Dr. Robert in the Pleasanton clinic on the appointment date. When I was in Dr. Robert's clinic, one of his nurses took me to the patient room. She measured my blood pressure and then asked me to wait for Dr. Robert. After a while, Dr. Robert came in and asked me about my problem. I explained to him that my chest bone had dislocated after my car accident and that Dr. Pono had pushed my chest bone back in for me. I also told him how my chest bone had twisted again when I lifted up Brain, how my right leg started swelling, and how the nerves of my neck seemed like tossing away to the left side after Dr. Wong pushed my right back with her hands. I also told him about the severe pain in my neck, chest, and the swelling in my right leg. Dr. Robert checked on my neck, chest bones, spinal cords, and legs. After he had finished checking my body, he advised me to push my two arms onto my body to see whether I had pain or not. I did the way he asked me to do. I did not feel any pain after I pushed my two arms onto my body, so I told him I had no pain at this moment. He said he would do the surgery only if I had a lot of pain when I pushed my two arms in the direction of my body. He advised me to go back to Dr. Pono to let him take care of me. I went back to Dr. Pono and checked up with him again. Both Dr. Pono and Dr. Wong tried their best to help me fix my body by continuously giving me machine massage treatments. When I have pains, I take Advil pain relievers myself. After many appointments that Dr. Pono made for me, he finally released me in February 2000. He had diagnosed me with costochondritis, sustained multiple soft tissue injuries, and damage to other parts of my body with contusion of my rib cage.

After Dr. Pono released me, I talked to my sister Holly about my pain in my twisted neck and chest bone and swelling of my right leg. I told her that Dr. Robert would do the surgery on my chest bone only if I had a lot of pain. She suggested that I check with the physical therapist to fix my body. I said to her that when my chiropractor could not even help me to fix my body to get rid of the pain, then how the physical therapist could help me to fix my body. Holly said they were different and the physical therapist was the medical doctor, but chiropractor was not the medical doctor of the medical field. She told me that it would not hurt me to checkup with the physical therapist, but I had lost the confidence in the doctors. I did not look for any physical therapist to fix my body. Every day, I kept calling my children, my sisters, and friends to complain about my car accident and the pain in my body. One of my cousin-in-laws told me about her father who had died on the roadside when he was hit by a car while he was walking on the sidewalk on his way home in San Francisco. She and her brother found her father's dead body lying on the roadside when they went out looking for him. She said she did not know who hit her father, and the car driver had also not called 911 to report the car accident to the police department. I felt very upset on hearing all these kinds of car accidents happening in our community.

After I kept complaining to Sirena about the pain in my body, she suggested that I go to New York to visit my brother Dr. Harvey Chu to let him check up on me. She bought me a two-way air ticket to go to King of Prussia, Pennsylvania, after Dr. Pono discharged me. So I flew to King of Prussia to visit my sisters and my brothers for two weeks. My sister Susong Thanse was working in New Jersey, and she came home every weekend. I lived in Susong's house alone. Rosie, Edward, and Susong took me to Harvey's clinic in New York to let Harvey check and take care of my body's injuries and to get suggestions from him on how to fix the discomfort in my body. After I was in Harvey's clinic, I told him about the pain in my body, how my neck nerves seemed like tossing away to the left side and how it made me very uncomfortable because of the great pain. After he heard about my body injuries, he suggested that I take pain-reliever pills when I had pain. He provided me Tylenol pain-reliever pills to take home. He drew my blood sample and sent it to New York laboratory. He received my blood test result within a day. He reviewed my blood test result and told me my cholesterol was a bit high and asked me not to eat too much fat meat. We commuted back and forth between New York and King of Prussia during weekends to visit Harvey when I was in King of Prussia. Rosie and Edward took me to different restaurants to eat different food to make me forget all my pain while I was in King of Prussia. After two weeks, I flew back to California.

After I came back from King of Prussia, I did not see any of my chickens at home anymore. I asked Sirena where all my chickens were. She did not tell me where she had taken the chickens away. She just said she felt bad for me to lose them and then went home. After I lost all my chickens and farm, I cleaned up my garage and put away all the birds' water and food bowls inside the coops in my garage. I spent my time watching television when I did not have anything to do. Sometimes I forced myself to learn to make bread and pastry to get some exercise at home. When I made bread, I had to knead hard to mix flour with eggs, water, sugar, and salt to make dough. This caused a lot of pain in my neck and my right chest. I took Advil pain-reliever pills to get rid of the pain in my body. I started to meditate at night by learning to concentrate and look at one small spot on the ceiling to forget all the pain in my body. At night, I used an electric heat pad on my body to prevent arthritis. I used pain-reliever pills whenever I had a lot of pain. Slowly, I was able to move around and walk regularly, but unfortunately, I was unable to lift and carry things over five pounds. When I did, it caused great pain in my right eye, right brain, and right back. Sometimes the lifting made my chest bone and vertebrae bones twist and slip, and this caused very bad headaches, and I started to lose my eyesight.

I was very upset at Sirena when she asked me to sign the release paper for the mechanic from Pleasanton Car Body Shop when he delivered my Cadillac to my house. When I test-drove my Cadillac to the supermarket, the front wheels of the car pulled to the right side. I had to be very careful while driving that car. So I took my car to the Cadillac car dealer in Pleasanton to request the mechanic there to check my car for me. I told the mechanic about my car accident and how I had let Pleasanton Car Body Shop fix my car and how when I test-drove it the front wheels of the car pulled to the right side. The mechanic at the Cadillac car dealer helped me to check my car. He test-drove my car. He found the front wheels of my car were pulling to the right side when he increased the speed to forty-five miles per hour. Then he checked the car's body. He found the alignment was out on the front left side of the Cadillac's body. He told me about the situation of my car and said it was very dangerous for me to drive the car again. He advised me to inform the other party, the insurance company, to let them know the condition of my car and how Pleasanton Car Body Shop had not fixed my car right. I thanked him and left.

I called Darren Chan from State Farm, an insurance agent, to let him know that I had taken my Cadillac car to the Cadillac car dealer in Pleasanton to have the mechanic check and test-drive my car. After the mechanic checked and test-drove my car, the mechanic advised me to let him know that Pleasanton Car Body Shop did not fix my car right, the alignment was out on the left side of my front car body, and it was very dangerous for me to drive this car. Darren told me State Farm Insurance Company was supposed to replace the car with another Cadillac car for Sirena as this car was registered in DMV under Sirena's name. He advised me to inform the lawyer Randy about my car's condition. When Sirena came home, I told her about the condition of the car and what the insurance agent had said. She suggested test-driving my Cadillac car, so we test-drove my car on the way to Walmart store. She found that the front wheels of the car were pulling to the right side when she drove more than forty-five miles per hour. She also admitted that it was very dangerous for me to drive this car, especially on a freeway. She suggested giving her 1998 new civic Honda car to me to drive and took my Cadillac car.

My lawyer Randy did not handle my case right. He had already set up the court date for me to go to the court. I did not know why he had called Sirena and suggested that she should not go to court after I checked in with him. When Sirena came home, she did not say the reason the lawyer Randy had cancelled the plan of suing Debbie Driscoll. She asked me to take the release form to the lawyer to sign the release form for the lawyer Randy. I asked Sirena again why he did so, but she did not say anything. I took the form to the lawyer Beverly Hoey in Pleasanton and signed the release form in front of him. Then I gave the release form to Sirena to turn it in to the lawyer Randy. The lawyer Randy settled the case with State Farm Insurance Company for Debbie Driscoll and released her from this car accident case. When I talked to elderly Catherine about this case, she suggested that I call the State Farm insurance agent in Pleasanton again. I called the State Farm insurance agent from Pleasanton and talked to one of the representatives of the Pleasanton State Farm insurance agent about my case. The lady representative suggested that I pull out all my car accident files from the lawyer Randy. I asked her the reason for pulling out all my files from the lawyer Randy. She told me just to do the way she had advised me to do. So I called the lawyer Randy's office to pull out all my files from him. After I pulled out my files from the lawyer Randy, I called back the lady representative of the Pleasanton State Farm insurance agent to let her know that I had already pulled out all my files from my lawyer. But she was not in her office, so I left a message to her. She called me back and suggested that I hire another lawyer to take care of my car accident case. She said the lawyer Randy should have proceeded with my car accident case instead of closing the case for me. I did not know what to do any more. I did not know where to get a lawyer to take care of my case. I talked to one of the lawyers from Villanova University about my car accident and requested him to refer me to a good lawyer to help me reopen my car accident case. After one week, he called me back and gave me Mr. Michael Greenberg's telephone number to call him in San Francisco. He told me Mr. Greenberg had graduated from Villanova University Law School and he could help me solve my car accident case. When I called Mr. Greenberg, he was not in his office. I left a message for him to call me back, but he did not return my call. I wrote a letter to Darren from State Farm insurance agent again about my car accident case. He advised me to let the lawyer Randy take care of the case and let it go to the court. I talked to Sirena about it. She stayed silent, so I did not call Randy to reopen the case. I believed this was not an ordinary car accident and that someone had set up that car accident on me. No matter where I went, I always had consideration for other people's safety. I liked the other people treating me with the same consideration and not hurting me. I was very upset at the lady driver, Debbie Driscoll, as she had failed to yield right of way by entering the main street at a high speed, leading to this kind of bad car accident. It was very unfair that because of this car accident I had to suffer severe injuries accompanied by severe pain for the rest of my life. I had lost my good Cadillac and also my bird farm.

I kept searching and looking for any techniques that could help me fix my body. I would try any techniques if it would help my body to get back to normal. Then I got an idea. I thought of finding a dance instructor for traditional western dances so that through the dance I could fix my twisted neck. Hence, in early January 2003, I started to look for a western dance instructor. When I talked to elderly Catherine about the problem of my twisted neck, I asked her for her suggestion for getting a dance instructor to fix my neck and body. She suggested that I look through the telephone book to find the name of the dance studio and call them to get introduced to the dance instructor. I looked through the telephone book to get the dance studio in Pleasanton. Then I called the dance studio, leaving them a message to call me back. The dance instructor Lois Hilton called me back. I talked to her about the twisted nerves of my neck and chest bone and my swollen body on the phone. She set up an appointment date for me to go to the dance studio in Valley Avenue, Pleasanton, and meet her there. I went to the dance studio that she had referred me to go. I met her there and talked to her about the problems regarding my neck and my chest bone. She said she would help me with her dancing experience, using the natural movement of the western dance to fix my neck nerves and my body. I set up an agreement to take private lessons with her once a week. Then she referred me to the shoe store in Dublin to buy dancing shoes for my dance lessons. When I was in the dance shoe store, I talked to the lady owner about Lois and told her that Lois was going to help me fix my injurious body with western dance lessons. The lady owner told me that Lois was a very popular dance instructor with great experience in the bay area and that she could help me fix my injured body. I was very pleased to hear the news from the lady owner about Lois. She helped me gain great confidence in Lois, who could help me fix my injured body.

I started taking private lessons with Lois once a week in the dance studio at Valley Avenue in Pleasanton. She patiently taught me the beginner's steps of the waltz dance first. Then she taught me the intermediate steps of the waltz dance and the movement of my body. I practiced my dance lessons at home to straighten my neck nerves and to get some exercise every day. I practiced all the steps that she taught me almost every day. She frequently tested my capability in the dance movements of my body with the help of her friend. Then she taught me certain hard dance steps and guided me on how to turn my body and dance. She carefully taught me how to turn my upper body slowly. I had a lot of pain in my right eye after a few days so I practiced turning my body slowly. After I had a couple of lessons with her on how to turn my body, the pain in my right eye got reduced and I felt much better. But my right leg was still swelling badly. Lois was teaching me the dance lessons carefully step by step. She was afraid to make my body get worse.

After three months, she taught me the steps on how to use forces to turn my whole body. After I went home, I practiced at home myself on how to turn slowly every day. Lois did not even believe that I could turn my whole body so well with great force after a few months. After I learned the turning dance steps, my neck started to get better. Lois reviewed the progress of my dance. Then she suggested that I go to different places to take dance lessons with her to get more practice on dancing and to get more exercise. I said OK to her. She took me to Rhythm Street Dance Studio in Dublin to learn how to dance cha-cha with a group of students. Then she took me to her East Coast dance class in Livermore, when she was teaching there. She advised me to go out to the dance studios to dance with other students to get more practice and experience on Friday nights. I registered in Rhythm Street Dance Studio in Dublin to take different western dance lessons with other instructors. I went to Rhythm Street Dance Studio almost every night to learn how to dance and practice the dance and to get exercises. I took West Coast dance lessons in Pleasanton Senior Center on Wednesday nights to learn West Coast dance. One Friday nights when I went to salsa dance class in Rhythm Street Dance Studio in Dublin, there were a lot of students in the salsa dance class and it seemed like all these students were enjoying learning this dance. At first, the dance instructor taught us the basic steps of the salsa dance. After I finished the beginner's salsa dance class, I joined the intermediate advance class of the salsa dance along with other students. The students said that the salsa intermediate dance steps were hard and complicated to learn, but I did not know what the students were saying because I was not in the intermediate salsa dance class before and I did not know how hard it was. I believed that once I learned the steps to do the intermediate salsa dance, I could overcome all the harder steps of the dance. So I joined the intermediate salsa dance class. The instructor advised me to get a dance partner to get in the intermediate salsa dance class. They introduced me to a dance partner for my intermediate salsa dance class. The instructor showed us how to adopt a sign to turn so that when the male partner threw his hand to signal the female partner, she would turn. When my partner threw my hand, signaling me to turn, I suddenly fell down on the ground. My spinal cord was twisted. I felt I had a lot of pain in my chest and my back, and my head went numb. I got up and stood there for a few minutes. All the students had seen me fall on the ground. When another partner came to me, he tried not to hold my hand to dance with me. When Mr. Gordon came to me, he held my hand, and he used little force to throw my hand to signal me to turn. I slipped and fell to the ground again. He realized I should stop for a while, so he suggested that I rest. I rested for a while and went home. After I reached home, I started thinking about the reason that made me slip and fall on the ground so many times even though my male partner just used little force to throw my hand, signaling me to turn. Then I practiced these steps at home to find the technique to protect myself from slipping and falling to the ground when my partner threw my hand, signaling me to turn. Then I found a technique by using my arm muscles to protect myself so as to not let the force of my partner make me slip and fall to the ground.

Next day, I went to my study room to take out the medical and health encyclopedia and look for the bone section to find the reason my spinal cord had slipped. In the book, it was written that "between the bones of one vertebra and the next is a piece of more resilient cartilage that acts as a cushion or shock absorber to prevent two vertebrae from scraping or bumping each other if the backbone gets a sudden jolt or as the backbone twists and turns and bends. These pieces of cartilage are the inter-vertebral disks. If they become ruptured and form slipped disks, they would cause great pain and misery." After I read this paragraph, I realized my vertebrae cartilage must have formed a slipped disk; when my partner used little force on my hand, I felt it and it caused me great pain in my back vertebrae bones. The movements in this intermediate salsa dance involved a lot of signaling forces from my partner; it hurt my chest bones and my spinal cord, but I decided to continue to take these dance lessons to find the technique to protect myself while I was learning the dance. I went to the dance studio every Friday night to learn the intermediate salsa dance. The students in the dance class must have seen me fall to the ground so many times; they took precaution for me when they danced with me. After I became familiar with intermediate salsa dance, I exercised to make my arms stronger, and I used my arm muscles to protect myself when my partner threw my hand, signaling me to turn on the dance. After this incident, I learned and practiced at home the movements of how to turn my whole body to prevent myself from the falling. After six months, I could protect myself and use the turning dance steps to straighten my twisted neck's nerves and bones when my neck and spinal cord got twisted. After I had learned all the western dance lessons, I stopped dancing. I spent most of my time taking care of my house and working in my backyard.

One night, while I was sitting in my family room, watching television, I suddenly had a bad feeling about the scene of a car accident, and the type of car that hit my car popped into my mind. I found this car was the type of car that would be parked in the main front street of Howard's farm in Livermore. When I realized it was an accident that was set up, I felt so bad. I tried to convince myself that it was just an ordinary accident. Then I remembered a couple of months before my car accident, a Jaguar car had pulled out from the same Pimlico shopping center in Pimlico Drive. As soon as I saw that car was pulling out from the shopping center, I had honked my car horn to alert the male driver in the Jaguar car, warning him to stop his car; at the same time, I stopped my car to prevent a car accident. The Jaguar car driver stopped his car after he heard my horn, but he was very mad at me. He was pointing his finger at me and shaking his finger to indicate that he was mad at me for using my car horn to alert him. I noticed that there were five men, including the car driver inside the car. I did not know them. I did not know why the driver was so mad at me when I horned at him to remind him to stop the car so as to prevent a car accident. I did my share as a good car driver to use my car horn to remind him so as to prevent a car accident. I ignored him and drove my car away. But I saw that this car kept on following me. The driver kept on pointing and shaking his finger at me to give out a warning to me. So I pointed my finger, signaling back to let them know I did not like the way he treated me. Then I took the 580 East Freeway to go to my farm. I could still see them following me in the freeway, so I changed my car lane to the fast lane, the left most side of the 580 Freeway, to stop them from following me. There were so many cars on the 580 Freeway that morning. After I changed the car lane to the leftmost fast lane, I did not see the car following me. Then I drove my car back to the right slow lane and went to my farm. Later on, I found out it was a car accident set up on December 20, 1998. I was really upset at the people who set up this kind of car accident for me. I could never believe people would do such kind of harmful thing to hurt anybody by setting up and creating a bad accident. I thought I had meant well in helping the people by using my car horn to warn them. I never suspected anyone would do such kind of things and set them up on me and make me suffer with pain the rest of my life.

On the way to my farm in Livermore, every morning I saw all kinds of drivers on the freeway. Sometimes the car drivers on the freeway were either doing something or they would fall asleep inside the cars, making their cars not run straight. When I came across such cars on the freeway, I usually followed the cars and used my car horn to wake them up, warning them until they saw me. People should not get upset at somebody who horns at them to remind them to drive carefully in the freeway. The drivers should check what is happening in their environment when they hear the car horns on the road or on the freeway. They should drive their vehicles carefully. Sometimes I also make a mistake while driving my car, but when I hear a car horn from other drivers on the freeway, I try to correct my mistake. If I find nothing wrong in the way I am driving my car, I continue driving my car cautiously and safely to my destination. I never get mad at the car driver who uses their car horn to horn at me. I usually wave my hand to signal to the other driver thank them for warning me. Whatever things happened on the road or on the freeway, I never recalled the cases after I came home. I did not have any intention to take any revenge on the other car drivers. Sometimes the police officer stopped my car and accused me when it was not my fault, but I never got mad at them. I just tried to explain to them. Sometimes they did not accept my explanation and issued a violation ticket to me. I went to the police department to explain to the police chief about the violation ticket that the police officer had issued me on the road when it was not my fault. In those cases, they cleared the violation ticket for me. If it was my mistake, then I had to go to the traffic court to clear out my violation ticket. I respected all the police officers quite a lot. I understood the nature of their uneasy jobs that they had to face every day. I hated so much to hear the news on the television that so many police officers got killed while they were serving their duties in Oakland. I disliked people using weapons to kill each other. I thought we should give them respect for safeguarding the community and take into consideration their uneasy duties to serve the community. We should help them, instead of using hatred to solve the problems by killing them. I believe we can solve any problems in our community if we are considerate to each other, back off a little bit with mutual understanding, and make correction by giving out an explanation if there are any misunderstandings or any mistakes. We can safeguard our community with great respect. There will be no argument and no killing, hence forming a respectful and safe community.

Chapter Two

Set Deal

Seasons passed, and my son Shaun graduated from the University of Davis. He got a job in Northern California. As usual, he came home every two weeks to cut the lawn for me. He always complained about the allergy every time he was done with the lawn work. After he would come inside the house, he would keep on scratching his face and complaining about the allergy. He showed me the rashes on his face after he took a shower. Sometimes his face had one big area of little pimple rashes, and sometimes his face had one big rash lump. Whenever I saw him scratching his face, I stopped him from doing that. I told him that I suspected the birch trees were causing the itching and allergy. This was the only type of tree that could cause allergy in our neighborhood. We usually cut down all the branches of the paper birch trees in our backyard during mid-fall and left only the trunks in the winter. The leaves would grow back in early spring. We faced so many problems while cutting the branches of these trees and while cleaning and dumping out all the leaves and branches each year. After Shaun would cut the paper birch branches and clean up the yard, he always complained about itching and allergies that he got outside in the yard again and again. Other than birch trees, we only had cypress trees and camellia bushes in our backyard. They were not allergic plants; hence, the only type of plants that could cause an allergy was the paper birch trees. So I suggested that Shaun should get rid of the paper birch trees in our backyard. He said OK. He cut down the two paper birch trees in our backyard in the late fall of 2000. After he cut down the paper birch trees, he did not complain about the allergy anymore after working in our backyard. However, he still complained about the allergy after he cut the lawn in the front yard. I felt bad that my son Shaun had to go through these kinds of allergies. I took over the responsibility from him of cleaning the dried white birch leaves and flowers from my neighbor's birch trees, which fell in my front yard. The dried birch leaves and flowers from my neighbor's trees flew all over my front and backyards when the wind blew, especially in the fall and in the winter when the leaves and flowers would start to turn yellow and fall onto the ground. They flew inside my garage all the year round when I opened my garage. I was getting tired of cleaning the leaves and flowers of my neighbor's white birch trees in my yards and inside my garage every week.

One day, while I was cleaning the birch leaves and flowers from my neighbor's three big birch trees on my front yard, I saw a lot of big and small pieces of fresh white birch flowers lying in front of my garage. I picked one of the fresh white birch flowers from the ground. Then I accidentally squeezed the fresh birch flower with my fingers. The flowers broke apart and the little fluid from the birch flower pieces stuck to my fingers. I tried to smell and taste the birch fluid on my finger. The fluid from the birch flowers was odorless and tasteless. After I tasted the birch fluid on my finger, my tongue started to itch right away. I went inside my house to wash my hands with soap and water first. I washed and rinsed my mouth with hot water again and again. Then I went back outside to my yard to clean all the birch leaves and flowers underneath the bushes on the right side of the garage near my neighbor's white birch trees. It took me more than a couple of hours to clean up all the birch leaves and flowers from my front yard. After I was done working on my yard, I went inside the house and took a shower. Then I prepared my dinner. After I finished my dinner, I went to bed early. That night, a small little pimple formed on my tongue. My tongue and lips began to itch, and I was very uncomfortably sick.

After I tasted the birch flowers, I started getting sicker and sicker. Both my legs started itching badly. I kept scratching my legs after I tasted the birch flower fluid on my fingers. Both my legs turned black when I stood up for long. I could feel that both my legs were itching badly and it felt like a needle was poking my left leg all the way to the end of my left toe. I found that my left toenail was turning black. Pale spots also formed on my knees and legs. Every time my legs itched, I had to keep my legs on the pillow to get rid of the itch. Once I kept my legs on the pillow, the itching and black color on my legs would be gone, but the pale spots on my knees and legs did not go away. My left ear started itching and it was infected badly. Sometimes I felt so dizzy that I could feel the whole ceiling of my house turning strongly when I laid down on my bed. Once I got sick and dizzy, I felt like throwing up. Usually I used my finger to tickle my throat to force all the food out from my stomach when I felt like throwing up. Sometimes I threw up undigested food, and sometimes I threw up black mucus. Most of the times, I felt so dizzy that I had to lie down on my bed. I talked to my sister Holly about my allergies and sickness that I had got at home from my neighbor's white birch trees. She did not believe when I told her that I had started itching after I came in from my yard and that I got my itching and my allergies from the birch trees. She knew I smoked cigarettes sometimes. She presumed that cigarettes could be the cause of the allergy that made my legs itch and turn black. I told her it was nonsense. I only smoked less than half a pack of light cigarettes a day. I had never heard of any smoker complaining about any allergy and sickness because of the cigarettes that they smoked. If the cigarettes could cause an allergy, all the smokers would complain to the consumer and no people would pick up cigarettes to smoke again. The consumer would find out the truth from the researchers, and they would ban the cigarette company for selling the allergic cigarettes in the market. After I talked to Holly, I felt very upset. I took out all my blood sample test results that I had saved for all these years and studied all the data from those results. I found my HDL good cholesterol data was very low when compared with the normal required data range. My bad LDL cholesterol data was very high when compared with the normal required data in my blood. I was getting very upset that my ears, lips, and legs were itching all the time after I came back from the yard outside. I did not know how to get rid of the itch in my ears, lips, and legs. Most of the times, I felt very sick and dizzy. I did not know how to get rid of all the allergies and sickness that I was getting every day due to my neighbor's birch trees. I decided to talk to my neighbor on the right side to request them to take care of their messy white birch trees that made me so sick.

When I was cleaning my front yard, I saw my neighbors Linsi and Tim Hoffman working outside. I went over to talk to them about their three big white birch trees. I requested them to do something about their three big white birch trees and their messy leaves and flowers lying in my front yard and inside my garage. Mrs. Linsi Hoffman promised me to take care of their white birch trees next year early spring. But they moved out in early winter to Texas and left their house empty with their real estate agent. The real estate agent came and put up the sale sign in front of their house. They brought in the buyers to look at my neighbor's house. After a couple of months, my neighbor's real estate agent sold their house. The new owner would not be moving in until the spring of next year. I talked to Bob Novel, my neighbor across the street, about my neighbor's white birch trees. He suggested that my neighbor should cut down their white birch trees if they were allergic trees. I told him the whole family of my neighbor had already moved to Texas and left their house empty. Then I heard another neighbor across the street complaining about the death of one of their cats due to poisonous chemicals in our neighborhood. I told them we had a lot of snails and slugs in front of our yards. I had seen a lot of cats eating the snails and slugs in our yards. We did not use any chemical insect killer in our yards; hence, their cat must have died because of the poisonous chemicals from the white birch trees, when they ate those snails and slugs in the bushes, which had the poisonous powder of the white birch flowers on their shells. I told them I had found a lot of dead birds with fat stomachs in our side yard, near my neighbor's white birch trees. I believed all those birds must have died because of the poisonous chemical powder from the white birch trees. The birds had been eating the snails, the slugs, and the insects that contained the poisonous powder of the white birch flowers and died. I called and complained almost every day to elderly Catherine about my allergies and sickness because of my neighbor's white birch trees. She listened to me patiently and advised me to call the city of Pleasanton to talk to them and let them know the problems that I had with my neighbor's white birch trees.

After I got the advice from elderly Catherine, I started to call the city of Pleasanton to complain about the allergies and sickness that I got from my neighbor's white birch trees. They told me to talk to my neighbor. I told them I had talked to my neighbor; they had promised to do something about their white birch trees in the next early spring, but they moved out from their house, and now no one was living in my neighbor's house. Then they advised me to call Mr. Hoffman's real estate agent to ask them to clean their trees' mess on my side. I tried to get their real estate agent's telephone number and called them to ask them to clean their white birch trees' mess in my front yard. When they came, they only cleaned their messy leaves and flowers around their house and in their yard, but they did not clean their messy leaves and flowers from their birch trees in my yards.

After I found out the birch leaves and flowers were causing me bad allergies and sickness, I started to talk to the people that I had met in my neighborhood and the people at the stores. I talked to one of the employees of Orchard Supply Hardware store in the gardening department. The employee told me his lips would itch all the time and he did not know what was causing the itching of his lips. I told him that if he had white birch trees in his surroundings, then the itching must be due to the white birch trees. I told him my lips had been itching too and I felt dizzy and sick all the time. I knew it was caused by my neighbor's three big white birch trees. He said he had so many trees like white birch trees, oak trees, maple trees, and different kinds of bushes in his backyard. Some people had told him the oak trees were the allergic trees. But he did not believe that oak trees could cause allergy and itching. He said he was confused and did not know the actual tree that caused the itching of his lips. I told him I had already found out that the birch trees were the allergic trees. I also told him that I had already cut down two of my paper birch trees in my backyard. I advised him to get rid of the white birch trees in his backyard. He said he would cut down the birch trees if the birch trees were really the trees that caused itching of his lips.

When I went to Pleasanton Stonebridge mall to look for a new microwave oven to replace my old broken microwave oven, I met a teenager in the appliances department in Sears store. He came to me and talked to me. I saw he had a lot of thick red rashes with blisters on his face. I asked him about the red rashes on his face. He said he did not know how he got all those rashes on his face. He had gone to see the dermatology doctor and had used the medicines that the doctor had prescribed to him. He had also bought and used the medicines that were advertised on television, but none of them worked for him to get rid of those bad rashes on his face. After I carefully studied his face, I told him all his rashes were external rashes caused by external allergy substances that had burned his face and formed the red rashes. I believed the medicines that he used for his rashes on his face had the ability to get rid of the rashes, but he did not give time to the medicines to get rid of the rashes from his face. He kept getting the allergy substances and burning his face again and again. This was the reason he could not get better. Then I asked him whether he took care of the lawn for his parents. He said yes. He had to cut the lawn every two weeks for his parents. Then I asked him if he had any white birch trees in his community. He said yes, there were a lot of white birch trees in his neighborhood. So I told him the allergy substances from the birch trees were the cause for the red blister rashes on his face. I advised him not to stay outside a lot before he got rid of all his rashes on his face and that he needed to clean his hands after he worked in his yard. He said OK and then left. The salesman of Sears store came to take care of me. I bought the microwave oven from the salesman and went home.

After I met the teenager in Sears store, I talked to a lot of people and teenage boys in my neighborhood who were getting blister rashes on their faces. Some of them had a lot of scars on their faces after they got the blister rashes on their faces. I tried to find the cause of the rashes on their faces and about their environment. After I found out they had a lot of white birch trees in their neighborhood, I felt very uncomfortable on seeing all those teenagers ruining their skin on their faces because of all the infectious blister rashes caused by poisonous substances from the birch trees. When I talked to my neighbor Susan on the left end corner of our street, she complained a lot about the allergies that they got from their lawn. She said they could not even lay their hands on their lawn. Every time her husband cut grasses and cleaned their lawn, he got bad blisters and rashes on his hands. They said they did not know how they got the bad allergies from their lawn. I repeatedly explained to them that all their allergies were caused by the chemical powder from their nearby white birch trees. When the wind blew, all the small broken pieces or the powder of the dried birch flowers and leaves would fly all over the place and land on their lawns. When they worked outside and laid their hands on their lawn, they got burned by all that allergic powder from their lawn, causing blister rashes on their hands. I told them about my neighbor's big birch trees that were causing me bad allergies and sickness. They told me they had no right to complain that they were getting allergies from my neighbor's white birch trees, because all my neighbor's birch trees were three houses away from them. I indicated to them that their neighbors who lived behind their house also had three big white birch trees. I told me we were surrounded by allergic white birch trees in our neighborhood, which made us very sick. They said they could not do anything about them. They told me that a lot of people had moved out from their houses to other places because of the bad allergies and sickness that they got from their neighborhood that they lived in. They said that instead of continuing to complain they would have to sell their houses to move out from this neighborhood. I told them that we did not need to move out from this neighborhood and that we could ask our neighbors to get rid of their bad allergic birch trees, but they said they had no right to complain to my neighbor who lived three houses away from their house. The only solution that they had was to move out from this neighborhood by selling their house. I told them if we sold the house and moved out from this neighborhood without getting rid of the bad trees, when another family moved into this house, they would suffer from the same kind of problems that we had. I told them that since I had already found out and proved the bad substances from the birch trees were causing the allergies and sickness in this neighborhood, we should advise all the people in this neighborhood to get rid of the bad allergic birch trees. Because I cared about the people and the environment in this community, I wanted the city of Pleasanton to take the lead in ordering the people of this neighborhood to cut down all the allergic white birch trees that caused bad allergies and sickness to the people in order to provide a healthy environment to all the people who lived in this city and in other cities. I kept calling the city of Pleasanton to complain about my neighbor's white birch trees that were causing the allergies and sickness in the neighborhood and requesting them to have my neighbor cut down their bad white birch trees.

After I talked to my neighbor, I called and talked to my sister Rosie in King of Prussia to tell her to get rid of her allergic birch trees in her side yard. She said there was no use in asking her to get rid of her white birch trees as all the neighbors around her were planting white birch trees in their yards. The neighbor behind her house had five big white birch trees in their yard. I reminded her about the herpes that she had got on her lips all the time. I told her she had never researched abut it to find when and how she got the herpes. She always liked to blame it on germs and said her herpes must be due to the germs. I asked her, "What are germs? Can germs survive without liquid or fluid in the air? Are germs the living micro-bacteria?" She did not say anything to me. I told her I knew how she had got herpes blister on her lips. I believed her herpes blister was caused by the broken pieces or powder of the birch flowers. I reminded her that she had two big white birch trees near her window.

The dining table was next to her window. The small broken pieces or the powder of white birch flowers possibly blew into her house when she opened her window and landed on her table. When she touched the table while she was cleaning it, those small sticky particles on the table must have got stuck on her hands. When she wiped her mouth with her hand, she would have got burned by those small sticky particles, causing herpes blister on her lips. Another possibility was she would have got herpes by direct contact with the birch powder that flew in through her screen window or when she was working outside in her yard. Sometimes those small pieces of sticky allergic particles were carried to other houses by humans, when those sticky allergic particles from the allergic trees landed on human bodies. Herpes blisters also formed on the lips of my two sisters in New Jersey all the time. They did not have any birch tree or poisonous plants in their houses or in their neighbors' houses. But when they came to visit Rosie in King of Prussia, they got herpes blisters on their lips after they went home. I tried to convince them to beware of the birch flowers from the white birch trees, which would cause bad allergies to them. Herpes blister is a kind of strong blister pimples that can spread if the blisters break. I told Rosie to beware of her white birch trees, and our conversation ended with her by hanging up our phone.

In early spring of April 2001, the new owner John Clark moved into my neighbor's house. As soon as I saw the new owner John Clark had moved in, I went over to my neighbor's house to talk to him. I knocked on his door. He came out from his house angrily when he saw me. I told him I had been very sick for three weeks after I cleaned up all the birch leaves and flowers that had fallen from his white birch trees in my front yard. He pointed his finger at me, yelling at me to cut down his white birch trees myself if I did not like the white birch trees. I told him I was not going to touch his trees; those were his birch trees, and he had to take responsibility for it to take care of his own trees. I got very upset after I talked to my new neighbor John Clark because of the way he treated me. Instead of talking to my neighbor on the right side of my house, I decided to inform the city of Pleasanton that my neighbor's birch trees were causing me bad allergies and sickness. I wrote a letter dated May 15, 2001, to Renee about the allergies and sickness that I got from my neighbor's white birch trees again. I explained in the letter that I was very sick over three weeks after I cleaned the messy flowers and leaves from my neighbor's white birch trees and that I had just got better. I also wrote that when I talked to my neighbor, he treated me badly and that he pointed his finger at me, asking me to cut down the trees by myself. I told her I did not know what to do anymore. After I finished my letter, I gave the letter to Renee's secretary in the city of Pleasanton and requested her to forward the letter to Renee for me.

Because I was very sick for three weeks, Sirena suggested I go and visit my sisters and brothers on the East Coast in July 2001. She bought me a round-trip ticket to go to King of Prussia, Pennsylvania. I flew to King of Prussia on August 2, 2001. I took this special trip to King of Prussia to get away from my allergic neighborhood. When I arrived in King of Prussia, I lived alone in Susong's house. Susong was working in New Jersey as usual, and she came home at weekends. Susong told me the people from King of Prussia were also suffering from bad allergies and sickness just like me. When I looked around their environment, I saw that almost every house in her neighborhood had planted white birch trees in their yards. Some of them were very big and over thirty feet high. One sunny day, when I was alone in Susong's house, I did not have anything to do inside the house, so I went outside the house to pull the weeds in the front yard. While I was pulling the weeds, I felt some small pieces of objects dropping from the air on my left arm. When I looked at my left arm, I did not see anything on it. I just wiped off my left arm with my other hand and went inside the house right away. After a couple of hours, my left arm felt very itchy. I kept scratching my left arm until my whole left arm turned red. Then I went to the kitchen sink to wash my left arm with soap and water. After a while, my left arm was covered with red rashes. When Susong saw my left arm covered with big red rashes, after she came home from New Jersey, she asked me what had happened to my arm. I told her that when I was pulling the weeds in front of her house outside her yard, I felt something land on my left arm and caused it to itch, and I kept on scratching my left arm; the more I scratched, the more I got a bad itch and rashes formed. She advised me not to go outside again. She took out Calamine lotion from her refrigerator and put it on my left arm to get rid of the itch. Next day, I went out again to the front yard to pull the weeds out of one of her front bushes near her car garage. I saw a small plant growing inside the bushes. I tried to pull the small plant out from the bushes. The plant did not come out, but the leaves broke, and part of the leaves came out from the plant. Then I held the small trunk of the plant and tried to pull the whole plant out with force, but I could not pull it out. I went inside Susong's garage and took out the screwdriver from the garage shelf. I used the screwdriver to dig the ground until the whole plant came out. I took out the plant from the bush. The plant trunk was really big. I did not know how long the plant had been growing underneath the bushes. After a while, my hands started to itch badly. I went inside the house. I washed my hands with soap and water. Then Rosie came to Susong's house to take me out for lunch in the King of Prussia mall. We went to the King of Prussia mall and had lunch. After we ate our lunch, she sent me back home. I told Rosie about the itch on my hands that I had after I pulled a plant out from the bushes. I showed her my itchy right hand. I kept scratching my right hand in front of her. A lot of rashes had formed on my right hand. I put Calamine lotion on my right hand to stop the itching, but it did not stop. She advised me not to go outside to pull the weeds. Then she went home. When Susong came home from New Jersey, I showed her the plant that I had dug out from underneath the bushes. She said it was poison ivy. She told me she had a lot of poison ivy plants in her yard. She warned me not to pull or touch with my hands any poison ivy plant in her yard. There was a pimple blister in my right middle finger and it was itching badly. The more I scratched, the bigger the pimple blister became. After a few days, the small blister pimple changed into a big blister. I had to take an allergy pill every four hours to get rid of the itch. After a couple of days, the big blister on my right middle finger broke, and the fluid kept flowing out from the blister. I had to keep wiping the fluid with tissue and put Calamine lotion to dry out the blister fluid. It took me more than a week to let the blister dry out. After the blister on my right middle finger completely recovered, it left a deep scar on my right middle finger. Even though I worked outside in my sister's yard the whole day, I did not feel a bit of itching on my lips, and I did not have any pale spotty on my legs and knees. But when I came back to California, my lips and legs started to itch badly. I could not even stand it for a long time.

While I was in King of Prussia, I compared and explained to my sisters and brothers that the types of burns caused by birch trees and those by the poison ivy plant were different. The burn from the poison ivy plant caused big blisters, because the poisonous chemical from the poison ivy was stronger than that of the white birch trees, but the burn from the white birch tree caused red blister rashes. I told them the rashes on my left arm were caused by the allergic powder from their neighbor's white birch trees. All of that small allergy powder was flying all over the neighborhood in the air. Susong told me she got bad allergy on her whole body after she took a shower at home every day. She did not know what was causing her to get this kind of red rashes and hives on her whole body after she took showers. She showed me her whole body that was covered by a lot of red rashes and hives after she took showers at home. She presumed her rashes and hives were caused because of the water that she used for taking showers at home. She said her whole body was very itchy. She kept scratching all over her body in front of me. I looked at her body and asked her what kind of towel she used to wipe her body after she took a shower. She said she used the towel that hung in her bathroom to wipe her body after she took the shower. I advised her not to use the towel that she had left inside her bathroom before she went to New Jersey for five days. I told her she should use a clean towel from her cabinet to wipe her body after she took a shower. I told her that the bad rashes and hives were not caused by the water at home when she took a shower. I explained to her that as most of her neighbors were growing a lot of white birch trees in their yards, all her allergies must have been caused by the dried birch flower powder that must have entered her room through her air conditioner. I suggested that she stop using the towel that would be hanging inside her bathroom when she came back home from New Jersey. When I observed her living style, I noticed that she liked to turn on her air conditioner inside her room after she came back from New Jersey. She left the air conditioner on in her room the whole day. All of that dry allergic powder from outside was carried inside her room through the air conditioner after she turned it on in her room. Then she took a shower at night. She used the towel that would be hanging inside her bathroom to wipe her body. This was the reason that her whole body would itching, causing big and small hives and red blister rashes. She took my advice and used a clean towel from her cabinet to wipe her body after she took a shower. She did not get any itching and red rashes and hives on her body. She was very happy and pleased that I helped her to solve her allergy problem that was making her so misery all these years. When she came back home from New Jersey on Thursday night, she told me Edward, Rosie, and she would take me to New York to see Harvey for my checkup. She asked me to get up early in the morning so as to be ready to go to New York on Sunday.

On Sunday morning, August 5, 2001, Rosie and Edward came to Susong's house to take us to visit Harvey in New York. It took us more than a couple of hours to arrive in New York's Manhattan, Chinatown. There was more traffic on the roads of Manhattan in the morning. Edward had to drive slowly to go to Harvey's clinic. We arrived at Harvey's clinic at 10:30 a.m. Edward dropped us in front of Harvey's clinic and left. Then we went up to the second floor in Harvey's clinic. When I was in Harvey's clinic, he helped me check my blood pressure. He drew my blood sample and sent it to New York laboratory to do a blood sample test. He asked Margaret to take me to New York C. P. Radiology Center (NYCPRC) on Bowery Street, a couple of blocks away from his clinic, for mammogram X-ray. Margaret, Rosie, Susong, and I went to the NYCPRC. Margaret registered me at the front desk counter for mammogram X-ray. We had to wait for a while in the waiting room. The technician came out and took me inside the mammogram X-ray room to take mammogram X-ray. After she took a mammogram X-ray of me, she asked me to sit on a chair outside the mammogram X-ray room, waiting for the films to be developed and printed out. Then she left. After a while, she came back looking sad; she'd reviewed the mammogram films and she exclaimed to me that I needed to retake the mammogram X-rays because the mammogram films showed two big plain spots on both my breasts. She said the machine must be broken and showed the two plain spots on the mammogram films. She assumed that I would be very unhappy to retake the mammogram X-rays. She tried to comfort me that those were machine errors. She took me back inside the mammogram X-ray room. She put the mammogram films on the light board and showed me the plain spots on my both breasts. I saw a big plain area on the top left side of my left breast and a small plain spot area near the bottom of my right breast in both mammogram films. After I saw those two plain spots on my mammogram films, I suddenly realized these two plain spots that showed on the mammogram films must be the cuts by the car's seat belts during my car accident in 1998. I had not driven my car anywhere after the car accident in 1998. Sirena was the one who drove me around the town, running the errands for me all these years. After she explained to me what happened on my mammogram films, she convinced me to retake the mammogram X-rays to make sure these were not caused by the X-ray machine errors. Then she retook the mammogram X-rays again on both my breasts. She asked me to wait for the mammogram films to be developed and printed out again. She said she wanted to make sure the mammogram films were developed and printed out right. After a while, she came back out and told me that both my mammogram films that I had just taken were showing the same plain spots on both my breasts. The doctor had compared the two plain spots from the mammogram films. Then the technician took me out to the waiting room. When she saw Margaret in the waiting room, she told Margaret that they had found two plain spots on both my breasts in the mammogram films. Then she released us. Margaret took us back to Harvey's clinic.

After the radiologist Dr. James Chang (M.D., FACR) read and reviewed all my mammogram films, he faxed a letter to Harvey's clinic to indicate that I did not have any significant abnormality on both my breasts, but there were some minimal nonspecific old inflammatory changes in the hilar regions of my breasts. Dr. Chang told Harvey to let me take the bilateral breast ultrasound screening test to make sure the plain areas on my breasts would not cause any breast cancer. After Harvey received the letter from Dr. Chang, he told Rosie and Susong about the two plain spots on both my breasts, which the doctor had found in my mammogram films. They were very worried that I might have breast cancer. They asked Harvey to set up an appointment for me to take the bilateral breast ultrasound screening test. Harvey made an appointment with the radiology clinic for me to take the bilateral breast ultrasound screening test on August 14, 2001. Then Margaret took us to dinner in Chinatown. After we had dinner, we went back to the clinic, waiting for Edward to take us back to King of Prussia. After 6:00 p.m., Edward came to Harvey's clinic to take us back to King of Prussia. Then we went back to King of Prussia, Pennsylvania.

On August 14, 2001, we went back to New York again for my bilateral breast ultrasound screening test in the NYCPRC. Harvey asked us to go with Margaret to the radiology clinic to take the ultrasound screening test. When I was in the ultrasound screening test room, Dr. Joan A. Kedziora screened both my breasts on the computer screen in detail. After she was done screening my breasts, she told me she was not too happy with the plain area on my left breast because it was too big to leave it alone. After she told me the result of the ultrasound test, she discharged me. We went back to Harvey's clinic. After Dr. Kedziora had reviewed my bilateral breast ultrasound test in detail, she faxed a letter to

Harvey, describing the result of my bilateral breast ultrasound test. After Harvey received the fax from Dr. Kedziora, he called and talked to her. She told Harvey that she had recommended to me to get surgery done on my breasts. Harvey said OK to her. Then he told Rosie that Dr. Kedziora had recommended to me to get surgery done on my breasts. He helped me pay for all my medical expenses at the NYCPRC. We went back to King of Prussia. Then Harvey requested the NYCPRC to give him the mammogram films for my breast surgeon to review. After he got my mammogram films, he asked Edward to take them to King of Prussia.

After I found out I had two plain spots on my breasts, I was very unhappy and did not want to perform breast surgery. I told my sisters that I wanted to go back to California, but Rosie and Susong insisted on me staying in King of Prussia to get my breast surgery done. They asked me to postpone the date of my air ticket to go back to California. They said they would take care of me. They called and asked Sirena to postpone the date of my air ticket to go back to California. Then they tried to find a good breast surgeon for me in Pennsylvania. Susong's daughter Sabrina was at home with me. She was practicing in the University of Pennsylvania for her undergraduate internship. She told her mother that her friend's father Dr. Thomas G. F. was a good surgeon. He was practicing in Bryn Mawr Hospital in Pennsylvania. She helped Susong to get the telephone number from her friend. Susong called and set up an appointment for me to see Dr. Thomas for my breast surgery, after she got his telephone number from Sabrina. On the appointment date, Rosie, Edward, and Susong took me to Dr. Thomas's clinic in Bryn Mawr Hospital. When we were in Dr. Thomas's clinic, Rosie and Susong went to the front desk clerk to register and check in for me. After they checked in, Dr. Thomas came out to take me to his office to talk about the procedures for my breast surgery. Rosie came in with me to the office. She gave Dr. Thomas the letters from the radiologists as well as the mammogram films for him to review. After Dr. Thomas reviewed all of the information in the doctors' letters and mammogram films for the two plain spots area that showed in them, he recommended me to only get surgery done on my left breast because the plain spot was too big and too dangerous to leave it alone. He said he would not worry about the small plain spot on my right breast at the moment. Then he asked for our opinion regarding him doing the surgery on my left breast to take care of the big plain spot. Rosie agreed to let him perform the surgery. Then she gave him permission to keep the mammogram films to study before the surgery. He took the films and told us he would call us after he had checked out which day the operation room was vacant in Bryn Mawr Hospital to do the surgery. The nurse called Susong after a few days to notify her that the surgery date was on August 30, 2001, in Bryn Mawr Hospital. The nurse instructed Susong to take me to Bryn Mawr Hospital to get an EKG test done and told her not to let me eat anything on the night before the surgery date.

On August 28, 2001, Rosie, Edward and Susong took me to Bryn Mawr Hospital to get an EKG test done. When I was in the EKG test room, I had to wait for the anesthetist to come and talk to me before the technician performed my EKG test. After half an hour, the nurse came into the EKG room first and asked me all the information she needed to know about me before my surgery. She filled up all of my information in the form. After she was done taking the information from me, the anesthetist came in and talked to me. After he got all the information he needed to know from me, he asked me to sign the paper for him. I signed the paper, and they both left. After a while, the EKG technician came in and asked me to lie down on the patient bed. He started to perform the EKG test on me. After he was done, he read the EKG results and told me the EKG test result was perfect and I did not have any problem in getting breast surgery done.

On August 30, 2001, Rosie, Edward, and Susong took me to Bryn Mawr Hospital early in the morning. When we arrived in the hospital, Susong helped me to register and paid for my surgery expenses at the front desk. The total cost of my surgery expense was over ten thousand dollars. Then the nurse took me to a room and asked me to change into hospital clothing. After I changed, one of the technicians came in and injected the relaxation medicine (I did not know the name of the medicine) in my left arm. After a while, the nurse took me to the second floor radiology room to wait for the doctor to perform the needle biopsy. Dr. John Stassi (M.D.) came in to perform the needle biopsy on my left breast, marking the size of the plain spot on my left breast, which showed on the computer screen. Then they took me into the surgery room and moved me to the operation bed. Then the anesthetist put the anesthetic mask on my nose. After a while, I fell asleep. I did not know exactly how many hours it took for Dr. Thomas to perform the surgery. I heard the nurse calling me to wake me up. Then I woke up and opened my eyes. I saw two nurses beside my bed. As soon as I saw the nurses, I asked one of the nurses where my sisters and brother were. The nurse told me they were waiting in the hospital waiting room. Then I went back to sleep. After a couple of hours, one of the nurses tried to wake me up again. I woke up again, and this time, I told the nurse I needed to go to the restroom. She took me to the restroom. Then she asked me to change into my regular clothing and discharged me from the hospital. Rosie, Edward, and Susong took me home. I stayed in Susong's house for another four more days after my breast surgery. After my breast surgery, Susong cooked chicken soup for me to eat with rice every day.

On September 5, 2001, I flew back to California. Sirena picked me up at San Francisco airport and took me home. I told Sirena about the nurse in Bryn Mawr Hospital. When I was in the EKG test room, the nurse had told me that she had graduated from Villanova University. She asked me about the red rashes on my left arm. I told her I got those rashes from white birch trees while working outside in my sister's yard. The allergy particles from white birch trees sprayed from the sky as if the angels had sprayed bad allergic particles from the sky. She thought I was joking. She laughed and said to me no. Instead of white birch trees, she wrote in my medical form that poison ivy was the cause of allergy and red rashes on my left arm. I was very uncomfortable and frustrated that the nurse did not believe me when I told her the truth that my allergy rashes on my left arm were caused by the white birch trees in Susong's neighborhood. I told Sirena that I had heard from either the doctors or the people everywhere that they all believed the pollens from the flowers were causing the allergies. They all were mistakenly misled by the doctors and the researchers. Sirena just looked at me without saying anything to me. Then I told her that one of my sisters' (Eileen) friends and her family had been complaining about the allergies inside their house after they came back from work every day. Eileen told me that the whole family of her friend had told her that when they just stepped inside their house, they would get the bad itch and the allergies on their body. No matter how they much they cleaned their house, they still could not get rid of the itch and the allergies from their bodies. They did not know what caused these kinds of itching and allergies. Sometimes they got big hives on their body; sometimes they got blister pimples on their uncovered body. They said they did not even know whether they should stay or move out from the house that they lived in. They were very frustrated to keep on complaining about their allergies and sickness every time they see their doctors.

On September 11, 2001, I woke up early in the morning. I was preparing myself to go out to do some errands. It was still a bit early, so I turned on the television to watch the news. I was shocked to see the scene of the first airplane hitting one of the World Trade Center (WTC) Twin Towers buildings in Manhattan, New York. The tower which the plane hit was on fire, and a lot of smoke was coming out from the tower. I did not know if this was a terror attack. I turned off my television when it was time for me to leave the house to run for my errands. I went out to the bank to deposit my check that my brother had given me. Then I went to the supermarket to buy some groceries. I came back home after I was done. I turned on the television again. I saw the second tower get hit by another airplane and catch fire. A lot of smoke came out from both WTC Twin Towers buildings. After a while, both WTC Twin Towers buildings collapsed and fell slowly to the ground. The people inside the buildings were very terrified and were running out from the buildings as fast as they could. I stayed in front of the television and kept watching it until it was dark. Two more terror attacks occurred in Pennsylvania and Washington DC. The terrorists blew up an American airline in Pennsylvania. The Pentagon military building in Washington DC was directly hit and attacked by the airplanes and a lot of people killed. I was so shocked and couldn't believe that we could get so many terror attacks in our country within one day.

Every week, I had to go out again to my front yard to clean the birch leaves and flowers. After I came in, my lips and my body would itch like insect bites. I kept cleaning my front yard. Finally, I stopped cleaning them after I got quite sick. Then I saw a big pile of dirt residing on the road in front of my car driveway. I did not know where the big pile of dirt had come from. The dirt kept washing down to my front road and residing in front of my house. I went outside to find out where all that dirt had come from. I found all that dirt was from my left-end corner neighbor Susan's house. They would wash their dirt to our side with water after they remodeled and replanted trees in their yard. All their dirt resided in front of my house. I called the city of Pleasanton to complain about the dirt and told them it was impossible for me to keep cleaning them. After I cleaned up and came back into my house, I got a bad allergy all over my body and I was getting quite sick again. The city

63

of Pleasanton told me to talk to my neighbors to move their cars that were parked on the street every Wednesday so that the city's truck could come and clean the street every Wednesday. I told the city that it was not my responsibility to tell my neighbors to move their cars from the street. This was the city's responsibility to notify my neighbors to move their cars from the street. But the city of Pleasanton did not take any action regarding my complaints. I kept calling the city of Pleasanton to complain about the dirt that resided in my front yard road. The city of Pleasanton advised me to call Pleasanton Police Department to complain about the dirt that resided in my front yard road and the messy birch leaves and birch flowers in front of my house. So I called Pleasanton Police Department to complain about the dirt and the dried leaves and flowers on the road of my front yard and in my yard, which were because of the three big white birch trees of the neighbors on the right side of my house. I was very upset as I had to keep on complaining about the dirt that would pile up on the road in front of my house, as well as the messy leaves and flowers from my neighbor's white birch trees in my yard. I was getting very frustrated living in this kind of neighborhood.

After the city of Pleasanton advised me to call the police department of Pleasanton, I kept calling Pleasanton Police Department again and again to complain about the dirt and the allergic birch leaves and birch flowers that were piling in front of my house. Five police officers came to my house at night after I kept calling to complain about the dirt and the messy leaves and flowers in front of my house. I showed them the dirt that had piled on the road in front of my house and told them they were from the neighbor Susan's house on the left side of my home. Then I showed them the big pile of dried birch leaves and flowers on my front yard, driveway, and underneath the right bushes next to my car garage. I told them those birch flowers were very allergic and they made me very sick. After the police officers saw a lot of the big birch flowers in the bushes and a big messy pile of white birch leaves and flowers in front of my house, they agreed about my complaints and said it must be very frustrating for me to live in this kind of neighborhood. Then one of the police officers looked inside the bushes. He picked up one of the big white birch fluid-like flowers. He suggested that I take pictures of these big birch flowers to show to the city of Pleasanton. I told them I did not have a camera to take pictures. At that moment, a drop of fluid from the birch tree dropped onto my neck. I wiped my neck off with my right hand.

After the police officers searched and looked around my front yard, one of the police officers said they would report the situation about my house to the city of Pleasanton, and they left. After the police officers left, I came into my house and was just about ready to go to sleep when I felt very dizzy and my neck was very itchy. I was just about to scratch my neck with my right hand when I felt a big, deep swollen lump on my neck. This deep swollen lump on my neck was formed by the fluid from the white birch trees, which dropped on my neck when I was under the birch trees with one of the officers. I was so upset I picked up the telephone right away and called the police department again to inform them about the big lump on my neck and that it had been caused by the drop of fluid that fell from the birch tree on my neck while I was talking to the police officers, showing them the big birch flowers under my neighbor's birch trees. The fluid was so poisonous that it caused the formation of a big lump on my neck right away. My hand was also itching badly after I used it to wipe out the birch fluid from my neck. I felt very dizzy after I came into my house. The operator from the police department promised they would report to the city of Pleasanton about this incident of poisonous fluid from the white birch trees. Then I hung up the telephone with a very heavy heart.

After that night, I kept calling the city of Pleasanton to complain about my neighbor's birch trees that were causing me bad allergies and making me so sick. I went over to the new neighbor on the left side of my home, Mrs. Linda Makjcour, who had just moved in. I requested them to clean their yard with a broom instead of using a water hose to wash the dirt on the road. I did not want all their dirt to wash down to my side and pile on the road in front of my house. I also requested them to move their cars on Wednesday to let the city of Pleasanton clean the side road in front of our houses. After I talked to them, every Wednesday, they moved their cars from the roadside to let the city's truck to clean the road. Then they started to clean their yard and plant a lot of roses on the right side of their house. After that, Mr. Makjcour cleaned up their yard with his two older teenage children. I saw their two older children working in their yard with their father. After a certain period of time, I saw the same size of spotty rashes scattered all over their faces. I felt very upset and frustrated to see those two teenage children's faces spotted with rashes after I complained to them to clean their yard. When I checked on their youngest daughter's face, I did not see any blister rash on her face because she was not involved in cleaning the yard with her father. After I saw spotty rashes over the faces of Linda's two older children, I went over to Linda's house to talk to her. When I knocked on their front door, her son Kurt Makjcour opened the front door. I saw his face was full of the same size of spotty rashes. I asked him whether he knew where the rashes on his face came from. He said he had gone to see a dermatologist. The doctor had told him the rashes on his face were caused by internal hormone change during his teenage period. I asked him about his sister's face. He said he did not know what the doctor had told her about her face. I told him I knew where all the spotty rashes on their faces were coming from. I told them that when they were cleaning the outside yard with their father, their faces were burned by the broken white birch flower pieces, causing the scattered red spotty rashes on their faces. He said he did not know. I asked him to give me permission to look at the rashes on his face clearly, but Kurt was shy and felt embarrassed when I asked him to let me look at the rashes on his face. He asked me to leave him alone. I said OK and I went back home. All of Linda's children had fair skins just like their parents. I did not believe all those spotty rashes on their faces were caused by hormone change or genetically carried on from their parents.

I kept calling and complaining to the city of Pleasanton about the allergies and sickness that I got from my neighbor's birch tree. Mr. Davis from the city of Pleasanton came over to my house to persuade me to have my neighbor John Clark clean the messy leaves and flowers of his white birch trees in my yard. I had to admit that Mr. Davis's idea was an excellent idea to have my neighbor clean their messy birch leaves and flowers falling from their allergic trees in my property. I thanked him for his generous idea to help me solve this problem. But I had to refuse, and I explained to Mr. Davis that his idea was an excellent idea, but just cleaning the mess would not solve the allergies and sickness problem long term. I told him that we needed to get rid of the allergic white birch trees totally from my neighbor's house to let me and my neighbors live in our houses healthily. He was a very understanding good man. He cared about the people who lived in this city. He went over throughout the neighborhood to count all the white birch trees and started to make arrangements to issue an order to cut down the birch trees. He also kept an eye on my house and informed me when one of my floral cherry trees died. I used gallons of water to water the floral cherry tree in order to save the tree, but the floral cherry tree died. I did not know the reason for the death of the floral cherry tree.

I was very upset with the allergies that I got every day because of my neighbor's white birch trees. I wrote a letter to the city attorney, Renee, dated October 26, 2001, to inform her about the allergies that made me sick because of my neighbor's birch trees. I also informed her about my trip to King of Prussia to get away from the allergic neighborhood. I told her that the people of King of Prussia were also surrounded by white birch trees and they were also suffering from allergies and sickness just like me. I requested her to tell my neighbor to cut down their white birch trees. I also wrote a letter dated December 2, 2001, to Darren of State Farm Insurance Agent, informing him that I had to go through surgery on my left breast, which was caused by the cut due to my car seat belt during the car accident. I enclosed all the documents from my doctors and sent out my letter to Darren.

After I kept on complaining to Renee about my allergies because of my neighbor's birch trees, Renee finally responded to my complaint. She indicated that she had discussed with her lawyer colleagues from the city of Pleasanton. All her colleagues had indicated that I had the right to tell my neighbor to cut down their trees if they were harmful to me. She also indicated that if they refused to cut down their allergic trees, I had the right to take them to court. She advised me to go to court to sue my neighbor if they disagreed to cut down their birch trees. I told Sirena the city attorney, Renee, had advised me to sue my neighbor if they disagreed to cut down their allergic white birch trees. Sirena advised me to see the doctor first for my allergy sickness before I filed a case in the court to sue my neighbor.

Sirena knew I was very upset on getting bad allergies because of my neighbor's birch trees. She felt that it was not good for me to stay alone at home. She suggested that I got a dog for companionship at home. Since I had a hearing problem, the dog would bark if somebody came to my house. So I agreed to get a dog for myself. Earlier, we had a short white hair male Pekinese dog, named Sir San Sha. We bought him from a family in King of Prussia, Pennsylvania, for Sirena when she was one year old. He was Sirena's best friend. He was a very beautiful and healthy dog. When we moved out from King of Prussia, Pennsylvania, to California in 1984, we brought him along with us. When he was fourteen years old, we had to force ourselves to put him to sleep because he had bad arthritis. He cried out very loud every day and night because of his arthritic pain. Siok used a blanket to cover him up to keep him warm at night. Then we gave him arthritis medicines to get rid of his arthritic pain. No matter how much we helped him to get rid of his arthritic pain, he still cried out very loud at day and night. We did not know how to help him stop crying. Finally, we made the decision to put him to sleep. I hate to say that this was the best way to help Sir San Sha from his pain. He did not have to suffer so much. My two children, Sirena and Shaun, cried a lot when we put him to sleep. We all missed him a lot. We remembered our good times and bad times together with him after we brought him home when he was only four weeks' old and he became one of our family members. We did not have anything to complain about him, but we did have a lot to talk about him. We all loved him so much that we were unable to describe our love in words about him. The only regret that we had about him was he did not leave any baby for us.

I still remember when we lived in King of Prussia, Pennsylvania my children went to Caley Road Elementary School that was behind our house. After school, some of the school children would climb up the wire fence of our backyard and come in to play with him. The children from our neighborhood knew him and played with him all the time. When they saw him, they kept calling him from a distance, "San Sha! San Sha!" He would wave his tail and bark at them. Sometimes they came to him and played with him. He liked to chase after and bark at the squirrels in our backyard. One time, I tied him with a dog's chain outside in our backyard porch. I did not know how he got out from the dog's chain, but he was gone for the whole morning. My neighbor who was one block away from my house brought him back to my house and knocked on my front door. When he saw me open the door, he showed me Sir San Sha and asked me whether he was my dog. I told my neighbor that Sir San Sha was my dog. My neighbor said he had found him sitting in front of his front porch the whole morning. Sir San Sha would not leave his house no matter how he much he chased Sir San Sha out from his front porch. Then he remembered seeing my children playing with Sir San Sha in front of our house and sometimes in our backyard when he drove his car by to go home or when he passed our house. So he brought him back to us. I thanked him for bringing Sir San Sha back home for me. I told him that I had put the chain on Sir San Sha this morning and let him stay in our backyard porch and that I did not know how he got loose from his chain from our backyard porch and was gone for the whole morning. Maybe Sir San Sha did not know how to come back home, so he just had to stay in front of his house to get help from him to take him home. When Sir San Sha saw me, he ran to me, wagging his tail. I helped him up on my body, and he was so happy to be home again.

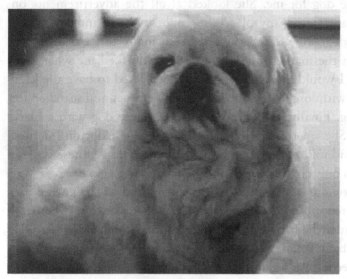

Sir San Sha

Sir San Sha liked to go out for a walk every day. Siok took him twice a day to go out for a walk. Every day when Siok came home, he would wag his tail and bark at Siok, asking Siok to take him out for a walk. After he came back from a walk, he would be tired and would rest in the kitchen. When he saw me, he would sit up and shake his both front legs and ask me for snacks. Most of the times, he got a snack bone from me. But sometimes, I would just give him a small piece of bread. He could predict the time when my children would be home after school, so he would stay near our front door, waiting for them to come home from school. Once my children were home, they liked to take him out to our backyard and play with him. Sir San Sha liked to play with softball. When Shaun threw the softball out, he would run after the softball to pick it up. Sometimes he would bring the softball back to Shaun, but sometimes he would disobey and take the softball to the place near the sliding door and would bite it. All the guests who came to our house said he was a very friendly dog and liked him a lot. He protected our family because of his sensitive hearing. He would bark and make a lot of noise when somebody showed up in front of our house. There were so many good things in our memories to talk about him. We have kept his picture in our family room to remember him.

Sirena knew I liked Pekinese dogs. She was on the lookout for another Pekinese dog for me. She looked at all the advertisements on Internet, newspapers, and any place she could look to find and study about Pekinese dogs. She found there were so many different kinds of Pekinese dogs in the market. She came home and asked me what kind of Pekinese dog I would like to have. I told her I liked to have the kind of Pekinese dog with long hairs. She looked on Internet and searched for the Pekinese dog. Finally, she found a baby Pekinese dog with a black face in Arizona. She saw the picture of the baby Pekinese dog on Internet. She called me and told me she had found a baby male Pekinese dog on Internet. He was only six weeks old, and his face was black; his eyes were big, his hair color was white mixed with brown, and his hair would be long when he grew up and became an adult. She asked me whether I wanted her to order the baby Pekinese dog from Arizona. I told her OK. She ordered the baby Pekinese dog from the Catering Pekinese breeder in Arizona. The breeder was an animal technician from Arizona. After one month, she sent the baby Pekinese dog to us on airplane. When the baby dog arrived at the San Francisco airport at the end of July 2002, Sirena picked him up and brought him home. I named him Sir Space after he arrived home. He was scared when Sirena brought him home. At night, I kept him on his bed that I had bought for him before he came. Next day, I found a lot of baby tapeworms in his bed. I did not know where the baby tapeworms came from. I kept cleaning those baby tapeworms from his bed. I tried to find where those baby tapeworms had come from. I picked him up and looked at his anus and found his stomach was releasing a lot of tapeworms from his anus. After the fourth day, I tried to get rid of all those baby tapeworms from his stomach by feeding him regular worm-releasing medicines from Walmart store. But I could not help him clear all the tapeworms from his stomach with Walmart store's worm-releasing medicine. I called Dr. Eliz S. from HAH to set up an appointment to take him to the HAH for a checkup. When I saw Dr. Eliz, I told her he had a lot of baby worms inside his stomach. Dr. Eliz checked him and said that he had a lot of tapeworms in his stomach and that she would prescribe tapeworm medicines for him to get rid of them from his stomach. She gave him all the shots that he needed to protect him. Then she prescribed him the tapeworm medicine and released him. After I came home from HAH, I fed him the tapeworm medicines that Dr. Eliz had prescribed for him. Next day, I took him out in my backyard for bowel movement. After he finished his bowel movement, I checked on his bowel discharge. I found out there were over a one-foot-long big female tapeworm and a lot of small tapeworms in his bowel discharge that had come out from his stomach. I did not know how long he had the mother tapeworm and all those baby tapeworms in his stomach. I continuously fed him the tapeworm medicines until all the tapeworms were gone from his stomach. I never let him out alone in my backyard, because there were so many wild animals in our neighborhood. I trained him to sit up in the plastic box and made him put up his two front legs together and shake his both front legs every day. He could sit up on the plastic box, but because his two front legs were short, he could not use his two front legs together and shake.

After Sirena advised me to see the doctor, I called Dr. David Chee to talk to him about my allergy that I had got from my neighbor's birch tree. He referred me to see Dr. Calvin L. from Tri Valley Physicians Group in VCMC in Pleasanton. I called Dr. Calvin's office to set up an appointment on August 8, 2002, to checkup with him. Before I went to see Dr. Calvin, I picked some fresh birch flowers from my neighbor's birch trees, washed them with clean water many times, and then saved them in a paper envelope to show to Dr. Calvin.

On August 8, 2002, I went to checkup with Dr. Calvin in Valley Care Clinic. Once I was in his office, I told him about the pain in my chest, brain, and body that I got from my car accident. Then I told him the main reason I had come to see him was about my bad allergy that I had got from the birch trees. I told him my lips itched after I came in from my front yard every time. I showed him the birch flowers in the envelope. I told him about the bad allergies caused by my neighbor's bad white birch trees, and my ears and my lips itched badly every time I came in from the yard outside. He referred me to take a blood sample test for my allergy. He set up an appointment for me in Valley Care laboratory on August 9, 2002, for my blood sample test. Then he set up an MRI test for my brain in VCMC on September 4, 2002. I went in to take my blood test and an MRI test for my brain at VCMC. Dr. Calvin called me to inform me that he did not find anything wrong in my brain after he received the result from Dr. R. Satterfield, Bay Imaging Consultant Medical Group, who had reviewed my MRI screen test. But he advised me to see the allergy doctor for my allergy after he received my blood test result. He referred me to Dr. Michael C. at Livermore Allergy Medical Clinic in Pleasanton. He gave me the telephone number to call Dr. Michael. I called Dr. Michael's clinic to set up an appointment on September 3, 2002, to see him. Before I went to check in with Dr. Michael's clinic, I put dried birch flowers in a plastic bag to take with me to show Dr. Michael when I went to checkup with him.

In early August 2001, I told Sirena to get another female Pekinese dog for Sir Space to have a playmate. I thought that maybe we could breed them later so they could have a baby to carry on their generation after they become adults. I was planning to give their babies to my sisters if they had any baby later. Sirena ordered by special mail another female Catering Pekinese from the same breeder in Arizona. She arrived home in late September 2002. I named her Lady Star. She was little, sincere, very cute, and a healthy baby. I had a lot of fun playing with her. They both had their own birth certificates. Sir Space was born on June 2, 2002. Lady Star was born on July 25, 2002. They kept me so busy every day.

I played with both my baby dogs. I taught them how to sit up and use their front legs to shake. I took both of them out with me in my car wherever I went. Sometimes I took them to supermarkets; sometimes I took them to visit Ada and Catherine. Catherine was a pet lover. She liked to hold both of them against her body and play with them. But Ada did not have the patience like Catherine to play with them. Ada always kept herself very busy, running around all over the places. Sirena loved to take them to her friends' houses, but they were not used to go out with her. They were a little bit afraid of going out with her. When I took them out in my backyard, they did not like to stay long because they were scared of wild hawks and wild animals in my backyard. Every day when I took them out to my backyard, they kept scratching their bodies after they came back inside the house. When I checked their bodies, I found they had a lot of red rashes on the underside of their bodies. I was very upset to see that they were also getting bad allergies just like me. I did not know how to stop them from scratching their bodies. I tried to give them bath twice a week to get rid of their allergies. I kept complaining to my children and elderly Catherine again and again about the allergies that my two baby dogs and I got because of my neighbor's birch trees.

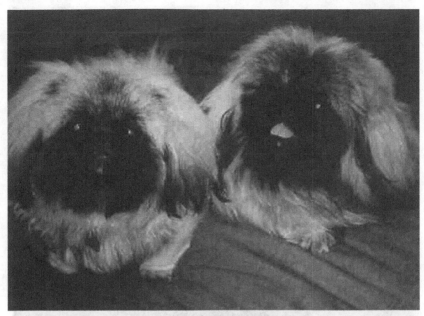

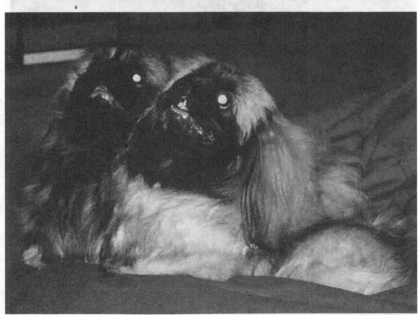

Lady Star and Sir Space

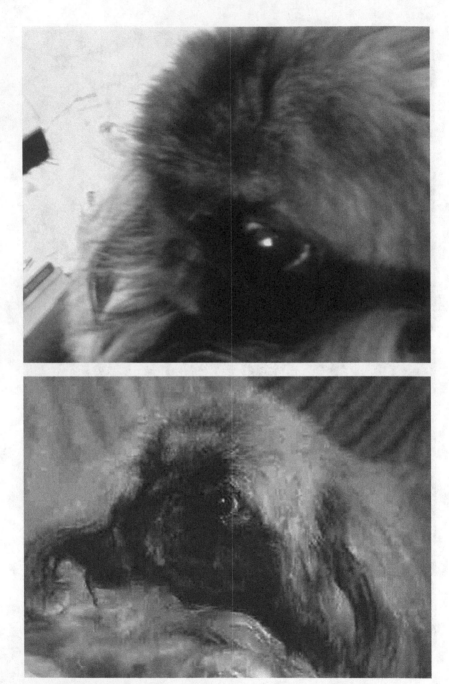

Sir Space and Lady Star's two years old pictures

On September 3, 2002, I took dried birch flowers in a plastic bag with me to checkup with Dr. Michael in Livermore Allergy Medical Clinic in Pleasanton. When I was in Dr. Michael's clinic, the front desk clerk gave me forms to fill up about my medical records. I filled in all the information that I knew in the forms. I skipped all the questions that I did not know. I did not know one single plant that was listed in the form. I felt the questions were strange. I did not eat or use any plants and meats that were listed in the form. I did eat a few types of fruits that were listed in the form, but it never caused me any allergy after I ate those fruits. After I finished filling my forms, I turned in the forms to the front desk clerk. Then the front desk clerk asked me to wait in the waiting room. I had to wait for a while in the waiting room for the nurse to take me to Dr. Michael's office. After a while, the nurse came out. She took me to Dr. Michael's office. She settled me in Dr. Michael's office and left. When Dr. Michael came inside the room, he asked me the reason for my visit. I handed out the plastic bag containing dried birch leaves and flowers to him. I told him I had got a bad allergy from my neighbor's white birch trees, my lips became very itchy, and I got very sick every time I passed the white birch trees and came inside my house. He did not take the plastic bag that I handed out to him. He did not ask me how I got an allergy from the birch trees. He just advised me to take the skin test before he could help me to diagnose my allergy and then left the room. Nurse Ann came in and asked me to follow her. She took me to another room and asked me to change into the patient clothing. After I changed into patient clothing, I sat on the patient's bed and waited for Dr. Michael to come in. After a while, Dr. Michael came in and checked my ears, eyes, throat, heart, and lungs. He said everything was OK with me. Then he told me the nurse would come in and talk to me about the skin test and then left the room.

After a few minutes, Nurse Ann came inside the room. She gave me the charts for the skin test and told me she was going to use the materials from the charts to test on the skin of my back for the allergy. I took the skin test charts from her, and I reviewed the charts. I was very upset after I reviewed the skin test charts. I told her I was not allergic to any food that was described in the charts. I did not understand the procedures and the purpose of using the fruits or meats listed in the charts to test on my skin to see whether I was allergic to them. In particular, I did not understand how they were going to use dog hairs to test on human body. I had so many questions to ask them about their skin test charts. I shook my head, and I asked her whether I definitely needed to take the skin tests because all the categories described in the charts had nothing to do with my allergy. Then she asked me what kind of plant had caused the allergy. I refused to tell her the type of tree that caused the bad allergy in me because I did not like Dr. Michael's behavior and the way he treated me by refusing to look at my birch flower sample. He did not even ask me about my allergy, what kind of symptoms that I had, and when and how did I get the allergy. He just told me I had to take the skin test first before he could diagnose me. I asked Nurse Ann whether I could skip the skin test. She said it was compulsory to take the skin test on my back. I was displeased as I disagreed with their unprofessional technique to test on human skin with food, plants, and meats that I had not eaten and complained about. They had nothing to do with my allergy. Nurse Ann gave me no choice, but I had to agree and asked her to set up an appointment for me to perform the allergy skin test. She set up the appointment for me and released me. I left Dr. Michael's clinic. My lips had been itching badly when I was inside the clinic. I wanted to find out what had made my lips itch when I was in the clinic. I looked around the surroundings of the clinic building after I came out from the clinic. I found two big birch trees were planted next to the entrance door of the front clinic. I did not know the reason which made my lips so itchy when I passed the birch trees at that time.

After I was home, I reviewed all the skin test charts. Then I called all the doctors from my family and friends to find out the reason they did the skin test for all those fruits, vegetables, plants, and meats listed on the skin test charts to test on the human body. I told them I did not even eat the fruits, plants, and meats described on the skin test charts. Every day I just made some steam chicken for my children and myself. I did not understand how they were going to make the assumption by using the skin test technique to test on my skin with food that I did not even eat and complain about. I told them I would send out the skin test charts to them for review and hung up the phone. Then I made the copies of the skin test charts given by Nurse Ann, Livermore Allergy Medical Clinic, and sent out a copy each to every one of them. After two weeks, I called all the doctors in my family and friends to ask them about the skin test charts that I had sent to them. They said they did not know and understand what the skin testing on human body was for, by using fruits, plants, and meats that was listed on the skin test charts. But they said they would talk to their fellow allergy doctors to check the purpose of testing on human skins with fruits, plants, and meats. I also called Dr. Calvin's clinic to complain about the categories that they had described on the skin test charts, which they were going to test on my skin. His assistant suggested that I cancel my skin test appointment if I did not feel good about the procedures at Livermore Allergy Medical Clinic in Pleasanton. After Dr. Calvin's assistant suggested that I cancel my appointment, I called Nurse Ann to cancel my skin test appointment and stopped seeing Dr. Michael again. When I received all my medical bills from VCMC and Livermore Allergy Medical Clinic, I sent all my bills to Blue Cross Insurance Company to let them take care of my medical bills for my visit to the physicians, the blood sample test, and the MRI test at VCMC, but Blue Cross Insurance Company refused to pay for my medical bills for VCMC. I had to pay all the medical bills for VCMC. I was getting very upset with Blue Cross Insurance Company. I cancelled my medical insurance with Blue Cross Insurance Company.

I kept calling and complaining to the city of Pleasanton and requesting them to ask my neighbor to cut down their birch trees. At the same time, I was trying to find a way to get rid of the allergies that I had got from my neighbor's white birch trees. I decided to clean my front yard to get rid of all the allergic birch flowers and leaves from my yard. First, I cut down all the bushes in my front yard all the way down to the ground. Then I dug out the old ground dirt from my front yard to get rid of all the old dirt soil that was filled with allergic birch flowers and leaves and refilled my front yard with the new dirt soil from Home Depot store. Unfortunately, I was still getting the same kind of bad allergies. Shaun was still complaining about the same kind of rashes and the allergies that he had after he cut the grasses from the front yard. Sometimes, it was so bad that I could not even stand up long because my legs would itch badly just like insect bites and many distinct pale spots formed on both my knees and legs. Sometimes I could feel my heartbeat was very fast and uncomfortable. I could not do anything except take the allergy medicines that Harvey gave me every day to get rid of the itching and allergies. I kept calling and complaining to the city of Pleasanton. I did talk to a lot of people about the allergies due to the birch trees, but no one knew the birch trees could cause allergies. Some people told me the doctors had verified that they had got the allergy from the dog hair after they did the skin tests, and then the doctor had advised them to get rid of their beloved pets by giving them away. I did not understand where the doctors were getting all those dogs' hairs from to use for testing on human skins. How did they make the assumption that the dog hairs could make the people get bad allergies? I never believed that dog hairs could cause allergy to any mankind because their hairs were just like human hairs and would never cause an allergy to mankind. This was the reason I refused to use the materials listed on the skin test charts to test on my skin and cancelled the appointment with Nurse Ann. Then I was thinking of the substance that caused itching on my lips after I passed birch trees. There must be some kind of bad substance from the birch trees that caused the itching on my lips. I did not know what kind of bad substances from the white birch trees were responsible for the itching and bad allergies and sickness.

I was getting very frustrated and upset about my allergy that I had got from my neighbor's birch trees. I kept complaining to the city of Pleasanton and to my children. No matter how much I complained to them, I did not get any reaction and conclusion from them. I was very much disappointed with the community that I lived in. It seemed like no one cared about the environment in this neighborhood. No one tried to dig out the truth about the allergies and sickness that we all were getting in this neighborhood. I was very much disappointed with my neighbor who did not take responsibility to get rid of their bad white birch trees to provide us a healthy environment. I decided not to complain anymore about my allergies that I got from my neighbor's white birch trees. I told Sirena that I had made the final decision to go to the court. Then I called my brother Harvey and Dr. Calvin to write letters for me, indicating that I got bad allergies from the white birch trees. Since they knew that I had bad allergies, I kept telling them my allergies were because of the white birch trees, but I did not know whether these both doctors knew what the white birch trees were. They both agreed to write the letters for me that I got very bad allergies because of white birch trees. They wrote the letters for me, but none of them indicated that my allergies were from white birch trees. Sirena did ask me whether the court would accept their letters the way they had been written. I told Sirena that I had told them to write that my allergies were caused by white birch trees. I did not know why they did not mention the white birch tree's name in their letters. I told Sirena that I was not going to tell the doctors what they should write.

If I asked them to rewrite the letters, maybe they would get mad at me. I was quite upset especially with my brother the way he had written his letter for me. He did not even describe the tree that I had got bad allergies from. He had just filled up his letter with general things that were totally different from the topic that I had told him to write about. He kept saying weeds had caused the allergies on me. I did not know whether he knew what kind of plant was weed. I did not want to call him again to tell him to rewrite the letter for me. I would not call Dr. Calvin to ask him to rewrite the letter either, because I had just checked up with him a couple of times. He knew I got bad allergies after I came in from outside my house. I kept repeatedly telling them the name of the trees that caused allergies before I requested them to write the letters for me. I did not know whether he wrote the tree's name as the causative agent of my bad allergies on my medical records. They were the doctors. They should listen carefully to the patients and write down the names of the trees in the patient's file about which the patients complain and describe to them, from which they get the allergies. So they knew what to write when patients requested them to write a recommendation letter to take to the court. I was very upset with both of them. Then I called elderly Catherine to request her to write a letter for me to indicate that I was very allergic to the birch trees. She agreed to write a letter to indicate that I was very allergic to the white birch trees. After she finished writing the letter, I went to her house to pick up the letter. After I got the letter from elderly Catherine, I went to Pleasanton Courthouse to get the small claim form. The front desk clerk gave me the form to fill up and told me that she would set up a court date for me after I turned in the small claim form. I took the small claim form from the court and went home. I reviewed all the information on the form, and I tried to fill in all the information in it. After I was done, I went to Pleasanton Courthouse to file in my small claim form to sue my neighbor for the allergies that I got because of their birch trees. I told her I had got bad allergies from my neighbor's birch trees. It seemed like no one believed my complaints about my allergies that were caused by my neighbor's birch trees. I indicated to her I was telling the truth. I also wanted to help all the teenagers in getting rid of the allergies on their faces that they got while they were working in their own lawns. She said she believed the birch trees were allergic trees. I asked her how much money I should put in to sue my neighbor. She said to just put in any amount, so I put in the maximum amount of five thousand dollars in the form. I told her since I had been complaining about the allergy from their trees so long I should get the maximum amount of money to offset my medical bills. After I turned in my small claim form to her, she set up the lawsuit court date on December 12, 2002, for me. Then she helped me fill in the small claim form to notify my neighbor, indicating that I had set up a lawsuit to sue him for five thousand dollars as the cost of my medical bills for treating the bad allergies and sickness caused by his bad white birch trees. Then she helped me to put it in the envelope and guided me to go to the post office and use registered mail to send out the letter to my neighbor. I took the letter and went to the post office to send it out in the registered mail. I received the return slip from the post office after one week to indicate that they had delivered my mail to my neighbor and my neighbor had received my lawsuit letter.

I called Marlene Peterson, the director of Pleasanton Senior Supporting Group, to let her know that I had filed in my lawsuit in Pleasanton Courthouse to sue my neighbor John Clark for the three big allergic white birch trees that were causing me bad allergies. The clerk from the courthouse set up the court date on December 12, 2002, for my lawsuit against my neighbor. She called me back to ask me to go to Pleasanton Senior Center to let her review my doctors' letters before I took them to the courthouse on the court date. So I set up a date to see her. I went to see her on the appointment date in Pleasanton Senior Center. I gave her all the doctors' letters and elderly Catherine's letter for her to review. She took the letters and looked at them. She did not see the name of the birch trees, which caused me bad allergies, in the letters. She reminded me I would lose the case if I went to the court without the doctor's indication about the name of the birch tree in the letters. Then she surprisingly asked me whether Harvey was my real brother. I told her he was my real brother and we had the same parents. In front of Marlene, I did not want to show my anger and frustration on my brother. I just kept quiet without saying anything to her. Then she said my neighbor had the right to sue me back for harassing him if I lost the case in the court. I told her I did not know the reason for not writing down the name of the birch tree in the letters. I had reminded them to make sure they included the name of the birch tree in their letters. I told her that I was telling the truth to let her know that I had really got the bad allergy from my neighbor's birch trees. I was not afraid of my neighbor suing me, because I had spoken out the truth to get rid of the allergies and sickness in the neighborhood. I did not want people to think that because I did not like the messy white birch trees I was asking my neighbor to cut down their birch trees. I told her I was tired of complaining, and I did not want to spend more money on my medical bills without getting any solutions or results by continuously seeing the doctors. I told Marlene that I would not cancel my court date and that I would go to the court to explain to them myself how I get the bad allergies from the birch trees. After Marlene found out that I would not change my mind for not going to the court, she just said good luck to me and released me. I went home.

After I talked to Marlene, she sent out two counselors, Charlene Swierkowski and Jody Landsittel, to my house to talk to me about my allergies. Jody told me she had a bad sinus allergy. She had been seeing the allergy doctor for quite long. The allergy doctor could not help her get rid of her allergies. She was still having a bad allergy problem. She did not know where her allergy doctor was now. When she described her allergy to me, she was very upset with her allergy doctor who could not help her get rid of her sinus allergy. I kept complaining to them the white birch trees were causing the allergies and sickness in our community. They must have been seeing a lot of allergy doctors before and had a lot of experience on how to find the allergy problems. They guided me to study the places and sitting positions in my house to find the real substances that caused me the bad allergy. I took them outside to my yard to show them all the trees and bushes. I told them we were carefully planting slow-growing trees like cherry trees and a lot of cypress trees in our backyard. Our whole backyard was surrounded with tall cypress trees to block all the objects outside from coming into my yard. I told them all the plants that we had in our yard were good plants. I told them I had already got rid of my two paper birch trees in my backyard after my son Shaun kept complaining about the allergies when he worked outside in our yard. Then I told them how I had squeezed the white birch flowers with my fingers and how I tried to taste the birch fluid on my finger. I got a bad itch on my lips and one little pimple formed on my tongue after I tasted the birch fluid on my finger. I told them both my ears were itching all the time. My left ear got infected again after I worked at home and I had to go through left ear surgery in 1994 by Dr. Lins in New York. After I told them about my ear infection and ear surgery, they told me to study the sitting position, to find out how I got my ear infection. I told them I spent a lot of time working in my study room with my window open before my left ear got infected. Now I spent a lot of times working in my yard and I got my left ear infected again. I showed them my neighbor's birch trees and described to them how the west wind blew in a lot of birch flower pieces from my neighbor's white birch trees. They said they believed what I told them, but they said that maybe people would think the cause of my allergy could be individual. They said they had never heard of people complaining about white birch trees before that it would cause allergies and sickness; in fact, a lot of people enjoyed the beauty of white birch trunks. They suggested that I get the doctors' letters before I went to the court to give out an explanation. I told them I put in five thousand dollars in the small claim form to offset my medical expenses. I told them this was the most I could get from my neighbor in the small claim court to sue my neighbor. I also mentioned to them the purpose of doing this was not to get money from my neighbor, but for good health for myself and for all the people in my neighborhood. I said I would represent myself inside the court to tell them how I found out my lips got a bad itch after I squeezed the birch flowers. After we finished our discussions about the allergy, they said they had to visit another family and they left my house. After that, Charlene visited me every two weeks. But Jody came with Charlene a couple of times to visit me; then she stopped coming to my house because she said she was allergic to my two dogs.

I went in the small claim court in Pleasanton Courthouse with my two children on December 12, 2002. When we arrived inside the court, I saw all the plaintiffs and the defendants come in with their relatives or friends to the courthouse. We all went inside the courtroom and waited for the court to start. They started the court at 9:00 a.m. All the people took the seats and waited for Mr. Judge Lee to come out. After a while, Mr. Judge Lee came out; he announced that he had given a chance to both the plaintiffs and defendants to discuss and settle their cases with the people who represented for the courthouse first. If they could not settle their cases after they discussed, they could go back to him. After he announced to both plaintiffs and defendants to talk over the cases in front of a group of people who represented the courthouse to help in solving the problems first, we went outside the courtroom to meet with a group of people that represented the court to settle the case. Then they took us inside a room to discuss my case. After we settled inside the room, they asked me about my case. I gave them all the letters that I had written to the city of Pleasanton and the doctors' letters. The people in the courthouse were speaking in very low voices, so I could not hear the conversation well enough to answer their questions. I had to keep asking them to repeat the conversation that they had with me. Because I had a bad infection on my left ear and had lost hearing in my right ear, I could not hear well when the people in the courthouse asked me about my case. That made me very frustrated to speak inside the courthouse. When I talked, I did not notice that my voice was very loud; it seemed like I was shouting and yelling at people. I was very concerned to explain about the allergies and sickness that I had got from my neighbor's white birch trees, but I did not have enough experience to explain how I got the bad allergies and sickness from my neighbor's white birch trees. I did not know how to explain except I insisted them to have my neighbor Mr. John Clark cut down all their white birch trees. My left ear was infected badly and I could not hear well. I used cotton to block the infectious black fluid from my left ear before I went in to the courthouse. I told them I would show them how bad my left ear was infected. Then I used the cotton swab to clean my left ear in front of the people in the courthouse to show them the black fluid from my left infectious ear. I insisted them to have my neighbor John Clark cut down his allergic white birch trees again and again. After the people in the courthouse saw the black fluid in my left infectious ear, they got upset and asked me to give them the doctor's letter which described that my ear infection and allergies were caused by the birch trees. I told them I had already given them the envelope with the letters from my two doctors and elderly Catherine. They took out the letters from the envelope. They read the letters and found that the doctors did not indicate that my allergies were caused by white birch trees. They said they could not have my neighbor cut down all their white birch trees without the doctors indicating in their letters that my allergies were caused by birch trees. I told them elderly Catherine's letter did indicate my allergies were due to the birch trees, but they insisted again that I needed the doctor to indicate my allergies were caused by the birch trees. Since I did not get any letter from my doctors to indicate my allergies were caused by the birch trees, I told them they could put me in jail if I had lied to them. I requested this group of people to have my neighbor cut down their white birch trees, but they kept saying that they could not make my neighbor cut down their birch trees without any notification letter from my doctor. I insisted and requested them again and again to have my neighbor cut down their birch trees. The lead man of this group of people in the courthouse made the final decision to ask my neighbor to cut down their two white birch trees instead of all his three white birch trees, and they dismissed the case. We went back to the courtroom to meet with Mr. Judge Lee. Mr. Judge Lee asked me whether I was satisfied the way the lead man and this group of people had settled this case for me. I was not happy and not satisfied the way they settled the case. They had ordered my neighbor to cut down only their two birch trees instead of all their three birch trees. I promised Mr. Judge Lee and the people of the courthouse that I would bring in the doctor's letter indicating that my allergies and sickness were caused by the white birch trees. Then I left the courthouse with my two children and went home with a heavy heart. I wanted to apologize to Mr. Judge Lee without saying anything and left the courthouse. I did not mean to be rude to him. I respected him a lot, and I understood his position was not easy being the middleman for solving and settling the problems for both the plaintiff and the defendant to make them satisfied with their cases, but I was very upset and disappointed that the people in the courthouse knew I was telling them the truth and they believed what I was telling them. But they could not order my neighbor to cut down all their three birch trees without my doctor's letter. However, they believed me that I was suffering from the allergies and sickness caused by the birch trees. They ordered my neighbor John Clark to cut down his two birch trees instead of all his three birch trees.

My heart was very heavy after I reached home. I felt very uncomfortable in this case. I had promised the court to get the doctor's letter that indicated that my allergies were from the birch trees. I understood I had to go through another round to see the doctors again. Next day, I took out the plastic bag with the dried white birch flower paper envelope from the drawer of my desk. I sat on the sofa. I took out the dried white birch flower paper envelope from the plastic bag. I opened the folding paper envelope. I transferred the dried white birch flowers from the paper envelope to the plastic bag. When I tapped the paper envelope to transfer all the leftover powder of dried birch flowers from the paper envelope to the clear plastic bag, I saw powder flying like smoke from the paper envelope. Suddenly, I felt the portion of my face near my upper lip all the way to my ear was itching quite badly right away. I scratched my face above my upper lip. I tried to finish transferring the dried birch flowers to the plastic bag. I rapidly sealed the plastic bag. Then I carefully put the empty old paper envelope inside another plastic bag and sealed it tight, throwing it in the garbage can. I washed my hands with soap and hot water first. Then I washed my face with soap and water and tried to get rid of the bad itch from my face, but it was too late for me to avoid getting red rashes on my face. I kept scratching my face until I felt pain in my face. Then I went inside my bathroom to look at the mirror. I saw a lot of small blister rashes on my face above my upper lip all the way to my left ear. I realized that even the dried powder that escaped like smoke from birch flowers could cause red blister allergic rashes. After I prepared a clear plastic bag with dried white birch flowers to show Dr. Calvin what the dried white birch flowers looked like, I called Dr. Calvin's clinic to set up an appointment on December 30, 2002.

On December 24, 2002, I took Lady Star to meet Dr. Eliz for her regular checkup in HAH. But Dr. Eliz was out from the office on that day. Dr. Larry S. was in the clinic, and he took care of Lady Star for Dr. Eliz. I told Dr. Larry about the allergies that we got from the white birch trees. I showed him the rashes on Lady Star's underbody and told him those rashes were from my neighbor's white birch trees. Dr. Larry looked at Lady Star's underbody rashes and responded to me right away that these were very common rashes for all the dogs and that all the dogs were getting this kind of rashes on their body from being outside all the times. I requested Dr. Larry to write a letter for Lady Star to indicate that she got all these rashes because of the birch trees. He wrote the letter right away for me, indicating that Lady Star got bad rashes on her underbody because of the white birch trees, and gave it to me. I took the letter from him and thanked him. I told him I would take full responsibility in this case if anything happened, but he told me that he already knew the white birch trees were allergic trees and he did not want me to take any responsibility for him writing this letter, indicating that the rashes on Lady Star's underbody were caused by birch trees. I thanked him, and he released me. I took Lady Star home.

On December 30, 2002, I took the letters from elderly Catherine and Dr. Larry, the dried birch flower plastic bag, and the information on the birch trees to see Dr. Calvin. When I was in his office, I took out the dried birch flower plastic bag to show him the dried white birch flowers inside it. I told him about the incident when I had got bad rashes on my face while I was transferring the dried birch flowers from the paper envelope to this clear plastic bag. I told him to take out the dried birch flowers from the plastic bag to test it on his skin to check whether he got the allergy. He refused to touch it. He said he still had a lot of patients waiting for him to see them. Then I showed him the letters from elderly Catherine and Dr. Larry, indicating my allergies were caused by white birch trees. He took the letters from elderly Catherine and Dr. Larry and reviewed them. I requested him to write a letter for me, indicating that I got bad allergies because of the white birch trees, but he hesitated. So I requested him to write that my allergies were possibly caused by the birch trees. I did not want to embarrass him when people asked him how he knew the birch trees were the allergic trees. I believed he did not know anything about the birch trees. He did not know what the white birch trees looked like, but I needed the doctor's letter to show to the court, so I suggested that he should trust me and requested him to write the letter for me, indicating that my allergies were caused by my neighbor's birch trees. We were family friends. I needed to protect him as a doctor by not letting the outsiders attack him. So I thought it was best for him to use the word "possibility" to describe the allergy from the patient was from the birch trees, because without knowing about the substance from the birch trees and the activity of the patient, it was hard for the doctor to write a letter for the patient. After he reviewed the letters from Dr. Larry and elderly Catherine, he took a few minutes to think it over. Then he sincerely agreed to write the letter for me, indicating that I had got the bad allergies from my neighbor's white birch trees. He went to the hallway, turned on the computer, and typed the letter. After he was done with the letter, he signed the letter and gave it to me. I was not too happy to see him write my allergies were possibly from the birch trees, but I did not want to force him to write the letter about the materials that he was not familiar with. I just had to accept his letter and went home with a heavy heart again.

After I was home, I called my brother Harvey to tell him about the letters that I had got from Dr. Larry and Dr. Calvin, and I asked him to allow me to fill up the name of the birch tree in his letter to indicate that I had got the allergies because of the white birch tree. He said OK to me. So I filled in the birch tree's name in his letter to indicate my allergies were from the white birch trees. I could not blame the doctors for being unaware that the birch trees were allergic trees. Most of the people that I talked to in Tri Valley did not believe that the white birch trees were the allergic trees. I was getting very frustrated when I talked to the people because I did not know how to give out the explanation to them as I did not know what kind of substances were in the white birch trees that caused the itch and the allergic reactions.

I received two letters from the court within a month after I was dismissed from the court. One letter was from Mr. Judge Lee to inform me to hire a lawyer to represent me for my allergy case if I still wanted to sue my neighbor. Another letter was from the lady clerk from Pleasanton Courthouse to inform me that my case was released. I took all the letters that I received from the courthouse and the letters from my doctors and went to the small claim court in Pleasanton to ask them the procedure of how to set up another court date for my lawsuit to my neighbor. After I went inside the small claim courthouse, I asked the lady clerk what I should do with the two letters that I had received from the court, and I handed out the letters to her. After she read the letters, she told me I was released from the court for my case. I thought she knew my case about the allergies and sickness that I had got from the white birch trees after she read the letters, and she suggested that I turn in to the city of Pleasanton all the documentation letters from my doctors that I had prepared for the court to review. I thanked her and asked her whether I could send out a thank-you note to Mr. Judge Lee. She said yes to me and asked me to send the letter to this court and that they would forward the letter to him. I said OK, and I left the courthouse.

After I came home, I thought of how I was going to find out more information about the birch trees to prove to the court that the birch trees were the allergic trees that were causing people to get sick. I started to find the solutions to prove the birch trees were responsible for bad allergies and sickness. I tried to read and studied the chemistry, biology, and medical books on my bookshelf, looking for information about the white birch trees and the type of chemical acid in the birch trees that might be the cause of bad reaction on the people, but I could not find any information about the birch trees in any book except the *Britannica Encyclopedia* that described a little bit about the white birch trees, their leaves, the cluster birch flowers, and the places that the birch trees grew. They did not mention any inner structure of the birch flowers and the chemicals of the white birch tree. I decided to get some birch flowers from my neighbor's birch tree to study and draw their structure after observing with my own eyes to show the city of Pleasanton and the court. I went out to my neighbor's birch trees. I picked the birch flowers and leaves and took them home. I studied the birch flowers and leaves and their structure generally and drew their pictures on the paper. Then I went outside to my yard to count all the trees and bushes that I had in my yard and listed the type of plants in the paper that I had in my yard. Then I prepared a three-page paper of "The Allergies and Sickness Exposed from the White Birch Trees." After I was done with them, I faxed them to my brother, my nieces, and my friends. After they received the paper about the birch tree that I had faxed them, I heard a lot of voices from them saying that they thought the birch trees had no flowers. If the birch trees had fruits, all the fruits could only have white meat just like any other fruits that we used in our daily life. After I heard them saying this and that, I realized no one actually knew about the white birch trees in detail; no one actually knew what the birch flowers and birch fruits looked like. After I found out a lot of people did not know about the birch trees and the structure of the birch leaves and flowers, it did not make sense for me to wait any longer to inform all the people of Tri Valley to get rid of the bad allergic white birch trees. When Sirena came home, I suggested that she took my three-page paper to publish in the newspaper. She advised me to wait till next week.

On Tuesday, when Charlene came to my house, I showed her what I had found from *Britannica Encyclopedia* about the birch trees and my three-page paper that I had written about the white birch tree. I indicated to her I would like to publish my three-page paper in the newspaper. She said she had friends in *Valley Times* newspaper and she would talk to them and help me find out how to publish my paper in the newspaper. I thanked her. Then I gave her one copy of my paper to review. She advised me to talk to my neighbor. I said OK, and I requested her to give one copy of my paper to my neighbor to let them review about their bad allergic birch tree and to request them to cut down their birch tree. She went over to my neighbor's house to give my paper to my neighbor John Clark and talk to him, asking him to get rid of their bad birch tree. But she came back to my house and told me my neighbor would not cut down their white birch tree after she had talked to them. She was very upset and left my house.

I prepared a letter, dated January 6, 2003, to Renee to indicate that I was still getting the bad allergies and sickness due to my neighbor's white birch tree; even my neighbor had cut down the two big birch trees in his yard. Then I indicated to her that this was not worth it as it made me and all my neighbors get bad allergies and sickness because of one particular type of birch tree. My neighbor had to get rid of their allergic birch tree. I also mentioned to her that I found out a lot of people in King of Prussia were getting bad allergies just like me, when I was visiting my sisters in King of Prussia, Pennsylvania. Then I enclosed inside a brown envelope the letter along with my three-page paper of "The Allergies and Sickness Expose from the White Birch Trees," all the letters from my doctors and the court, air tickets, some medical bills, and the plastic bag with the dried white birch flowers that I kept in my drawer, for Renee to review them. Next day, I took the brown envelope to the city of Pleasanton to give it to Renee for review. When I was in the city of Pleasanton, I did not see Renee in her office. I requested the office secretary, Kim, to forward the brown envelope to Renee and went home.

When Charlene came to my house, she told me she had talked to her friend in *Valley Times* newspaper regarding publishing my paper about the white birch trees that caused bad allergies and sickness to the people, in which I requested the people to get rid of them. The *Valley Times* newspaper had agreed to give me one small column to publish my short warning note. I said OK to her. I prepared a short warning note to inform the people that the birch trees contained acid, causing the people to get allergies and sickness. I requested all the people to get rid of the birch trees in their neighborhoods. After two weeks when Charlene came over to my house, I gave her my short warning note that I had prepared to be published in the newspaper. She took my paper and helped me to turn it in to the *Valley Times* newspaper to publish my short warning note. After the *Valley Times* newspaper published my short warning note in the newspaper, requesting the people to cut down the allergic birch trees in the neighborhood, I got two phone calls from Pleasanton and Tracy, asking me to send them more information about the birch trees. I sent a copy of my three-page paper about the birch trees to the people of Pleasanton and Tracy for them to review. I also got many phone calls from other people, but I did not get a chance to answer their calls, because of my bad ear infection, which caused bad hearing in both my ears.

I was getting very frustrated that I kept getting the allergies and sickness because of my neighbor's birch tree. I decided to find out about the ingredients in the birch tree and how those ingredients caused bad allergies and sickness in the air of our environment. I started to look up the chemistry, biology, medical, and health chapters in *Britannica Encyclopedia*. I read and studied them. I made some copies of the chemicals and their reactions from the encyclopedia book, which I thought might be important and helpful to the people to understand the chemical reactions. Then I realized I need a laboratory to analyze the ingredients from the birch tree. If I could analyze the ingredients from the birch flowers and know the type of chemicals from the birch tree, we would be able to tell how the chemicals from the birch tree were causing bad allergies and sickness. Even though I did not have the money to build an analytical laboratory, I was willing to borrow the money to rent a place to use it as an analytical laboratory to find about the ingredients from the birch tree, so I called Dr. Calvin to ask him where I could find an analytical laboratory to analyze the birch flowers' ingredients and the type of chemicals that are contained in the birch tree. He said he did not know any laboratory where I could analyze the birch flower ingredients in this neighborhood. Since I could not find any analytical laboratory, the only solution that I had was to use my own skin to test the birch flowers. Before I used my skin to do the testing with the birch flowers, I went outside and walked around at different times in my neighborhood to make sure I got the allergy. I purposely took Lady Star with me daily at different times to pick up the mails from my mailbox in front of my left-side neighbor's front yard.

One windy day on April 4, 2003, I came back inside my house with Lady Star after I had picked up my mails from my mailbox. I sat on my sofa and watched the television. Then I saw Lady Star scratching her body, near my sofa. A few hours later, suddenly, my neck, left face, and ear started itching badly. I scratched and scratched. The more I scratched, the more I had the itching. After a while, I felt pain in my face. So I picked up a small mirror and looked at my face. I saw my face was swelling and there were rashes on my left ear all the way to my upper lip. The rashes on my face were getting worse and thicker. The red rashes kept spreading to the sides near my lips and there was swelling. I called elderly Catherine and told her about my incident. She suggested that I go and see the doctor. So I went to see Dr. Calvin again. He suggested I get a cortisone shot after he checked my face and asked me whether I would be ready to take a cortisone shot. I said yes to him. He asked his assistant, Eliviver, to give me a cortisone shot. He advised me to come back the next week if the rashes on my face did not get better. I told him I would come back again next week to take a cortisone shot to get rid of all the itches on my body, and I said I would also like him to see what they looked like after they healed and what kind of scars they left on my face. I also indicated to him the red rashes on my face were just like the kind of rashes on the boys' faces that I had met in the stores and in my neighborhood. Then I left his clinic and went home.

After I took the cortisone shot, I felt much better, but my ears, lips, and legs were still itching. My left ear was infected badly, so I went back to see Dr. Calvin again after a week. When Dr. Calvin's assistant, Nonette, saw me, she asked me what was wrong with me again this time. I told her the same thing—that I was still getting a bad itch from my neighbor's birch tree. After Dr. Calvin checked me, he asked Nonette to give me another cortisone shot, and she advised me to keep calling the city of Pleasanton to complain about my neighbor's white birch tree. It took a couple of months for the red rashes to disappear from my face. In early September 2003, I went out to my backyard to plant spring flower bulbs near one of the cypress trees on the right side of my yard. I fell down accidentally on the ground near the cypress tree. Some dry pieces of substances from the trees dropped onto my hand and body. I got up from the ground using both my hands on the ground to support my body to get up. After I got up, I tried to shake both my hands to clean the sticky pieces of substances and the dirt and soil from my hands and body. Then I cleaned both my hands again. After I cleaned my hands, I found there were some oily sticky substances left on my hands. I rushed into my house and washed my hands with soap and warm water to get rid of the sticky substances. That night, both my hands felt very itchy. I kept scratching until the skin on my left hand opened. Next day, my left hand swelled up with thick rashes. The heat that was produced from the rashes on my hand made me feel very uncomfortable. I knew the cypress trees did not contain the kind of substances to burn the skin. I believed all those allergic substances had flown in from my neighbor's white birch trees with the strong wind, and some of them had landed on the cypress trees. My hands itched and swelled up on and off after I cleaned my yard all the time. My ears and lips itched on and off. My left ear was infected badly and getting worse. Since I could not make my neighbor cut down their birch tree, I felt very frustrated that I could not help myself and my baby dogs in getting rid of allergies. I just had to stand near my two baby dogs restlessly, looking at them as they scratched their bodies. Sometimes when they drank the water from the plant trays outside my backyard, they threw up yellow mucus bubble after they came back inside my house. One time when Sirena saw Lady Star throwing up the yellow mucus bubble, she asked me again and again what was wrong with Lady Star. I told her they were drinking the water from the outside plant trays that contained the poisonous ingredients from the birch flowers, which blew in from my neighbor's birch trees, and that was the reason they threw up the yellow mucus. I told Sirena that there was nothing I could do to prevent them from drinking the water from the plant trays when I let them go stay outside in my backyard and that I could not keep an eye on them all the time. I felt bad that my neighbor kept refusing to cut down their allergic white birch trees to clean the environment for us.

No matter how much information I sent about the allergies and sickness to the city of Pleasanton, all I got from them was "silence." I called elderly Catherine again and asked her why the people did not take any action to cut down all their allergic white birch trees and why they wanted to keep the trees that made the people suffer with allergies and sickness. Then I asked her whether she had seen the birch flowers before. She said she did not know that the white birch trees had flowers and she had not seen them before. I told her I would bring fresh birch flowers and the letter that I had written to the city of Pleasanton for her to review. She said OK. Next day, I took fresh birch flowers and the letter to her house to let her review. After she saw the birch flowers, she told me unpleasantly to take the birch flowers away from her and advised me to leave the letter that I had written to Renee to her. She said she would review later. I gave her my letter and left. Next day, I called her again to make sure whether she had reviewed the letter. She said she did not get a chance to review it yet. She wanted me to give her time to review the letter and then to call her back after a week. After a week, I called her back. She advised me to rewrite my paper more clearly so that it was short. I told her I would do it. I realized before I rewrote my paper that I needed to know in detail the structure of the birch flowers and the ingredients in the birch trees. Only then I could answer all the questions which the people would ask me about the birch trees. I was looking for a person who could tell and advise me what was inside the birch flowers and how to find the ingredients in the birch flowers. Then I remembered my brother-in-law, Richard Thanse, was a chemical engineer who had worked for a rice bran oil company in Burma before. I called to ask him about the ingredients that were in the rice. He told me the rice bran contained bran oils and bran acids. When they produced pure bran oil, they needed to separate the bran acids from the rice bran in order to get pure bran oil. He told me they could not use the rice bran oil without taking out the acids from the rice bran. I called Richard several times to talk to him about the substances in the rice bran. Then I realized that the birch leaves and flowers must contain birch oils and birch acids just like the rice bran. But I needed an analytical laboratory to analyze the ingredients from the birch tree to find out the type of acid in the birch tree, which caused the allergies and sickness to the people.

I called Renee in late October 2003. Renee's secretary, Kim, picked up the phone. I indicated to her to tell Renee that I believed the birch flowers contained the acid. I suggested that Kim should tell Renee that I would like to set up a deal with the city of Pleasanton to pay me five million dollars if I could find out the type of acids in the birch trees that had the capability to cause bad allergies and sickness in the people. Kim said she would tell Renee. Then I hung up the phone. After one week, Charlene came to my house. She told me the city of Pleasanton had agreed to my deal of paying me five million dollars if I could find and give out the proof to the city of Pleasanton about the type of acids in the birch tree that caused the allergies and sickness to the people. I said OK to Charlene. We set the deal at five million dollars for me if I could give out the type of acids in the birch tree, to prove that acids from the birch tree could cause the bad allergies and sickness.

Chapter Three

Confirmation

After I set up the deal with Counselor Charlene from Pleasanton Senior Supporting Group to represent the city of Pleasanton to find the type of acid in the birch tree, for proving the birch family trees are allergic trees that caused people to get bad allergies and sickness, in October 2003 I went to my neighbor's yard to get birch flowers from their white birch tree. After I picked some leaves and flowers from the birch tree, I took them back to my backyard porch, washed them with fresh water, and studied them in detail. I found there were two types of fruit-like birch flowers, male and female flowers. In my backyard porch, I cut both types of white birch flowers into half and studied what was inside the flowers and took pictures of them with the camera that Sirena had bought for me. I used a small portion of each type of the young birch flowers to rub softly on my left hand, but it did not show any sign of rashes on my hand. I rubbed softly again the whole piece of the small young male flower on my hand because I was scared something would happen to me if I rubbed them strongly on my hand, breaking my skin. I did not feel any itch or see any rash on my hand. Then I rubbed with both types of birch flowers on my hand again and again. I did not see any sign of rashes on my hands again. After I tested by rubbing the male flowers on my hands, I cleaned and packed the rest of the male and female flowers and the birch leaves that were full of small insects and eggs inside the plastic bag and threw them away in the garbage can. Then I sprayed and cleaned my porch carefully and came back inside my house. I cleaned both my hands with soap and water thoroughly. I decided to collect more birch flowers for testing again tomorrow.

Next day, I went to my neighbor's birch tree to pick more birch flowers, cleaned them with fresh water, and then tried to use different sizes of white male birch flowers to rub on my hands in the porch again. I found the smallest male birch flowers caused red rashes, which were so small you could notice it only when you observed them carefully. The skin also became very smooth after rubbing male birch flowers on it. I believed the ingredients in the birch flowers contained bad acids and oils. I did not know what kind of acids were in the birch flowers. I predicted the birch acid must be strong and very toxic because they had the ability to burn the skin and form blister rashes. Then I packed and saved all the big male birch flowers inside the plaster bag and took them inside my house. I threw away all the leaves and smaller birch flowers in the garbage can. Then I cleaned my backyard porch with water carefully.

A few days later, one evening, I sat on my sofa. Lady Star was sleeping on the sofa near me as usual. Sir Space was sleeping on the floor at a distance from where he could see me. I took out the birch flowers that I had saved in the plastic bag. I took out one big male flower from the plastic bag, and then using both my hands, I pressed hard the big male birch flower. Both my palms started to itch within a few minutes. I kept scratching my palms and then I saw some small red pimple rashes on my palms. I got up and washed my hands with soap and warm water. Then I pressed three birch flowers together in my fingers and rubbed them on my left hand skin. I kept continuously rubbing the male birch flowers on my skin. After fifteen minutes, my fingers started itching badly. I got up quickly and washed my hands with soap and warm water many times. Then I checked my hands and fingers. I found a red burned spot on my right hand middle finger and a small blister pimple. My fingers were itching badly. I kept on scratching my fingers. The small blister pimple on my middle finger was getting bigger and it formed a big blister.

On that night, Lady Star wept in a low voice and kept scratching her face on the carpet floor, and she was scratching her lower body with her back leg. I got up and comforted her a little bit to let her go to sleep. Next day, when I got up, I checked on Lady Star's whole body. I found her body had a lot of red rashes. She had been with me all the time when I had tested my skin with the birch flowers. I believed the fresh juice from the male birch flowers must have splashed on Lady Star's body and caused a lot of red rashes on her body. After I found the blister rashes on Lady Star's body, I figured out the birch tree and their leaves and flowers must contain a strong acid that could burn the skin badly and form blister rashes. One of the blister rashes that I found on Lady Star's underbody is shown in the picture.

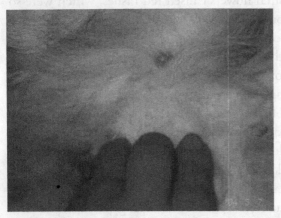

The yellow liquid blister was formed on top of the rash on Lady Star's underbody.

On Saturday, November 15, 2003, around three o'clock, I went outside to my neighbor's birch tree to get more white birch flowers from the white birch tree. I washed them thoroughly outside on my porch and left them on my kitchen counter. Then I cut and took pictures of the birch leaves and flowers on my kitchen counter. While I was cutting the birch flowers, as usual, Lady Star stayed near me, barking at me for food. I looked at her and yelled at her not to bark at me. I indicated to her that I did not have any food for her and asked her to go away to let me work. But she did not go away. Instead, she moved her body closer to my legs and put her face up, looking at me while I was busy cutting the birch flowers. Sir Space was near the sliding door next to the bird cage, looking at me. After I yelled at Lady Star, I continuously cut the male and female birch flowers into half to observe how to take pictures. Then I transferred those on a white paper and took pictures of female flowers. After I was done with the female flowers, I transferred the male birch flowers onto the white paper. Then I took the pictures of male birch flowers. After I was done taking the pictures of the birch flowers, I put all the birch flowers and the papers in the plastic bag and cleaned up the counter. When Lady Star saw me cleaning the counter, she moved away from me. I wiped the kitchen counter with wet towels. Then I prepared chicken and rice for my dinner at 5:30 p.m. After I was done with my cooking, I fed my two baby dogs with chicken and rice first. Then I had my dinner. I washed all the dishes after my dinner. I sat on my sofa and watched television for a while. I felt very dizzy and nauseous, so I took both my dogs and went to my bedroom. Usually, I hand-fed them snacks and played with them for a while before I went to bed in my bedroom, but on that day, I went to bed without giving them any snacks because I did not feel good. I felt so dizzy and sick. Then I heard Lady Star crying in a low voice. I did not know what was happening to her. I yelled at her to stop crying and asked her to go to sleep. Then I told her I did not feel good. Lady Star was a very good understanding dog. After she heard me telling her I did not feel good, she stayed quiet and went to sleep. Next day, after I woke up early in the morning, I took my two baby dogs out to my backyard. Then I made myself a cup of hot milk. After I drank the hot milk, I felt dehydrated and dizzy. I went to my bathroom. I put a finger in my mouth to tickle my throat to force all the food out from my stomach. After I threw up, I felt better. Then I came out to my family room and rested on my sofa. Then Sirena came home. I told her that I did not feel good and asked her to take care of the dogs for me. Then I went to my bedroom and took an antibiotic pill. I slept the whole afternoon. After I woke up, I cooked a chicken and rice dinner with Sirena. I ate some chicken with rice. Sirena gave me company. After our dinner, she fed the dogs with chicken and rice. I told her I did not feel good and I was very sick. She said she would not go back home since I was so sick. She stayed with me at home that night to take care of the dogs for me.

On Monday morning, I was still very sick after I woke up. I heard Sirena had taken the dogs out in the backyard. After a while, she settled the dogs in the family room and left home about seven o'clock in the morning to go to work. I did not feel like getting up. I went back to sleep for a while. I came out to my living room at 10:00 a.m. to check on my two baby dogs. I heard Lady Star was weeping in a low voice again in front of the sofa that I usually sat on. Then I picked her up and checked her. She looked very sick. I saw her entire left eye was filled with white thick soft tissue like soft white meat. I did not know what the white soft tissue in her left eye was. I went to the kitchen to get a paper towel and wet it with water. I tried to clean the soft white tissue out from her left eye, but the soft white tissue did not come out. I stopped cleaning the soft white tissue from her left eye. I took her in my room, and then I called my brother Harvey to tell him about Lady Star's left eye. He suggested that I feed Lady Star one-third portion of Tetracycline antibiotic medicine every four hours. I continuously fed her one-third portion of Tetracycline antibiotic medicine every four hours. I fed Sir Space one-third portion of Tetracycline antibiotic medicine to prevent him from getting sick because he had thrown up a small amount of yellow mucus bubble last night. I took Advil and Tetracycline antibiotics for myself after I had taken care of my dogs. I called Holly that night. I told her about the soft white tissue in Lady Star's left eye. She suggested that I put a few drops of Ocuflow ophthalmic solution eyedrops in Lady Star's left eye. I went to my room and took the Ocuflow ophthalmic solution eyedrop bottle out from my medicine box. I applied a few drops in Lady Star's left eye. After a while, I checked her left eye. I saw the soft white tissue had started to come out from her left eye. I cleaned the soft white tissue with a wet paper towel time to time, but there were still some small pieces left in her left eye corner. I could not totally clean it out, so I just left it in her eye. I was afraid she would hurt her eye if I tried to pull it out with force.

On Tuesday morning, I saw a big piece of thick soft white tissue coming out from Lady Star's left eye again. I cleaned it for her with a wet paper towel. I saw a bubble-like deep burned sign in the middle of her left eye. I realized that she must have got the burn from one small drop of juice or small piece of the birch flowers in her left eye while I was cutting and taking pictures of the birch flowers on the kitchen counter. Then I called my brother Harvey to ask him what I should do with Lady Star's left eye, whether I should continuously give her antibiotic medicine or not. He told me to go ahead and feed Lady Star antibiotic medicine every four hours. Then he asked me to take Lady Star to checkup with her vet doctor if she did not get better after a week. So I continuously gave her antibiotic every four hours.

On Tuesday night, I put Lady Star on the sofa in the family room with Sir Space. I went to the bathroom to brush my teeth. Lady Star jumped down from the sofa and ran after me with Sir Space to the bathroom. Then I heard Lady Star crying in a high pitch, "Ah!" I ran out to the hallway from the bathroom to check on her. I saw she was in the hallway between the washing machine room and the kitchen. She looked like she had got hurt and turned back to the kitchen that she had just come out from. I picked her up and checked on her. I saw another big piece of thick soft white tissue coming out from her left eye again. It seemed like she had accidentally hit her left eye with the corner edge of the washer room's wooden door. But her left eye still had some small pieces of soft white tissue. She looked very sick and was in a lot of pain. I took both of them into my room, turned off the light, and let them sleep. Then I called my two nephews, Dr. Danny Chu and Dr. Felix Chu, and Susong to tell them about Lady Star's left eye accident. Susong suggested that I take Lady Star to see her doctor. I told her I would take her to her doctor tomorrow.

On Wednesday morning, November 19, 2003, I checked Lady Star's eyes after I woke up. A big piece of soft white tissue in her left eye came out again. This time after I cleaned the soft white tissue, I saw aqueous fluid in Lady Star's anterior chamber of her left eye; it seemed like her left eye's corneal layers were ruptured and broken. I became so scared. I was afraid she would have a lot of pain, so I gave her small portions of Advil pain reliever to help her get rid of her pain. Then I called HAH and told them Lady Star's eye seemed like it was broken and fluid was coming out from her eye. The front desk clerk asked me to take her to the clinic right away. I took her to HAH right away without having a second thought. When we arrived in HAH, Dr. Eliz was in the clinic. She asked me what was wrong with Lady Star. I told her about Lady Star and the burn in her left eye, which she must have got from the birch flower acid when I was cutting and researching the birch flowers. She must have accidentally hit her left eye on the washing machine room door's corner edge and hurt her left eye. She said to me that we never knew until things happened, and all these Pekinese dogs had the same kind of problems. Then she checked Lady Star's left eye. After she looked at Lady Star's eyes, she said in a very unpleasant voice, "Ah! This case is out of my hand. Only the eye specialist can help her fix her eye." She referred me to take Lady Star to check with an eye specialist in Fremont to fix her eyes. I said OK to her. She went back to her office and contacted Dr. Deborah S. F. of Animal Eye Care Hospital (AECH) in Fremont. Then she came back out to me and told me she had already contacted Dr. Deborah, and she asked me to take Lady Star to checkup with Dr. Deborah. I asked her to give me the direction to go to Fremont city to see Dr. Deborah. She said OK, and she went back inside her office. Then she asked her assistant Judy to give me Dr. Deborah's business card, which had the directions for Dr. Deborah, Animal Eye Care Hospital (AECH) in Fremont. Her assistant came out to me and said she would give me Dr. Deborah's business card and told me Lady Star needed a collar to put on her neck to protect her eyes from getting hurt again. I said OK to her. Judy went back inside the clinic. After a while, she brought out a collar and put on Lady Star's neck. Then she told me Dr. Eliz did not want to charge me anything for this visit. She just wanted me to pay for the dog's collar fee. I thanked her and gave her my credit card. After a while, Judy gave me back my credit card and receipt slip. Then she told me to follow the directions given on the back of the doctor's business card to go down to AECH clinic in Fremont to checkup with Dr. Deborah. I took the doctor's business card from her and went down to AECH with Lady Star and Sir Space right away.

After I was in AECH, I checked in with the front desk clerk first. Then the medical assistant took me and Lady Star inside the clinic patient room. Dr. Deborah came in. She checked Lady Star's eyes carefully. After she checked Lady Star's left eye, she told me Lady Star had the dry eye syndrome and she had a very deep ulceration. She needed a corneal surgery to repair her ulceration that had ruptured her left eye. She asked me whether I agreed to let her perform the surgery on Lady Star's left eye. I said yes to her without any hesitation. Then I asked her to do whatever she said she needed to do for Lady Star. I did not know what to say and what to do. I just wanted her to do something to help Lady Star to get better and requested her to do the best for Lady Star to help her get back her eye vision. Then I said to her that they were good doctors, and they were the only persons who could help Lady Star. She explained to me all the procedures about how she was going to perform surgery on Lady Star's left eye. Dr. Deborah then asked me whether I would like to use corneal tissue from Lady Star's left eye or from other animals to repair her eye. She showed me a big dog's picture and explained to me that if we used her own tissue to repair her left eye, her eye would look like this big dog's repaired eye, which would show some reddish color in her eye. If I used tissue from other dogs, no reddish color would show in her repaired eye. I told her to use tissue from other dogs to repair her eye. Then I requested Dr. Deborah to follow the best way to repair Lady Star's left eye. She asked me to sign the agreement form before the surgery could take place. I said OK to her. Then she asked her assistant to give me the form to fill in Lady Star's information and the agreement form for me to sign for allowing Dr. Deborah to perform the surgery. I studied and filled in all the information in the form and signed the paper for them. Then they asked me about the medicines that I had given to Lady Star. I was so upset that I even forgot the name of the eyedrop medicine that I had put in Lady Star's left eye, and I did not write the medicine as I had forgotten the name. After I was done filling the form, I turned in my form. I told her assistant that I did not remember the eyedrop medicine's name and that I would tell the eyedrop medicine's name for them after I came back to the hospital to pick up Lady Star. Dr. Deborah asked her assistant to give me the paper on which the cost of surgery was written for review. I took the paper, and I did not even look at it. I said OK to them right away as I agreed to pay Dr. Deborah the cost of the surgery to fix Lady Star's left eye. I asked her assistant whether they wanted me to wait in the hospital while the doctor performed Lady Star's eye surgery. She said I did not need to stay in the hospital to wait while Lady Star's eye surgery was done. She advised me to go home and wait at home for them to call me after the surgery was done. So I left Lady Star in AECH and went home with Sir Space.

After I was home, I took out the Ocuflow ophthalmic solution and other medicines that I had fed Lady Star that morning. I kept them inside the plastic bag to take them to AECH to show Dr. Deborah. After I organized the medicines that I had given to Lady Star, I sat on the sofa with Sir Space, waiting for the hospital to call me. After an hour, I received a telephone call from Dr. Deborah's assistant, Stella. She kept pressurizing me to tell them the kind of medicines I had applied in Lady Star's eyes. I told her I had used a few drops of Ocuflow ophthalmic solution to apply in Lady Star's eyes, and I had fed her one-third pill of Tetracycline antibiotic pill and a small piece of Advil to help her get relief from pain in the morning. Stella asked me to bring all the medicines I had given to Lady Star to the hospital to let Dr. Deborah look at them. I said OK to her. I did not know how many hours it would take for Dr. Deborah to repair Lady Star's left eye with corneal transplant surgery. After the surgery was done, Stella called me to indicate that Lady Star's eye surgery was done successfully and that I could pick her up and take her home from the hospital.

After I received the telephone call from Stella to pick up Lady Star at 5:30 p.m., I took all the medicines that I had given to Lady Star that morning and drove down to AECH with Sir Space to pick up Lady Star. When I was in the hospital, I gave the medicines to Stella as soon as I saw her. Stella told me to give the medicines to Dr. Deborah when I saw her.

While I was waiting for the doctor to release Lady Star to go home after the surgery, I saw Dr. Deborah come in from the front main door of the hospital. As soon as she saw me, she yelled at me and said Lady Star had got a very deep ulceration in her left eye. She advised me not to feed the dogs any medicine. She said if I fed them the medicine, it would be like I was feeding them poison. She suggested that I inform their doctor first before I gave any medicine to them, if anything happened to the dogs. I said OK to her. Then I gave her the medicines that I had fed Lady Star in the morning to look at. I told her I had only given her very little of Advil pain reliever to get rid of her pain. I showed her the Ocuflow ophthalmic solution bottle, the Tetracycline pill, and the leftover big portion of Advil. Then I asked her whether she used human medicines on animals or not. She took the medicines and looked at them. Then she said Ocuflow ophthalmic solution eyedrop was a good eyedrop medicine to apply in eyes. She also indicated that sometimes she did use Tetracycline pills for the dogs, but the ratio that she used on animals was different from human beings. Then I told her Lady Star's left eye must have been burned by the acid of the birch flowers while I was doing research on the birch leaves and flowers at home. I told her I had gotten very sick after I cut and studied the white birch flowers. Then I handed out to her my paper "The Allergies and Sickness Expose from the Birch Trees" to let her review it. She took the paper and went inside her office. After a while, Stella brought two sheets of discharge papers and gave them to me. One sheet of paper had the description of the surgery and discharge information of Lady Star; another sheet had a list of the medicines that Dr. Deborah had prescribed for Lady Star. The medicines that Dr. Deborah had prescribed for Lady Star were Baytril 22 mg antibiotic pills and Clavamox antibiotic liquid medicine to take in orally and four different kinds of ophthalmic solutions to apply on Lady Star's eyes, such as Neo/poly/gram, Ciloxan, Atropine Sulphate, and Cyclosporine 2 percent ophthalmic solutions. Then her assistant Stella set up an appointment for the next day on November 20, 2003, at 10:00 a.m. for me to take Lady Star back to the hospital to let the doctor check up on her operated left eye. I paid them with my credit card for Lady Star's visiting and surgical payments. She gave me the receipt, all the paperwork and the medicines. I took all of them from her, and she released Lady Star from the hospital. I brought Lady Star home with a very heavy heart, because I was afraid Lady Star might lose her eye vision after this surgery.

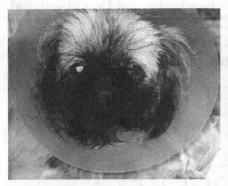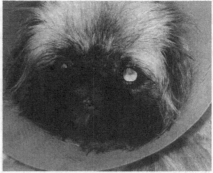

Left: After surgery, Lady Star could not open her left eye.
Right: Lady Star opened her left eye the first time after surgery.

After I arrived home, I took Sir Space out from my car and brought him inside the house. I came back out to the garage to carry Lady Star from my car and took her to my family room and placed her in the bean bag. Sir Space was scared and kept following me and Lady Star from the kitchen all the way to the family room. Then he stayed near Lady Star, quietly looking at her after I put Lady Star down on the bean bag in the family room. I gave both of them water to drink. Then I prepared food for Sir Space and myself. After I fed Sir Space, I fed a little chicken soup to Lady Star. Then I ate my dinner. After I ate my dinner, I went to my car in the garage to get the paperwork and medicines that I had brought home from AECH. I sat down on my sofa and took out the description sheet of the discharge information of Lady Star and Dr. Deborah's medicine prescription sheet for Lady Star and read them. Dr. Deborah had described on the discharge sheet that Lady Star's left eye was ruptured and had been diagnosed with several types of deep ulceration known as a descemetocele. She had to repair her deeply ruptured corneal of her left eye by transplanting with new corneal tissue from another dog. Keratoconjunctivitis (dry eye syndrome) had also formed in her eyes. Dr. Deborah had explained to me the cause of Descemetocele and Keratoconjunctivitis diseases on the sheet in detail. After I finished reading Lady Star's discharge sheet and prescription sheet, I studied all the medicines that I needed to give Lady Star and the number of treatments given on the treatment sheet, which I needed to apply on Lady Star's left eye daily. After I studied all the medicines for Lady Star, I divided the times for her eye drop medicines to apply on her left eye within the twenty-four hours of each day. Then I listed all the prescription that Dr. Deborah had prescribed for Lady Star on the medication organizer chart from AECH and marked down the times that I had to apply the type of medicine and number of drops on her eyes on the chart as shown in Chart 3.1.

O'clock a = am, p = pm		1	2	3	4	5	6	7	8	9	10	11	12
a	Ciloxan		x				x				x		
p	Left,1		x				x				x		
a	Neo/poly/				x				x				x
p	gram, left, 1				x				x				x
a	Clavamox						x						
p	Liqd, mth, 1						x						
a	Atropine Sulp, left, 1									x			
p										x			
a	Cyclospo-						x						
p	rine, both, 1						x						
a	Erythromy				x						x		
p	cin, right, s				x								
a	Sod.Chloride, left, s				x						x		
p					x						x		
a	Baytril								x				
p	1 tablet								x				

Chart 3.1: Lady Star's eyes' daily medication organizer chart

After I was done listing the prescriptions on the medication organizer chart shown in Chart 3.1, I started to give Lady Star one tablet of Baytril 22 mg tablet first. Then I applied one drop of Ciloxan ophthalmic solution eye drops in her left eye and a small amount of erythromycin ointment in her right eye at 8:00 p.m. as instructed by the doctor on the first day. Then I took both Lady Star and Sir Space to my room. I cleaned Lady Star's left eye with distilled water. I applied one drop of Neo/poly/gram ophthalmic solution eye drops to her left eye at 10:00 p.m., then I cleaned her left eye with distilled water again. I applied one drop of Atropine ophthalmic solution eyedrops in her left eye at 12:00 p.m. I cleaned her eye again with distilled water. I applied one drop each of Cyclosporine 2 percent ophthalmic solution eye drops in both her eyes at 2:00 a.m. next day.

I took Lady Star back to AECH to check up with Dr. Deborah the next day, November 20, 2003, at 10:00 a.m. Dr. Deborah was not in the clinic. Dr. Patty S. was in the clinic and she took care of Lady Star. She checked Lady Star's eyes with laser machines and told me Dr. Deborah had done a good surgery on Lady Star's left eye. She indicated that Lady Star's left eye would be fine after this surgery. After Dr. Patty checked up on Lady Star's eyes, she discharged Lady Star. I went out to the front desk clerk to set up another appointment on November 24, 2003, at 11:45 a.m. for Lady Star to come back to the hospital to check up. Then we went home. After I was home, I readjusted the times to make myself more convenient to take care of Lady Star and marked down on the medication organizer chart as shown in Chart 3.1. I used distilled water to clean her eyes before I rotated and applied the medicines, as marked on the medication organizer chart, on her eyes day and night.

Dr. Deborah called me after she got Lady Star's left eye's culture result from the laboratory. She indicated that Lady Star's left eye was infected with three kinds of organisms, such as a few *Citrobacter koseri*, a few *Pseudomonas aerusinosa*, and 2+ *Beta Hemolitic Streptococcus*. She advised me to continue the medicines that she had prescribed for Lady Star. She said the medicines that Lady Star was using could also treat the diseases given by the culture result. I told her I knew nothing about the diseases that she had described to me. I requested her to help Lady Star get back her vision. I did not know how to help her get back her vision, and I had to depend on her. She told me just to do what she had asked me to do. Then she told me to follow the instructions as listed on the sheet every day to treat Lady Star with the medicines that she had prescribed for Lady Star. I said OK to her and thanked her on the phone. Then I told her I did not know any of the disease that she had described on the telephone and requested her to give me a copy of Lady Star's left eye's culture result that she had received from the laboratory. She said she was off on November 24, 2003, but Dr. Patty would be in the clinic to take care of Lady Star. She suggested that I ask Dr. Patty on my next visit to get the culture results and print them out from the computer for me. I told her that I would request Dr. Patty to give me a copy of Lady Star's left eye's culture results on Lady Star's next doctor visit. I thanked her again on the telephone, and we ended our conversation. I made Lady Star sleep on the bean bag in the family room after she came home. At nights, she would sleep on her pillow bed in my room. I had to clean her urine discharge for her for the first three days. She was a very disciplined dog. She cried when she wanted to urinate. I did not let her out until she could control to get up and go herself. I hand-fed her until she could eat herself. It was hard for Sir Space to get little attention from me. He would not eat the food from his own bowl. He preferred to eat Lady Star's food, and he kept following me every single step that I took inside my house.

Next day after Lady Star's left eye surgery, I called my children to inform them Lady Star's left eye had ruptured accidentally and she already gone through her left eye's corneal transplant surgery. I told them she was very sick and could not open her eyes after her left eye's surgery. My children asked for my permission to come home and look at Lady Star. I told them to come home on the weekend to look at Lady Star. They came home on Saturday. Usually, when my children came home, they would hear Sir Space and Lady Star barking. They would make a lot of noise when my children would come home, but that day, when they were home, the whole house was quiet. They did not hear a single sound from those two baby dogs. Lady Star was so sick and had to stay on the bean bag day and night. Sir Space was scared. He stayed near Lady Star. He would not even go to the kitchen to drink or eat his food. I had to feed him from a separate bowl, as he sat near Lady Star while I fed Lady Star. After they both came home, they went to see Lady Star in the family room. When they saw Lady Star, they felt so bad to see her suffering from pain following her left eye's corneal transplant surgery. They stayed with Lady Star in the family room. They asked me whether Lady Star could lose vision in her left eye. I said yes to them. Lady Star would lose her vision in her left eye after surgery. This was a terrible strategy to see a healthy baby dog getting eye surgery and becoming blind. Then they held Sir Space and tried to comfort him and played with him. They saw the way I was taking care of Lady Star, which was not an easy job. Every hour, I had to apply different kind of medicines in Lady Star's eye. It was hard for Lady Star to get hurt like this. They felt bad and upset that they could not do anything to help Lady Star get better. Sirena helped me by making dinners for all of us, and then they both went home.

After a week, I called Counselor Charlene and told her about Lady Star's accident. She was very upset and unhappy to hear this bad news. She came to my house right away to see Lady Star. She was a pet lover and always liked to play with them when she came to my house. She felt very bad after she heard Lady Star's left eye had to go through eye corneal transplant surgery and suffered after an accident. She asked me how Lady Star had got hurt. I told her that Lady Star had got hurt when I was doing the research on the white birch trees at home. She had told my neighbor so many times to cut down their birch tree. Each time she went over and talked to them, they refused to cut down the birch tree. She felt so bad that she could not help a bit to get rid of my neighbor's allergic birch tree.

I took Lady Star back to AECH to checkup with Dr. Patty on November 24, 2003, at 11:45 a.m. Dr. Patty said Lady Star's left eye was in good condition after surgery. She prescribed one more sodium chloride ointment to be applied for a small amount four times a day on Lady Star's left eye. She reduced erythromycin ointment from three times to one time a day to apply a small amount on lady Star's right eye. Before she released me, I told Dr. Patty that I did not know and understand any disease that Dr. Deborah had described to me on the telephone. I requested her to print a copy of the Lady Star's left eye's culture result for me. Dr. Patty said yes to me and released me. I went to the front desk clerk to set up another appointment for Lady Star on November 29, 2003, at 11:00 a.m. After I set up the appointment, Dr. Patty's assistant gave me a new medication instruction sheet to apply on Lady Star's eyes and the copy of the printout of the Lady Star's eye culture result. Then she released me. I bought sodium chloride ointment from AECH. I went home with both my dogs. I applied all the medicines on Lady Star's eyes as instructed by the doctor every day. On Saturday, November 29, 2003, I took Lady Star back to the AECH at 11:00 a.m. to checkup with Dr. Deborah again. After Dr. Deborah finished checking Lady Star's eyes with a laser machine, she reduced neo/poly/gram and Ciloxan ophthalmic solutions from six times to four times a day to apply one drop each and reduced Atropine eyedrops from twice a day to one time a day to apply one drop in Lady Star's left eye. She indicated to me to use all of the Cyclosporine 2 percent ophthalmic solution and Clavamox ophthalmic solution until all the ophthalmic solutions were over. After she was done, I went to the front desk clerk to set up another appointment on December 2, 2003, at 2:15 p.m. Her assistant gave me another new instruction sheet to follow. I took the instruction sheet and left with Lady Star and Sir Space from AECH and went home.

In the night, I called my friend Theda Tan to talk to her about Lady Star's accident and the allergies and sickness that I had got from my neighbor's white birch trees. I knew Theda since I was in the first year of university. I remembered she had told me earlier that her son was attending Stanford University, majoring in biochemistry. He was doing very well at school. He liked to read and study all kinds of books. I asked her whether her son had already graduated from Stanford University. She told me her son had already graduated from the university and was working in Stanford Hospital. So I asked her to let me talk to her son to look for an analytical laboratory to analyze the birch flowers and their ingredients. She suggested that I call her son directly to talk to him. Then she gave me her son's name and telephone number. Next day, I called her son Dr. Thomas Tan (PhD) after I got his telephone number from his mother. I told him about Lady Star's accident and that I needed his help to find an analytical laboratory to analyze the ingredients of white birch flowers. He suggested looking on Internet first, as sometimes all kinds of lists of the plants and chemicals that are contained in the plants are posted on Internet. I told him I had a computer, but I did not have Internet connection to search for the plants. He said he would help me to look for the plants on Internet. He asked me to wait for him while he searched on Internet first. He said that after he found the information on Internet, he would call me back and let me know if there was anything about the birch trees. I said OK and waited for him to call me back. I knew he was the one who could help me to find and solve this problem for me.

3-O-(3',3'-Dimethylsuccinyl)-betulinic acid; Betulinic acid, 3-O-(3',3'-dimethylsuccinate)

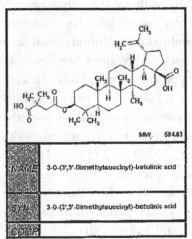

3-O-(3',3'-Dimethylsuccinyl)-betulinic acid is one of the most active betulinic acid derivatives (1,2).

MW. 584.83

NAME: 3-O-(3',3'-Dimethylsuccinyl)-betulinic acid

SYN: 3-O-(3',3'-Dimethylsuccinyl)-betulinic acid

The chemical structure of betulinic acid

Next day, December 1, 2003, Dr. Thomas Tan called me back after he had searched through the Internet to inform me that he had found a list of all different kinds of plants and trees and their chemicals. He asked me the type of plant that I needed to know. I told him about the white birch tree and their biological family step by step for him to search through the Internet. Then he found American Cancer Society (ACS) had posted the description about the white birch trees. The ACS stated that the birch trees contained betulinic acid. Then he said he would send me the chemical structure of betulinic acid.

Dr. Thomas Tan suggested that it was not necessary for me to get a laboratory to analyze the ingredient of the birch leaves and flowers again and that I could use the information from the ACS website to show the city of Pleasanton, the judge in the court, and the people that the birch trees contained the type of acid that was strong enough to cause the people get allergies and sickness. I told him I needed the information to show the city of Pleasanton and the judge in the court to prove that the birch trees contained betulinic acid and that the acid had the ability to cause burning and itching, thus making the people get sick. He said he would fax all the information about the white birch trees and the structure of betulinic acid to me right away. But my fax machine was broken. I requested him to print out the copies about the birch trees and mail them to me. He said OK and then hung up the phone.

I took Lady Star to checkup with Dr. Patty in AECH on December 2, 2003, at 2:15 p.m. After Dr. Patty checked up on Lady Star's eyes, she reduced Ciloxan ophthalmic solution from four times to three times a day to apply one drop a day in Lady Star's eye. Then she told me to stop using erythromycin ointment on Lady Star's both eyes. She indicated to me to use all the Baytril 22 mg tablets and Neo/poly/gram ophthalmic solution until all the medicines were finished. Then she discharged me. I set up another appointment. Then we went home. I received the mail dated December 5, 2003, from Dr. Thomas Tan, enclosing all the copies of information about the birch trees on December 8, 2003. After I received the copies from him, I called him back to inform him I had received his letter and thanked him for his help. I reviewed all the information about the birch trees and the structure of the betulinic acid from the paperwork that he had sent out to me.

I took Lady Star to check in at AECH on December 12, 2003, again at 11:45 a.m. Dr. Deborah was in the clinic. She told me Lady Star's left eye was in good condition, after she checked up Lady Star's eyes with a laser machine. She gave me the treatment instruction sheet that indicated to discontinue using erythromycin ointment and changing sodium chloride ointment on Lady Star from four times to four to five times a day. Then she discharged Lady Star. I set up another doctor visiting appointment on December 22, 2003, at 11:30 a.m. with the front desk clerk for Lady Star.

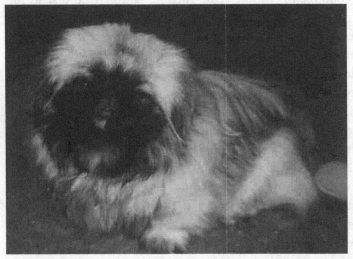

Lady Star recovering after her left eye's corneal transplant surgery.

On December 22, 2003, when I took Lady Star to AECH, Dr. Patty checked Lady Star's eyes with the laser machine. Then she used her finger to move around in front of Lady Star's eyes to check whether her left eye's vision was lost. Lady Star's left eye was not moving. She indicated that Lady Star's left eye's vision was lost. After she checked up Lady Star's left eye, she gave me the treatment instruction sheet. She reduced Ciloxan ophthalmic solution from three times to two times a day and sodium chloride ointment from four times to two times a day until all the medicines were finished. She also indicated to me to stop using Atropine ophthalmic solution. After she was done, she released Lady Star, and we went home. I made two more follow-up appointments on January 22, 2004, at 11:45 a.m. and March 13, 2003, at 9:00 a.m. with Dr. Patty. Each time I took Lady Star to check in at AECH, Dr. Patty checked Lady Star's left eye carefully with an electronic laser machine. Then she told me her left eye was in good condition and she released us.

On March 13, 2003, at 9:00 a.m., I took Lady Star to checkup with Dr. Patty. After Dr. Patty checked Lady Star's eye, she said Lady Star's left eye was totally healed. She advised me to take Lady Star back to see her after one year. Then she released Lady Star. I went to the front desk clerk to set up an appointment on March 19, 2004 at 9:00 a.m. for Lady Star to check with her after one year. I left AECH with Lady Star and Sir Space with deep appreciation for the two eye specialists, Dr. Deborah and Dr. Patty, for helping Lady Star recover from her ruptured left eye, and we went home. I was happy to see Lady Star getting better.

Prescription Changing Date		11/19	11/20	11/24	11/29	12/02	12/22
1	Ciloxan L,1	1	6	6	4	3	2*
2	Neo/poly/gram L,1	1	6	6	4	3*	2*
3	Clavamox M,1			2	2	2	2*
4	Atropine L,1	1	2	2	1	1	stop
5	Cyclosporine B,1	1	2	2	2	2	2
6	Erythromycin Sm	1	3	1	1	stop	
7	Sodium Chloride Sm			4	4	4	2*
8	Baytril 1 tablet	1	2	2	2	2*	

Chart 3.2: Lady Star's eyes' prescription treatment chart

I have prepared Lady Star's daily prescription treatment chart for the readers to see more clearly how many times a day she needed each type of the medicines to apply in her eyes and the dates when the doctor was adding or reducing the medicines to apply on Lady Star's eyes in Chart 3.2. The symbol (*) in Chart 3.2 indicated that all the medicines were to be used until (*) finished. "stop" indicated to discontinue the medicines on the dates that were shown in Chart 3.2. During Lady Star's doctor visits, I used the medication organizer chart as shown in Chart 3.2 at home. I applied all the medicines, which were marked on the medication organizer chart separately, on Lady Star's left eyes every one to six hours daily. When Lady Star's left eye started improving and stayed in good condition, the doctor started reducing some of the eyedrop medications. Then I crossed out the old mark and divided the number of eyedrop medications used by the number of times for me to apply on Lady Star's left eye. I rearranged the medication organizer chart and marked the new instructed medication time on the medication organizer chart. I applied the medicines in Lady Star's left eyes with new marks for time. I cleaned her eyes with distilled water before I applied any medication in her eyes. I fed her the medicines on time every day. I did not put her down on the floor until she got better. I did not keep her out of my sight. I took care of her day and night according to the doctor's instructions.

While I took care of Lady Star, I kept asking myself every day, "Why did I do this research on white birch tree? Was this worth it to dump in a healthy dog, making her eyes get blind?" I prayed to God every day to help Lady Star get back her vision. I called my sisters, brothers, nephews, and friends again and again, trying to take my frustration out on them. I could do nothing but keep telling them that Lady Star had accidentally become the victim of my experiment. I did not purposely experiment on her; it was just an accident that a small piece of birch flower dropped in her left eye and burned it, while I was cutting and taking the pictures of birch leaves and flowers. I was very upset with my neighbor after Lady Star's left eye got blind with my neighbor's birch tree acid. She would not have ruptured her eye corneal if I knew the birch tree contained acid, and if I knew she would get the accident, I would prepare a collar for her to protect her eyes, but she would still be blind because her ulceration was so deep due to her accident. When Lady Star got this incident, I was in the middle of taking treatments for cleaning my teeth. I was so upset and cried. I even lost a couple of my teeth. After this incident, I decided to get an analytical laboratory to find out the white birch flower ingredients and their acid that could cause burn, damaging Lady Star's left eye. When I called Dr. Thomas Tan on November 30, 2003, to ask him about birch acid, he looked through the American Cancer Society website on Internet. On the American Cancer Society website, he found that the white birch tree contained betulinic acid. He indicated that I did not need to get an analytical laboratory to search the type of acid in white birch trees. This was enough for me to prove birch trees could cause allergies and sickness to human beings. Then I called Renee to let her know that the birch trees contained betulinic acid that caused bad allergies and sickness in people. She said she did not know the birch trees contained acid. She felt bad about Lady Star's accident and that she had to go through the eye surgery.

During the time, I took Lady Star to Dr. Patty for checkup. I asked Dr. Patty about the cause of rupture of Lady Star's left eye. Dr. Patty said that the rupture of her left eye was possibly caused by the inflammation from the ulceration, or less likely, glaucoma could have caused loss of vision. I disagreed with Dr. Patty's assumption in Lady Star's case based on her daily activities and the food she ate. I fed my dogs nothing but fresh meat and dog snacks. The meat would never cause inflammation in animals leading to burns or form any allergy on their body. If the meat could inflame the dog's body, all the dogs would get very sick, and no dog would survive in this world. It was impossible for us to make such a kind of assumption to say that Lady Star's left eye was ruptured because of internal inflammation. If it was true that Lady Star's left eye was caused by internal inflammation, it would cause both her eyes to get burned and infected. It was impossible for Lady Star to get internal inflammation just in her left eye. I knew Lady Star's left eye must have been burned by a drop of acid from birch flower pieces while I was cutting and taking pictures of the birch flowers on the kitchen counter. According to Dr. Deborah's description that Lady Star had got real deep ulceration in her left eye, then only the acid had the ability to burn the eye's corneal layers so deep. Her eye would never be burned so deeply if it was caused by any other chemical. There are so many corneal layers in our eyes. The clear corneal layers of the eyes had enough strength to protect human and animal eyes. If our eyes did not have enough strength in the clear corneal layers to protect our eyes, our eyes would be ruptured by just scratching our eyes. The only possibility of rupture of her left eye was an external object containing acid or some acid must have dropped onto her left eye, causing very deep burn, severe itching, and formation of a blister. When her left eye hit the corner edge of the washing machine room door, the sharp edge of the door cut and broke the blister in her left eye. I did not keep or use any chemical inside my house. I had not worked on anything but birch leaves and flowers inside my house in the past before Lady Star's left eye was ruptured. The only possibility was the bad acid from the birch flower pieces must have dropped onto her eyes when she was sitting near me, as she lifted her head up and looked at me while I was cutting and taking the pictures of the birch flowers.

I told Dr. Patty that I had already found the type of acid in the white birch flowers from the ACS website. I explained to her that while I was researching the white birch tree at home Lady Star must have accidently must have come in contact with the birch acid, which burned her left eye. After I gave out enough reasons to explain and convince Dr. Patty, she told me to fax all the information about the white birch trees to her. I told her I would fax the copies of the birch trees from ACS to let her study. She promised to write a letter for me to indicate that Lady Star's left eye was burned by the chemical acid after she reviewed the papers and the structure of betulinic acid of the birch flowers on the ACS website. Then she gave me the fax number. I took her fax number and went home. After I reached home, I faxed all the information about the white birch trees and the structure of the betulinic acid to her. On my next visit, Dr. Patty wrote a letter for me to indicate that Lady Star had lost her eyesight because of the chemical substance that burned her left eye. But she did not indicate the type of chemical and the name of the white birch tree in her letter. So I called Dr. Patty to ask her why she did not indicate the name of the birch tree in her letter and that Lady Star had got her eyes burned because of the birch flower acid. She said she did not have the time to go through the whole thing, so she just wrote down in general that the chemical was the reason for the rupture of Lady Star's left eye. Then I showed Dr. Patty's letter to Charlene and Marlene. I told them Dr. Patty had not mentioned the birch tree's name in her letter. Maybe she thought she had not seen with her own eyes, as she was not in the place when the accident happened, but she did agree with me that Lady Star's left eye was burned by the chemical in the birch flower. Then I told her this was enough to prove that the birch trees were the bad allergic trees that could cause allergies and sickness to mankind and animals. It also could make the people's eyes get burned or blind just like Lady Star if the birch flower pieces or powder accidentally came in contact with any human eyes.

After Lady Star was discharged from AECH, I had to deal with the problem of fleas on my dogs' bodies at home. I did not know how Lady Star got fleas at the AECH clinic. I tried to kill the fleas on her body every night as much as I could by pressing the fleas with my two thumbs.

I did not want to use any flea-killer medicines on Lady Star's body when she was so sick. Then the fleas from her body transferred to Sir Space's body. I found Sir Space also had a lot of fleas on his body. I bought the flea-killer medicines from Costco store to spray on both their bodies to kill fleas. But I could not get rid of all the fleas from their bodies with the flea-killer medicines from Costco store. I had to call HAH to set up an appointment with Dr. Eliz on January 29, 2005.

I took Sir Space and Lady Star to HAH on January 30, 2005, to checkup with Dr. Eliz for their flea problem. Dr. Eliz explained to me that we cannot just use the medicines from Costco store to get rid of the fleas. These dogs needed to take flea-killer medicines to get rid of the fleas from their bodies. After the dogs took the flea-killer medicines, the fleas died when they sucked the blood from the dogs. She prescribed flea-killer medicines for six months for both Sir Space and Lady Star, and she asked me to give them one pill in each month for six months. Then she suggested that I get canine shampoo that contained sulfur, salicylic, and trilosan to be used during the dogs' bath to get rid of the fleas and their eggs from the dogs' bodies. I bought canine shampoo from HAH, and I took both of my dogs home. I used the canine shampoo every week when I gave bath to both of them. It took me more than six months to get rid of the fleas completely from both Sir Space and Lady Star's bodies. I had to spend so much time on both my dogs when they got sick. I just worried about their health and safety every day, just like my own children.

After Lady Star's left eye accident, I blamed myself a lot every day. It had been very hard for me to see Lady Star lose her eyesight. I did not like the way she got hurt. I did not want her to lose her vision. I felt sad every time I thought about it. I just wanted her and Sir Space to be perfect just like my own children. I told myself that if I had got the information about the birch trees a bit earlier I would not have to search and test at home. If she had stayed far away from me on the day when I was studying the birch flowers in the kitchen she would not have had the accident and burned her eye, losing her eyesight. If my neighbor had listened to me and cut down the white birch tree, she would not have got hurt and we would not have suffered from the allergies and sickness caused by the birch tree. If my neighbor had cut down their birch tree, all the people in our neighborhood would have followed him to cut down all the birch trees to clean up the environment. But, unfortunately, my neighbor refused to cut down his birch tree. I was still getting bad allergies and sickness. Lady Star and Sir Space were still throwing up a lot of yellow mucus bubble and getting a bad allergy after they came back in from my backyard. In particular, Lady Star's underbody had a lot of rashes which caused itching because she ran around in my backyard. Sir Space was also suffering allergy from the birch tree just like Lady Star, but he did not get a lot of rashes on his body because of his long fur hairs. After Lady Star was discharged from AECH in Fremont, I developed all the pictures that I had taken before Lady Star's left eye's corneal transplant surgery. I have summarized the information that I collected about the birch trees as follows:

Birch trees:

Birch trees belong to the "Betulaceae" biological family, and their scientific name is Betula. There are white birch, paper birch, gray birch, yellow birch, sweet birch, and river birch. They are well known and quick-growing trees. They have mostly pointed and toothed margins on their triangular-shaped leaves. They have two kinds of flowers: male and female flowers. The male flower is slimmer than the female flower. The female flower is bigger and fatter. There are many bird-shaped shells inside the female flower. The male flowers form corn-like clusters in the birch tree. The female and male flowers have one middle screw-shaped long stem holding a lot of sets of four bird-shaped shells or round pollens at the different meeting points (b, c, d, . . .) as shown in Diagram 3.3.

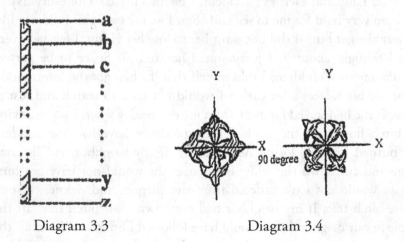

Diagram 3.3   Diagram 3.4

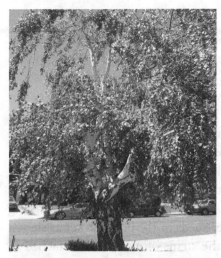
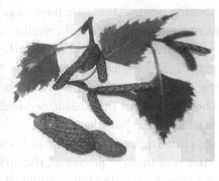

Left: My neighbor's allergic white birch tree
Right: Slim male, fat female allergic white birch flowers and leaves

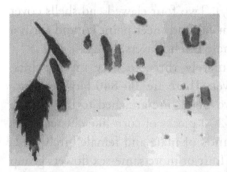
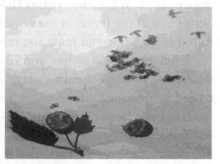

Left: Fruit like male birch flower
Right: Bird shape nut-let shells in female birch flower

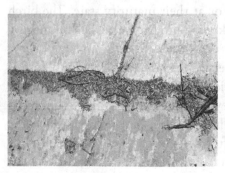
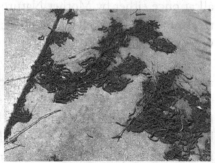

Messy dried white birch leaves and flowers

A female flower can hold eight to twenty-four pieces of one seed with two colorless petals of bird-shaped shell and all their petals overlap each other tightly in each sector. One sector is the distance between two meeting points. The male flower can hold four to twelve pieces of small round pollens. Each fruit contains white meat in the young stage, but transforms into small yellow fruits in their maturity stage. The bird-shaped shell from the female flower has a layer of skin and tissue. When the shell dries out, the tissue layer breaks into big or small dry particles. The skin layer of the bird-shaped shell forms brown hard shells. The head portion of the bird-shaped shell and the half of two top portion feathers are curled upright naturally and sealed tight with each other, forming outer skin shells to protect all the inner seeds of the birch flower as shown in Diagram 3.4. The tail portions of the stems of nut-lets are attached to the middle main long stem of the fruit-like flower and the two bottom tail portions of the stem of nut-lets attached to the middle long stem at different meet points act as the divider shell and are approximately ninety degrees apart at the meet points (b–y). Two four clawed end shells cover both ends of the flower at meet point (a) and meet point (z) and form a round-shaped body for male and female birch flowers.

Each birch flower has approximately three to fifty meet points, depending on their ages in each flower. There are 24–840 pieces of one-seeded bird-shaped nut-let shells (two petals are attached to the middle seed) in each female flower, and 12–200 pieces of corn-like cluster fruits inside the male flower. Many thousands of male and female birch fruit-like flowers bloom each year. Two to four or more same-sex flowers group together on the branches. The male flowers bloom more than female flowers. When some or all the pieces of the flowers disintegrate from the tree, either they release the pieces of the birch flowers sector by sector or all at once either by Mother Nature or at their maturity state. The birch trees not only cause allergies and sickness but also make the community very messy and toxic.

The trunk, bark, leaves, and flowers of the birch tree contain betulinic acid, oil, and fluid. The betulinic acid is a highly aromatic hydrocarbon acid compound and is very toxic. They have the strong ability to burn and form pimple rashes and blisters on human skin and tissues. When the birch fruit-like flowers disintegrate from the birch tree, all the fruit-like flowers break apart, the nut-lets from the fruit-like flowers fly all over the places, and some of the nut-lets from the birch trees break into different smaller sizes and fly all over the places. If your skin comes in contact with these breaking pieces, they can expose blister rashes on your skins. If you breathe into your internal system the powder or broken pieces of the birch flowers or smoky gas or the moisture of birch acids, it can cause different kinds of allergies and sickness with high fever; sometimes it can lead to infections like cancer inside your system. The worst part is it can possibly cause death of the people. If your eyes or ears come in contact with these birch substances, it would get infected. Sometimes these infections may become very complicated and can cause blindness and deafness.

The scientists from ACS had posted in their website that they are still testing and researching for using this birch acid to treat on skin cancer and HIV in the laboratory. The scientists from ACS also posted in their website that Native Americans are using birch leaves as tea to treat diarrhea and dysentery. When you put birch leaves in hot water, the acid from the birch leaves dissolves in hot water. The birch acid could burn the tissues in your stomach if you keep drinking the birch leaf tea. They could burn any portion of your internal organs like heart, lungs, livers, kidneys, stomach, etc. Sooner or later, it could cause serious sickness to the people who keep drinking birch leaf tea. The doctors blamed germs and virus instead of the bad chemicals in the air or in the food that they are using every day.

I went to Pleasanton Library to look for more information about the birch trees. I requested the librarian at Pleasanton Library to help me find more information about the birch trees on Internet because my eyes were not too clear to look at the computer. The librarian helped me find more information about the birch trees on Internet. After she found the information about the birch trees on Internet, she let me look at it. While I was reading the information about the birch trees on Internet, I told her how the people were getting leukemia and why children were more susceptible to leukemia than adults. I explained to her that the reasons were that the roads, sidewalks, and the garage driveway concretes heated up in day time due to the sun. If there were a lot of birch trees in their neighborhood, the sun heated up all the birch trees, birch flowers, and birch leaves on the roads, sidewalks, and garage driveway concretes. In the hot weather, all of the chemical acid from the birch trees and their flowers and leaves vaporized. If the people breathed in all these vaporizing chemical acid moistures or smoking gases into their internal organs, their internal organs would burn and get destroyed. Because the children were shorter than the adults, the possibility of them breathing in the vaporizing chemical acid moisture from the ground were higher than the adults. This is the reason the children were more susceptible to leukemia than adults. After I explained to her about leukemia, I requested her to help me print out all the information about the birch trees to take home to review. She helped me to print out all the information about the birch trees that she could find from Internet and gave them to me. I took the papers, thanked her, and went home.

After I was home, I studied the papers from the library. I found some of the papers were written by the people using the name of God to make people believe the birch trees were good trees, but they never thought that the birch trees contained a bad chemical acid that could cause allergies and sickness. One of the papers, "My White Birch and the Will of God," written by Robert McQueeney really made me upset after I read his paper. He did not even know what he was talking about. I presumed he did not have any knowledge of science, as he was misleading the people in the wrong direction using the name of God by describing that God created the beauty of the white trunk of the birch tree for the people. Another paper was written by Alien Earth. He had described that the barks of white birch tree could burn quickly, but it was not a good idea to use white birch barks as firewood to burn in the residential areas because the white birch bark contained strong betulinic acid. If you use the birch bark to burn in your house, that would be very harmful to the people who lived in the neighborhood. I found that birch wood was very light. The Red Indian people used the birch wood to build canoes in Canada. I found some industrial companies were using birch oil to make chewing gum, breath mints, and skin lotions. The Russians used birch oil to soften their leathers and to protect the leather from the insects, and they also used birch oil in the book industry to protect the books from the insects. The businessmen did mention in the papers that they used 100 percent pure birch oil in their products. I can only clearly explain here that even though the birch oil is useful to produce products for the business people, the birch acid is not good. The business people cannot use all the ingredients from the birch trees. The chemists from those companies have to go through so many steps in order to get the pure birch oil from the birch trees. First, they have to get rid of the birch acid completely from the birch oil before they can use the pure birch oil in their products. The chemists in the production line do not even allow 0.0000001 mg of birch acid in the products. This could cause itching and allergy to the people who used their products that they made with birch oil. Sometimes people get itching after they use some products on their skin, causing them bad allergies, if the company does not completely get rid of the acid from the ingredients of the plants that they are using. People should report to the consumer if they get any allergy due to the products that they are using. The reason for the businessmen using pure birch oil from the birch trees in their industries is they take advantage of the fast-growing birch trees to bring down the costs of their products. The people are planting birch trees in the residential areas all over the United States without knowing the effects of the chemicals in the birch trees. We must set the rule of law to ban the growing of certain bad plants that are harmful to the people in residential communities.

Other types of plants you should get rid of from your environment are as follows:

Both poison ivy and poison oak have three shiny leaflets, greenish white flowers, and clusters of berries. Poison sumac's branches usually contain nine leaves, four rows of two leaves, and one leaf at the end, but they can contain seven to thirteen leaflets as shown in the pictures. Both poison ivy and poison oak plants usually grow in shrubs, vines, or small plants all over America. Poison oaks are widespread in California and other southeast and western states of America. Poison sumac plants grow in most of the eastern states of America.

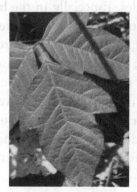 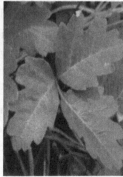 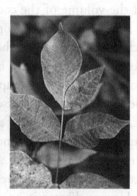

Poison Ivy   **Poison Oak**   **Poison Sumac**

Poison ivy, poison oak, and poison sumac belong to Anacardiaceae family. They are the strongest untouchable poisonous plants and contain their relative urushiol oil and their relative anacardic acid. If you come in contact with any one of these untouchable plants, your skin and body will develop bad itching, swelling, and burning and form bad blister rashes. We should get rid of them if we have these kinds of poisonous plants in our neighborhood.

The allergies and sickness:

A lot of people do not really know and understand the definition of allergy and burns of chemical compounds. They are misled by the doctors and researchers. The people are so much dependent on the doctors when they get sick. The doctors believe that sickness is carried on to another person by germs and bacteria through the air. But they are not aware that germs and virus cannot survive in the air without fluid. People are having problems in dealing with their lives as they do not know from where all the allergies and sickness come from and how the chemical compounds relate to the allergies and sickness.

Allergy means burning and itching that form pimple, rashes, and blisters. When any portion of the human body comes in contact with any particle or powder that contains chemicals having the ability of causing burning and itching any kind of redness rash, pimple, lump, hive, or blister can form. Sometimes the contacting body forms one or more spotty rashes, lumps, hives, or blisters because the contact areas of the body produce various heats depending on the strength of the chemicals and the volume of the contacting object particles. Especially in the late fall and early spring, people get bad allergy, flu, and hay fever because of the chemicals from those dried and rotten flowers of the bad trees or bushes like the white birch tree, poison ivy, poison oak, and poison sumac. If the body temperature exceeds 102 degrees, your body can experience pneumonia disease and cause inflammation, making you very sick. The various kinds of allergies depend on the allergic substances, such as age, size, weight, volume, time, weather, and distance. Sometimes these allergic substances cause various kinds of diseases and sickness that the doctors and the people are not aware of.

Herpes disease is one of the allergy diseases. The researchers claim that Herpes disease is formed by the germs in the air. Actually Herpes disease is caused by the burning of the small sticky powder or particles from the trees that contain chemical substances with a strong burning ability. Sometimes a concentrated white or yellow fluid will form on top of the Herpes pimple. Sometimes you lay your hands on the tables or the chairs that have the powder or the particles that contain the chemical substance with the burning ability and these particles get stuck in your hands, and when you wipe your mouth with your hand, then your lip gets burned and Herpes pimple rashes or Herpes blisters are formed.

The chemical compounds:

The chemical compounds are the materials that can transform into four different states, such as gas, moisture, liquid and solid states. Maybe one kind of chemical reacts with another kind of chemical and forms another kind of chemical compound with the help of heat or water (sun or rain), with or without metals. Carbon dioxide, carbon monoxide, oxygen, hydrogen, nitrogen are the chemical gases you can find in the air. Acids, alcohols, esters, and ethers are the chemical compounds that we deal with in our daily life. Among all the chemical compounds, acids are the worst compounds. The strength of the acids depends on their number of hydrocarbons and acid symbols. Most of the acids are very toxic and have the ability to burn and cause a high explosion if we do not handle them correctly. Hydrochloric acid is the strongest acid among all acids and very useful in pharmaceutical industries to make medicines.

If you review the contents of the ophthalmic solution medicine, the scientists from the pharmaceutical company showed how much of the individual chemical solutions are in this medicine. Mostly they use dilute hydrochloric acid in ophthalmic solution medicines to adjust the PH and let the excess hydrochloric acid burn the infectious layers of the skin tissues. Usually, they use sodium hydroxide as a base to neutralize hydrochloric acid and mix with purified water to absorb the infectious fluid from the wounded areas and let the excess acid burn and clean the bad tissues from the infectious skin. Then they use other ingredients in other medicines like antibiotics to heal the wounded area. Hydrochloric acid is the strongest acid among all acids. If you use 100 percent hydrochloric acid, they will burn and eat all of your skin deeply. Mostly we use fruits like lemons, limes, orange, and tangerines that contain citric acids and acetic acids in our daily life to enjoy their sour taste and to digest the food in our body. Citric acid and acetic acid are not highly aromatic hydrocarbon compounds. They do not have the strong ability like acids from the birch trees to cause either burn or itch on our body, but they can cause diarrhea in our system if the intake exceeds the body limit. We need to be careful regarding the food that we eat every day. Following are some of the arguments that I disagreed with the doctor's concepts.

Arguments:

The insect killers that are sold in the stores are ether chemical compounds, not chemical acid compounds, which are employed as insecticides to kill insects (*Britannica Encyclopedia* P804). If you swallow them accidentally, they can either make you throw up or cause diarrhea.

Mostly people claim that it's due to the insect's sting when there is a red rash on their body. You can distinguish the rash that is caused by an insect bite due to the burn that is caused by allergic powder. If the rash is a sting by the insect, you will find a little hole on the pimple rash immediately after the sting, which turns into a small black hard shell if you do not scratch the rash. The size of the red rashes is smaller and it will not itch like it does for the allergic substances. Sometimes bacterial fluid forms on top of the sting area because these insects suck blood from other living things (dogs, horses, or sick people) or juices of plants that contain bad chemical bacteria. The bad chemical bacteria can get into your blood system through their suckers (different insects have different names for the suckers) and the sting areas get infected. The insects that contain bad chemical bacteria also get infected and die. The insects can also get diseases similar to human beings. The only difference between the human beings and the insects are the tissues and the sizes. Some spiders contain very strong poison in their bodies. If the people get stung by a spider having strong poison, it could lead to the death of the people.

Pollens from any plants could cause allergy if the plants contain chemical acids with burning ability; otherwise, the pollens from the plants will never cause any allergy if the plants does not contain any chemical substances that may cause burning. All the researchers should indicate the type of the plants that may cause allergy and indicate which portion of the plants has the ability to burn. A lot of birds and insects eat pollens from the flowers for food. If all the pollens are allergy pollens, then there would not be any birds and insects.

Dog's hairs are just like human hairs and can never cause allergy to human beings. But when your pets come in from outside, there is a possibility your pets could carry in all these allergic particles or powder from outside into your house if you have allergic bushes or trees in your areas. After the dogs come in from outside, when they shake their body inside your house, these allergic particles or powder could fly all over the places inside your house. They can even get into your uncovered food and cause you allergy after you eat the food that contains allergy particles, or the allergy particles can enter the body while breathing and can cause allergy. Sometimes if you open your window, these allergic gases can come into your houses through the window screens, change to solid state, forming fine powder, and drop on your uncovered food or anywhere inside your house, especially during night when the weather is cold. If you eat the uncovered foods that contains the allergic substances, it can cause allergy and form blister rashes inside your body and show up as pale spotty allergy on your skins. If your hands or your body come in contact with the places that have the allergic powder inside your house, you can get bad allergy on your hands and skin; sometimes it may cause pimples or blister rashes on your hands and skin. If there is allergic powder inside your house and when the temperature inside your house increases during the day time, it can make this allergic powder to vaporize and change back to moisture or gas state. When you breathe in these moistures or gases inside your house, you get bad allergy. The bad chemical substances in the air burn your internal organs, cause diabetic disease, and form pale spots on your body. Sometimes the bad chemical substances burn your internal organs which can be infected badly inside your body and possibly form cancerous diseases.

The sugarcane and sugar can never cause healthy people to get diabetic diseases because they do not contain the type of chemical compounds or their relative chemical acid that have the ability to burn the human skins. Only the people who already suffer from diabetic diseases are not allowed to eat sweet food made with sugar. That would make the diabetics get worse.

The inflammation of eyes can be caused either by poisonous substances from plants or burned by hot liquids. It can cause inflammation of your eyes with deep ulceration, and there is also the possibility of losing eyesight. If the eyes are accidently hit by an outer object, inflammation of eyes can occur, but the possibility of losing eyesight is less, because the eyes have so many corneal layers to protect the eyes and do not form deep ulceration inside the eyes.

The tobacco leaves contain nicotinic acid. The nicotinic acid contains only one aromatic benzene ring, nitrogen, and acid. The property of nitrogen is to kill the fire. When the cigarette lights up, the cigarette produces smoke and forms nicotine oil, nicotinic acid, and fluid. When people smoke, the smoke gets into the lungs. Then they blow the smoke back out from the lung. In this case, the possibility of nicotine staying inside the body is less when compared with those who take nicotine pills or injection. The possibility of smoke from cigarettes that produce strong heat can possibly burn the throats and lungs and form emphysema in your lungs, depending on the size of the cigarette and the number of cigarettes that the people smoke. It is similar to drinking hot water. If you keep drinking hot water every day, the hot heat from the hot water can burn your throat and your lung, causing infection inside your throat or your lung.

Nicotine   Nicotinic acid

Some tobacco companies give out the warning label on the side of cigarette packs that smoking can cause emphysema, lung cancer, and heart diseases and can cause complicated pregnancy. The smokers should read the warning label on the cigarette packs of the brand that they choose to smoke. The nicotinic acid from the tobacco leaves do not cause any burning and itching after you squeeze the fresh leaves or their fresh flowers. The possibility of getting cancer by the nicotinic acid from the tobacco depends on the number of cigarettes that you smoke and the burning heat from the cigarette when you light up the cigarette. The strength of nicotinic acid in the tobacco does not cause your skin tissue to itch and burn if you use their leaves to rub on your skin to experiment whether they cause itching and form blister rashes just like betulinic acid chemical compound of the birch trees. The vegetables that we eat every day also contain vegetable acid and oil, but the acid from the vegetables can never cause you any allergy. Only when these vegetables absorb the poisonous chemicals from the water can it cause you allergies and sickness.

People like to drink and enjoy alcoholic beverages in their daily life. Alcoholic beverages have the strength to get rid of infections inside their body. But the alcoholic beverages can cause drowsiness in people and lead to all kinds of accidents depending on the percentage of alcohol levels that they consume. A lot of people drink alcoholic beverages without eating any food. This is the wrong way to drink and enjoy alcoholic beverages without eating any food. The human body produces uric acid to digest the food inside your stomach. If you drink alcoholic beverages without eating any food, the uric acid that produces inside your stomach can burn the tissue layers of your stomach if there is no food or not enough food for the acid to digest inside your stomach. This can cause infection leading to stomach cancer because the acid that produces inside your stomach needs food substances to burn and digest. If there is no food or not enough food inside your stomach, the acid would just burn the tissue layers of your stomach, and those areas would become infected. These infectious areas would cause cancer in the long run and would spread to the nearby areas inside your body if you do not get help from the doctors on time. All of us must know and understand the danger of drinking alcoholic beverages. We must learn how to use alcoholic beverages wisely to enjoy and prevent ourselves from getting sick.

Other organs of the human body, such as livers, kidneys, and hearts, can also suffer from cancer, just like stomach cancer. The doctors' explanation to the patients of leukemia that the white blood cells eat out all the red blood cells inside the blood system is a wrong concept. One portion of the liver transfers the oxygen to the bones to produce the red blood cells for blood and spread the oxygen all over the body. The Peyer's patches are the place in the bone that produce white blood cells and send it to the blood veins inside your body. The white blood cells absorb carbon dioxide from the blood veins and carry carbon dioxide to the lungs. Then the lungs blow out carbon dioxide to the air. When people breathe in a lot of these bad acid gases into their internal system, some portions of human system can burn and be damaged. If they damage the portion of the liver of the human body that sends oxygen to the bones to produce the red blood cells, the production of red blood cells would be decreased, but the Peyer's patches will continuously produce the white blood cells in the blood system of human body; thus, white blood cells take over the whole blood system of the human body. They call this kind of cancer as leukemia.

Why and how women are getting breast cancer? Can we prevent breast cancer? Yes, we can. All human beings have tiny little holes on the skin and the breast nipples. All women have milk or fluid in their breasts whether they are married or not. When this milk fluid flows out from the women's breasts through the nipple holes, sometimes they dry out fast on the nipple holes and form small solid white crystals on their nipple holes. These crystals from their nipples would block the milk fluid from flowing out of their breasts. The milk fluid that is inside the breasts would change into white human cheese if you keep them long inside your breasts. Sometimes because of the body heat, the milk fluid or white human cheese from the breasts will rot and get infected. If the breast is infected badly, the infection will spread all over the breasts and nearby areas of the body.

I used one gallon of cow milk plastic bottle with the expiration date marked on the bottle and kept it inside my refrigerator to do the experiment to find out what would happen to the milk after the expiration date. When they exceeded more than four weeks from the expiration date that was marked on the milk bottle, I found the formation of soft white cheese inside the plastic bottle in my refrigerator. These soft white pieces of cheese inside the plastic bottle were rotten and had a bad smell. This proves that the white spots that are seen in the women's mammogram films are rotten human cheese in women's breasts. All the women should clean their nipples when they take showers every day to avoid the formation of crystals on their nipple holes. This way they can let the fluid from their breasts flow out constantly to prevent themselves from getting breast cancers. In particular, women who have excess milk should clean their nipples every day when they take showers. They should get the advice from their doctors to take mammogram X-rays every year to check on their breasts to protect themselves from breast cancer diseases.

There are so many ways we can get allergies and blister pimples on our body from the heating areas and the areas that have bad chemicals with which our skin comes in contact. One of the worst allergies that I got in the past was from the milk cookies that I bought from Chinatown, Oakland. After I ate half of the box of those cookies from Chinatown, my legs burned and started to itch. I scratched and there were rashes on my legs. After one week, the itching on my legs disappeared and slowly the allergies moved up to my upper body and started to itch. I scratched and there were red rashes on my upper body. After one week, the itching in my body disappeared. The allergies moved up to my neck and both my arms, burned, and started to itch. I scratched and there were red rashes. The rashes on my neck and arms disappeared after a week. I could not do anything with this kind of poisonous allergy that I got from the cookies, but I had to take allergy medicines and I kept drinking a lot of water to get rid of the bad allergies. After a few weeks, all the itching and rashes on my body disappeared. This was really amazing that the allergy substances in the cookies could cause burn, itching, and rashes and could migrate from one section of my body to another section within a couple of weeks. This was my favorite brand of cookies that I usually bought from Chinatown. I never got any allergy from this specific brand of cookies before. The ingredients in the cookies were nothing but flour, butter, oil, sugar, and milk. The ingredients in the cookies would never make people get any bad allergy. I did not believe the cookies could cause me any allergy. Since I still had half a box left, I tried to eat and finish the remaining cookies again. I got the same kind of allergies again. The burns, itch, and rashes formed, starting from my legs, then my body and my neck and arms in different weeks and days. I believed at the time when I bought that batch of cookies that the allergy substances must have got into the cookies when the company was mixing all the ingredients and making this batch of cookies. After I got bad allergy from these cookies, I stopped buying the cookies of that name brand from Chinatown.

I got another type of allergy that formed external pimples on my back, caused by heat that was produced from the contact of my body back against the wooden floor in hot weather. When we were young, my parents used to let us sleep on the wooden floor with bamboo mats at night in our house when the weather was really hot. We did not have any big trees in our surrounding neighborhood that we lived in. Sometimes a lot of external type of pimple rashes formed on my back and got very itchy when the weather was very hot. These pimple rashes formed because of the heat that was produced in our skin when our backs came in contact with the wooden floor in the hot weather. My parents would turn on the fan for us to cool down the air in our environment to prevent us from getting pimple rashes on our backs when we slept on the wooden floor. This kind of pimple rashes would go away after a few days when the weather cooled down.

I tried to collect as much information I could get to help people understand the allergies and sickness that they could get from different sources in their daily lives. I hated to see people become victims of allergies and sickness. I found out the birch trees were the worst allergic trees that could cause the people and animals bad allergies and sickness in the residential neighborhood; sometimes it would lead to the death of people and animals. This was the reason I requested the people to get rid of the birch trees from our environment in the residential community. I would not make people to do things only for my interest. In this case, I have been patiently persuading people to get rid of the birch trees over many years. The best way for all of us to get rid of allergies and sickness is by cutting down the bad allergic birch trees. It has been more than a decade I searched the allergies and sickness in my own time in the community. I started from raising fish, then raising chicken, and I built the chicken farm. After I got involved in a bad car accident, I lost my chicken farm. I stayed home and studied the plants.

When I was researching the birch leaves and flowers at home, my female dog Lady Star had met with an accident. She had to go through her left eye's corneal transplant surgery. I got very upset at myself. I knew Lady Star's left eye was burned by birch acid. I wanted to protect the people from accidents just like Lady Star. I prepared seventeen pages of the report about our allergies and sickness caused by birch trees in early January 2004. I included my seventeen pages of the report paper, six pages of the papers from the American Cancer Society, letters from three doctors, twelve page copies of chemical reactions from the *Britannica Encyclopedia* book, four pages of sample copies of the eyedrop medicines, five copies of the picture of my swollen hands, twelve copies of Lady Star's pictures after she had her left eye's corneal transplant surgery, six copies of the picture of Lady Star's body rashes, ten copies of pictures of my neighbor's birch trees, and four copies of the birch flowers, a total of thirty-seven copies of the pictures that I enclosed each inside three brown envelope packages. I gave one brown envelope to Marlene from Pleasanton Senior Supporting Group in Pleasanton Senior Center dated February 10, 2004. I turned in one brown envelope package to the city attorney Renee dated March 7, 2004, and one brown envelope package to the city of Pleasanton dated March 8, 2004, to review about the allergies and sickness caused by birch trees, how my dog Lady Star had ruptured her left eye, how she suffered after her corneal transplant surgery in her left eye, and how the blister rashes formed on my both hands, causing swelling by the acid from the birch tree. After I turned in the brown envelope package to the city of Pleasanton, I did not hear anything from the city of Pleasanton, except Charlene coming to my house and visiting me every two weeks.

My neighbor's white birch tree was growing so big each year and our allergies were getting worse. I was unable to leave my windows open. If I left my windows open, a lot of those strong allergic particles got into my house through the screen windows, making my allergy get worse and make me very sick. I had to close my windows all year round. I used antibiotic pills to protect myself and my family. Sirena got pimple rashes on her right hand quite often when she came home on Sunday to take the garbage cans out. We kept our garbage cans next to our garage near the white birch tree. She would push the garbage cans with her right hand to the sidewalk in front of our house. Her right hand got a lot of pimple rashes, and she kept scratching her hands, causing the formation of a big area of pimple rashes after she took out the garbage cans. When she went to the doctor to check the pimple rashes on her right hand, the doctor told her that the pimple rashes on her right hand were due to the heat produced by the sun. How could she get all those pimple rashes because of the sun's heat? She did not even stay under the sun. I indicated to her that the pimple rashes on her right hand were not caused by exposure to the heat produced by the sun, but they were exposed to the dried powder of my neighbor's white birch tree that resided in the garbage cans. When she pushed the garbage cans with her hands out to the sidewalk, the birch powder from the garbage cans flew and landed on her hands, burned her hand, and formed pimple rashes. As usual, Shaun came home and cut the lawn for me every two weeks. He would complain after he cut the lawn that he got bad allergy rashes on his face. He showed me the red blister rashes on his face. I felt very upset, and I could not do anything, but I just had to ask Shaun not to clean our front yard again, because I did not want him to get the allergies and get very sick. So I took over the cleaning job from him. I cleaned the messy birch leaves and flower discharges in my front yard. After I cleaned them, my whole body got a bad itch and I was very sick.

I continuously complained to Renee about my neighbor's white birch trees by calling her. When I complained to Charlene when she visited me, she told me a lot of people were complaining about the allergy in

Pleasanton Senior Center. She said the people were blaming on the big city tree that was planted in front of Pleasanton Senior Center. I told her the city trees were not the allergic trees and their white flowers bloomed very prettily in the spring. The city of Pleasanton had planted white birch trees in the backyard of Pleasanton Senior Center. The dried birch flower powder of the white birch trees from the backyard of Pleasanton Senior Center blew out to nearby areas by the wind, causing these people to suffer from bad allergies and itching when they were in Pleasanton Senior Center. I told Charlene about Lori H. When I was in Pleasanton Senior Center, I had met Lori H. in the hallway. She had been working with Marlene all these years. I thought she knew about the search for the allergies and sickness from the birch trees. I took her to the backyard of Pleasanton Senior Center and I showed her the big white birch trees that were planted in the backyard of Pleasanton Senior Center. I told her the birch flower powder from these white birch trees was responsible for the allergy complaints from the people who came in Pleasanton Senior Center. Lori just looked at the white birch trees. She did not say anything. It seemed like she did not know anything about the allergy complaints from the people. Then we went back to Pleasanton Senior Supporting Group office.

After my family and I had been through so many allergies accidents caused by the white birch trees, I did not want the people to get the same kind of allergies and sickness from the birch trees just like me and my family. I wanted to let all the people know about the bad allergic birch family trees and request them to get rid of the bad allergic birch family trees from their neighborhood. We could expand our search if we could form a research center to search more about the ingredients and the chemicals in the other plants in the analytical laboratory. I got the idea to extend my paper and publish it as a book to warn the people who owned the white birch trees to get rid of them from their neighborhood to clean up the environment for all the people in the community. Then I planned to sell my book for twenty-five dollars, if people agreed to buy my book. I would use that money to build an analytical laboratory research center to hire a lot of scientists to research on more ingredients of all the plants and trees that have not been analyzed yet. I told Charlene about my idea when she came to my house. She said she agreed with my idea. She said she would let Marlene know it. After I talked to her, I called some of my friends and talked to them about the book. They all agreed to pay twenty-five dollars for my book. So I extended my paper about the allergy and sickness from three pages to twenty-nine pages with the book title of *The Scaring Birch Trees*. After I wrote the twenty-nine-page book, I printed out hundred copies of *The Scaring Birch Trees* book at home. I gave one book to Charlene and asked her to read it and to make corrections if there were any mistakes in the book. She read it again and again to find mistakes and made corrections in my book. Then she said there were a lot of places that needed rephrasing of the sentences so that it could be in perfect English. I told her I had just written the main points to make people understand the contents of this book. Then she said OK. She paid me twenty-five dollars for the book. I gave the money back to her and asked her to keep the money at the moment. I told her she could pay me later at the same time when other people paid me. She said OK. I mailed out some books to my sisters, cousins, and friends. I received the books' money from my sisters and cousins. I used that money to pay for my monthly mailbox fee. But I did not get any money from my friends after I sent out the books to them.

When Charlene came to my house and visited me, I told her about Renee. I told her that every time I talked to Renee to complain about my allergies and sickness due to my neighbor's white birch tree she always recommended me to go to the court. She knew I had enough reason and confidence to go to the court and could win this case. Charlene advised me not to go to court because one of her friend's doctors had already confirmed her friend's allergy was due to the birch trees. She told her friend about my book and let her friend read it. I told her since I did not have any allergy to food or medicines I refused to let any allergy doctor perform any skin test on me. The idea of testing on the patient's skin with food products was either to find out the type of food that could cause allergies or to test out whether the type of foods that they were complaining were really causing them allergy or not. But I never complained about any food or medicine that was allergic to me. I did not use or eat any vegetables, plants, or meat that they had described on the allergy skin test charts given from the allergy doctor's office. She knew I was exposing the allergies and sickness due to my neighbor's birch trees. Every time she came to my house, she felt so bad that my dogs and I were suffering from severe allergies and sickness. Sometimes she saw me all the red rashes and hives on my hands and legs. Sometimes she saw pale white spots on my knees and legs. She also saw that my legs were swelling and turning black, slowly spreading up to my knees when I stood up for more than five to ten minutes. She offered to me to go over to my neighbor's house to talk to my neighbor John Clark and ask him cut down his white birch tree. She gave him my paper or book when she went over to talk to him about my allergies caused by his birch tree and requested him to cut down his white birch tree for me. He refused to cut down the birch tree and gave her all kinds of excuses each time she went to talk to him. All the excuses he gave out to her were unacceptable to me. He said they were also getting the same kind of allergies and sickness from his right-side neighbor's white birch trees. He wanted me to solve this problem rapidly. I told Charlene to tell him, "If I can have his right-side neighbor to cut down their birch trees, will he cut down his white birch tree?" Another time when Charlene talked to him, he had said a lot of people owned white birch trees in this community, and if they did not cut down their white birch trees, why did he have to cut down his white birch tree? The last time when Charlene had talked to him, he had said to her that he would not cut down his white birch tree because people still owed me money. They all had to pay me because I had proved the allergies and sickness were from the white birch tree. If he cared about me, he would cut down his white birch tree first. But he kept refusing to do it. I do not know how to describe all his excuses he continued to tell us. People still owed me money; he should have thought of me suffering from bad allergies. It was his responsibility to plant good trees in his house to provide a healthy environment for the people who lived in our neighborhood. If he cut down his bad white birch trees, it would be good for him and for all the neighbors to keep the environment healthy for the people who lived in this community. If he got sick, he had the right to blame his right-side neighbor if he did not own the birch tree. But if he himself owned a big white birch tree in his own house, how was he going to complain to his neighbor if he got sick and died? I did talk to his right-side neighbor about their white birch trees. They said they would not cut down their trees unless John Clark cut down his white birch tree. I did not know who would be the first one to cut down the birch tree. I told Charlene I did not know what to do anymore. She told me the members from the Rotary Club had offered to help people to trim and cut their trees for free. They had also offered free cleaning service in the people's yards. I told Charlene that I did not have any tree to cut or trim at this moment and that I would let them know when I needed help from them.

I told her about how my Honda car had got hit by the Safeway and 99 Ranch supermarkets shopping carts in front of the supermarkets while their employees were carelessly working in front of their supermarkets. When I went in and complained to their managers, they refused to fix it for me. I showed her my car that was damaged by the shopping cart. She said I had bad luck after she looked at my car. I told her that when I called both supermarkets to complain about my car, they refused to fix it for me. When I talked to my sister's friend, Ann Kyu, she suggested that I should not go to the court. She said 99 Ranch supermarket had promised to replace my car with another car for me. But I did not hear from the employee of 99 Ranch supermarket about this case. When I talked to Ann about this case, she said she was very upset with 99 Ranch for not taking care of this case for me.

In late 2005, my left ear was infected badly. A lot of black fluid came out from my left ear. Charlene knew I had a sister and brother who were doctors, and they had provided the allergy medicines for me for my ear infection. But the infection in my left ear did not get better. So Charlene tried to get California medical insurance for me to see the doctor for my ear infection. But I did not accept it. Then she asked me to give my son Shaun's telephone number to her so that she would talk to him. I gave her Shaun's telephone number. She called Shaun to talk to him about my ear infection and asked him to get insurance for me. Shaun got Kaiser Permanente Medical Insurance Company for me. After I joined Kaiser Permanente Medical Group, I chose Dr. Ma Aye Myint to be my adult medicine doctor. I told her about my allergies that I had got from the birch tree, when I first went in to check up with her. She examined me and asked me to take a blood sample test first. I went into Pleasanton Kaiser Permanente Medical Center (KPMC) laboratory department to take a blood sample test on May 3, 2006. After Dr. Ma received and reviewed my blood sample test result, she indicated that I was pre-diabetic because my glucose fasting data was 175 mg/dl. She prescribed me hundred tablets of Metformin Hydrochloride 500 mg pill, hundred tablets of Fexofenadine 60 mg pills to be taken twice a day, and hundred tablets of Lovastatin 40 mg pills to be take once a day. I started to take medicine pills as instructed by her every day. She asked me to use "OneTouch UltraSmart" blood glucose monitoring system to test my blood sample at home every day. I refused to use it after a couple of times. I felt very uncomfortable with the pain that I got on my finger after I used the needle to poke my finger to get blood for measuring the diabetic data on the meter. I told her I'd rather go to the laboratory department to take a blood test if she allowed me to take the blood sample test in the laboratory. Then I went to the laboratory department on September 12, 2006. I received my blood sample test result from Dr. Ma. My diabetic HGBA1c data was 6.9 percent, and my glucose fasting data was 147 mg/dl. Dr. Ma indicated that my diabetic data range was very high. I told her I had been using hydrogen peroxide to clean and whiten my teeth a couple of years before I checked up with her. I would keep hydrogen peroxide in my mouth and let it stay in my mouth for a couple of hours a day; sometimes I used it twice a day. My glucose meter would show the glucose data would be a little bit higher than the required normal data range all the time. Then she asked me how. I explained to her the concept of marinating the meat with salt, sugar, and wine. If we kept the meat marinated with salt and sugar and let it stay for half a day, the ingredients would spread through the meat, leading to tasty, sweet, and salty meat. I told her I would stop using hydrogen peroxide to clean my teeth. Then she told me to checkup with her every three or four months until my glucose data went down to the required normal data range.

Every three months, I checked up with Dr. Ma and took a blood sample test to check on my diabetic HGBA1c, glucose fasting data range, and my lipid data for my blood test results. Dr. Ma persuaded me to take the allergy skin test every time I checked up with her and complained to her about the bad allergy that I got from my neighbor's birch trees. She advised me to go and see the allergy doctor to perform an allergy skin test. I told her I had refused to take the allergy skin test from the allergy doctor because I had not complained I got any allergy from the food that I ate. I did not eat the food that was listed on the charts that the allergy doctors gave to me. Then I told her about my bad ear infection. She gave me the ear doctor's telephone number to call and set up an appointment to see the ear doctor.

Because my left ear infection was getting worse, I called Pleasanton KPMC head and neck surgery clinic to set up an appointment with Cara T. for my hearing test on June 9, 2006, and set up an appointment with Dr. Glenn S. to check up my ear infection on June 11, 2006. I went in the head and neck surgery clinic to checkup with Cara T. on June 9, 2006, for my hearing test. After the hearing test, she told me the hearing in both my ears was very bad. Then I checked up with Dr. Glenn on July 11, 2006.

Dr. Glenn checked both my ears and said I had lost hearing in my right ear and my left ear was infected badly, so I needed to perform surgery on my left ear. He advised me to take CAT scan X-ray in the radiology department before my ear surgery. I called the radiology department to set up an appointment for my CAT scan X-ray on July 20, 2006. I went in the radiology department to take CAT scan X-ray on the appointment day. Dr. Glenn called me after he had reviewed my ears' CAT scan X-rays. He told me my left ear was infected badly. He had to operate my left ear to clean up all of the bad infectious area inside my left ear. I said OK to him. I agreed to let him operate my left ear. He suggested I set up another appointment to see him before the surgery, because he wanted me to sign the contract paper for him to operate. I said OK to him. I told him I will call to set up an appointment to see him to sign the contract that would allow him to operate my ear. Then we ended our conversation. After he hung up the phone, I felt that he was afraid something might happen to me during my ear surgery. So I called Pleasanton KPMC to set up an appointment with another doctor. They referred me to Dr. Cornelius J. and set up an appointment with him on October 25, 2006, for me.

I went in the head and neck surgery clinic to checkup with Dr. Cornelius on the appointment day. Dr. Cornelius checked my ears. He referred me to Dr. Kato of the Fremont KPMC head and neck surgery department to operate my left infectious ear. I told Dr. Cornelius that I did not want to go to Fremont KPMC to checkup with Dr. Kato. There were some misunderstandings with Dr. Glenn. I said I would go back to Dr. Glenn and let him operate my left infectious ear. I set up an appointment with Dr. Glenn on November 28, 2006, with the front desk clerk before I left the head and neck clinic. Then I left Dr. Cornelius's clinic at 9:30 a.m. and went to the parking lot in front of the Pleasanton KPMC main building.

I walked carefully to the handicap car parking lot in front of the Pleasanton KPMC main building. When I walked carefully down the sloping concrete curb from the sidewalk to my car, I took out my car key and bent my body to get ready to open my car door. Suddenly, I could not balance my body. I slipped and fell down on the sloping concrete curb beside my car. I could not get up right away. When I looked around the parking lot, I saw a car stopping behind my car a few minutes and the male driver looking at me. When the driver saw me trying to get up, he drove his car away. I tried to get up in spite of the pain in my left foot and got into my car. I did not think of going to the KPMC minor injury clinic, because I thought this was a minor fall; I even had a lot of pain in my left foot. I drove my car and went back home. On my way back home, I remembered I needed to go to Home Depot store to get some accessories for my garden. I drove my car to Home Depot store. I parked my car in the parking lot in front of the store. I opened my car door. I put my left foot down on the ground and I tried to step down from my car, but my left foot caused a lot of pain. I could stand on my left foot. So instead of going into Home Depot store, I drove back home. I leaned on my left ankle to get down from my car and went inside my house. I went to the kitchen to take out the blue jelly cool comfort pack from my refrigerator. I used a rubber band to tie around my left foot with the jelly cool comfort pack. I went in my room and laid down on my bed. Then I called Shaun. He did not pick up the phone. I left him a message to inform him that I had met with an accident and fallen down in the parking lot of the Pleasanton KPMC main building and hurt my left foot badly. Then I called Charlene, but she was not in her office. I left a message in her answering machine to inform her I had fallen and hurt my left foot in front of the Pleasanton KPMC main building. After an hour, Charlene called me back. She suggested that I call my doctor right away. I said OK, and I hung up the phone. Then I called Dr. Ma's office. But the KPMC operator referred me to talk to the emergency nurse after I told him about my accident in front of the KPMC main building. He switched my telephone line to the emergency nurse so that I could talk to her. The emergency nurse asked me about my accident. I described to her how I had slipped and fallen and hurt my left foot in front of the Pleasanton KPMC parking lot. I told her I could not put my left foot down on the ground. She said my left foot bones must have been broken after she heard the way I described the accident. She referred me to go in Pleasanton KPMC minor injury clinic right away to take an X-ray of my feet.

I called Charlene and told her that the emergency nurse had advised me to go to the minor injury clinic in Pleasanton. I could not drive my car. I requested her to take me to the KPMC minor injury clinic in Pleasanton. She said OK, and she came to pick me up right away to take me to Pleasanton KPMC minor injury clinic. Charlene helped me to check in with the front desk clerk after we were in the minor injury clinic. The head nurse arranged me to take an X-ray of my left foot in the radiology department. After I was done taking the X-ray, she took me back to the minor injury clinic and settled me in the patient room to wait for the doctor to come. One of the nurses came to check on my left foot. He did not believe that this was a fresh wound on my left leg. He kept asking me if I had used an ice cube on my left foot because it did not look like a fresh wound and it was not swelling up like a freshly wounded foot. I said no to him. I told him I had used Jelly type of cool comfort pack to put on my left leg after I reached home. He said I had taken good care of my wounded foot. He asked me when and how this accident happened. I told him this accident had happened in front of the Pleasanton KPMC main building on the left side of the handicap parking lot after I left Dr. Cornelius's clinic at 9:30 a.m. Then he put a water cool pack on my left foot and asked me to wait for the doctor to come. After a while, an employee from KPMC came into my room and asked me how that accident had happened. I told him I had fallen on the side sloping concrete curb in front of the main Kaiser Permanente handicap parking lot. I did not see anything on the sloping concrete curb that would have made me fall when I had walked down it to my car. When I arrived on the left side of my car, I took out my car key from my pocket, and then I bent my body. Just about to open my car door, I slipped to the left side on the sloping concrete curb. My left ankle twisted and hit the roadside ground and my whole body fell on the ground. I drew the picture for him to show him the place that I had fallen, and I explained to him how I slipped and fell. I blamed it on the structure of the sloping sidewalk concrete, as they had built it too straight down on both edges of the sloping sidewalk concrete. When my left foot slipped from sloping sidewalk concrete, my left ankle twisted and I fell from the edge of the sloping sidewalk concrete and hit the ground. I was upset with the engineers who had built this car parking lot without giving any consideration of what could happen to the people after they slipped and got into an accident. He wrote down all the information that I had mentioned to him. Then he asked me was there anybody at the time I had fallen on the ground. I told him there was a car that had stopped behind my car on the driveway and the driver looked at me after I fell on the ground, and then he drove away. Then he said he was done taking the information from me and he left. Charlene and I were in the room, and I was telling Charlene about the accident that I met with in front of Pleasanton KPMC while we were waiting for the doctor. Then the doctor came in. He turned on the computer to examine the X-ray film of my left foot. He said there were two fractures on the fifth bone and one fracture above the fifth bone of the left foot, after he reviewed my left foot's film on the computer. He asked me about my accident. I told him how I had met with the accident and how I had fallen on the ground in front of KPMC. Then he held up my left foot and twisted it to the right side, which hurt me so much. I cried out loud. After he was done, I asked him why he had twisted my left ankle to the right side instead of the left side. He said he had just wanted to make sure my left foot was in the right position by twisting my left ankle to the right position. I said to the doctor that he twisted my left foot in the wrong direction and caused me more pain. The doctor laughed and said, "It's right." After he was done fixing my left foot, he told me I needed to wear a special cast shoe and use crutches to help me walk until all my broken bones healed. He put the socks and cast shoe on my left foot carefully for me and advised me to wear the cast shoe even at night when I slept. Then he told me to come back after five days to check in the minor injury clinic. He set up an appointment for me on October 30, 2006. Then I left the minor injury clinic with Charlene, and we went home. Charlene settled me inside my house and left. I could feel my left foot swelling at night, which made my cast shoe really tight and gave a lot of pain. I adjusted my cast shoe to the right size for my left foot so as to reduce my pain.

Sirena took me back to Pleasanton KPMC minor injury clinic on October 30, 2006. Dr. Dyke E. checked my big swollen left foot. He provided me cam walker shoes and advised me to wear the cam walker shoes instead of cast shoes which would support me to walk better. He prescribed thirty tablets of Hydrocodone/Acetaminophen 5–500 mg pill for me to take two tablets every four hours. Then he told me to set up another appointment to come back to the podiatry clinic and left. Sirena and I went to the front desk clerk to set up an appointment on November 20, 2006, to check in with the podiatry clinic. Then we went home. Sirena settled me at home and left. After I was home, I took one tablet of Hydrocodone/Acetaminophen 5–500 mg pill, but I felt dizzy after I took it. I stopped taking Hydrocodone/Acetaminophen pills. I changed to Advil pain-reliever pills on the second day. I took Advil pain-reliever pills twice a day for six days. Every night, while I slept, I felt the forces from my lower body pushing down to my left foot and all the way to my left toe. I felt the forces pushing down all the way to my left foot toe while I slept almost every night.

On November 20, 2006, I checked up with Dr. C. J. Hanson in the podiatry clinic. She told me my left foot was progressing. She told me to wear the cast shoes instead of cam walker shoes to help me walk better if I did not have so much pain. She suggested that I come back after one month to take an X-ray of my left foot again. She said she wanted to make sure all my fractured bones had healed before I took an X-ray. She arranged another appointment on December 28, 2006, for me to go back to the podiatry clinic to take an X-ray of my left foot. Then she released me, and I went home. When I got home, I changed my shoes from the cam walker shoes to cast shoes and tried to test whether I had pain or not. I felt more convenience in wearing the cast shoes. I changed to cast shoes on my left leg every day. I soaked my feet in warm water as instructed by the doctor to make my feet heal faster.

On November 28, 2006, I checked in with Dr. Glenn to sign the paperwork for him to operate on my left infectious ear. When I was in his office, Dr. Glenn asked me which ear I wanted him to do the surgery. I suggested that he operated my right ear first, because my hearing in it was the worst and I could not hear any sound. I wanted him to operate my right ear first and then operate my left ear. He said if I wanted him to operate my right ear first, he would operate my right ear first for me. He put the information on the surgery agreement paper to operate my right ear. Then he let me sign the paperwork. I signed the surgery agreement paper for Dr. Glenn to let him operate my right ear. After I signed the paperwork, Dr. Glenn set up the surgery date on December 7, 2006, and he released me. I went home and called Shaun to ask him to take me to Pleasanton KPMC head and neck surgery clinic for my ear surgery on December 7, 2006, because Sirena was very busy and unable to take me in that day.

On December 7, 2006, Shaun came home from Davis and took me to Pleasanton KPMC head and neck surgery clinic. We arrived at Pleasanton KPMC head and neck surgery clinic at 7:50 a.m. and checked in with the front desk clerk. After I checked in with the front desk clerk, the nurse took me inside the room. She asked me whether it was the right side of the ear that I would let Dr. Glen operate. I said yes to her. She marked down on the paper, and she asked me to change into my patient outfit. Then she measured my blood pressure, pulse, and glucose data. Then she asked me to lie down on the patient bed and told me to wait for the anesthetist.

141

The anesthetist came and injected the anesthesia medicine into me. I fell asleep on the patient bed. After a while, two nurses came and pushed me inside the surgery room. They moved me to the surgery room. I did not know how many hours it took for Dr. Glenn to finish my right ear surgery. I heard the voice of the nurse trying to call me to wake up. I opened my eyes. I felt I was in a big room, and I heard a lot of voices coming from nearby inside the room. When I turned my head to both sides of my bed and looked around, I saw Shaun and Dr. Glenn were on both sides of my bed and talking in very low voices to each other. As soon as I heard their voices, I told them that I could hear what they were talking. Then I went back to sleep. I woke up again after the doctor woke me up. I heard a lot of voices in my surroundings again, including the nurses and the doctors' telephone conversations as well as the patients' voices talking to the doctors and the nurses. When I saw Dr. Glenn again, I was very happy to see him. I told him that I could hear everybody's voices in this room now, and this was my first time I could hear low voices since I was a baby. He was very happy and said to me with a smiling face, after I told him I could hear so much better, that he had found the old ear bone inside my right ear was disconnected from my right eardrum. He said the artificial bone in my right ear had been placed in the right position by my previous ear doctor. So he did not need more time to locate the center point to attach the artificial bone inside my right ear. Then he said he had used a new longer artificial bone to replace the old artificial bone to make my hearing better. I thanked him with deep appreciation, and I closed my eyes to go back to sleep. Then the anesthetist came and woke me up and asked me how I felt. I told him that I felt very dizzy, and I felt the whole ceiling was turning very fast. I explained to him the dizziness that I felt now was just like I felt at home. The whole ceiling was turning fast just like now. Then I went back to sleep again. I did not know how long I went back to sleep. The doctor woke me up again. This time I told the nurse I needed to go to the restroom. The nurse told me to stay on bed and she would take care of me. She took care of me after I was done. I told the doctor I did not have any more dizziness, but I still felt like throwing up. I told the doctor that I usually put my finger into my throat to tickle my throat to force food or mucus out of my stomach. After I threw up, I felt better; sometimes I saw black mucus coming out from my stomach. Then the doctor told me not to worry. She had the medicine to get rid of this symptom. She injected the medicine (I do not know the name of the medicine) in my Ivory plastic pipe. Then I went back to sleep. The doctor woke me up again. This time after I woke up, I told the doctor that I felt much better, and I did not feel like throwing up anymore. I asked the doctor the permission to go home. The doctor said yes to me. I jumped up from my bed to change into my regular clothing with the help of the nurse. After I got dressed, the nurse gave me the paperwork and asked me to follow the instructions after I got home. Then she asked me to sign the discharge paper. I signed the discharge paper for her. Then I took the paperwork from her. The nurse took me down to the front main door in front of my car to let Shaun take me home. I got inside the car and went home with Shaun. We saw Sirena was waiting for me at home. She was pleased and happy to see me come home. Shaun cooked rice soup for me, and my two children settled me on my bed.

On December 14, 2006, I went in the KPMC head and neck surgery clinic to checkup with Dr. Glenn after my ear surgery. Dr. Glenn took out all of the cotton from my right ear and checked it. He said my right ear condition was good. He advised me not to let water get into my right ear when I took the shower. He asked me to come back after two weeks for my hearing test and checkup with him. Then he released me. I set up both appointments with the doctor's assistant for my hearing test with Cara T. and the doctor's visiting appointment with Dr. Glenn on January 30, 2007. Then I went home. On December 28, 2006, I went and checked in the podiatry clinic. Dr. Randall K. T. was in the podiatry clinic, and he advised me to take an X-ray of my left foot. Then he checked my X-ray film on the computer and told me all my fifth metatarsal fractures were healed fine and I could wear my regular shoes, and he discharged me.

On January 30, 2007, I went to Pleasanton KPMC head and neck surgery clinic to see Cara T. for my hearing test. After my hearing test was done, I checked up with Dr. Glenn. He looked at my hearing test result and said my right ear condition was in good shape. The hearing was good in my right ear. He indicated to me that he could help me to get better hearing than now if I wanted to make my hearing better later. Then he suggested that he wanted to do the surgery on my left infectious ear in the coming September in 2007. But I did not get a chance to go back to him to let him operate my left ear. I decided to wait for my neighbor to get rid of his white birch tree first, and then I thought I would call him to perform surgery on my left infectious ear. After my right ear was fixed, I was very happy that I could hear a lot better than before. I realized I made a mistake by not accepting the Pleasanton KPMC doctor's offer in 1988 to fix my right ear to gain better hearing. I did not know the procedure would be that simple and only need one day to operate my ear to get better hearing.

After my ear surgery, I stayed inside my house with all the windows and doors closed. I did not want to make my ears get infected again. I tried to work outside my yard only early in the morning before 10:00 a.m. or in the evening after 7:00 p.m. Depending on the weather, I went out and watered the plants. After I came back in, I got a bad allergy. My ears, lips, and legs were itching. I complained to my children again about the allergies on my body. I did not have any choice not to go outside to water my plants. My two dogs were suffering from the same allergy just like me. They threw up yellow mucus quite often. I had to clean Lady Star's left eye discharge every day. If I did not clean her eyes for her, the discharge from her eyes dried out and formed thick black layers in both her eyes. I used antibiotic eye drops that Holly sent to me to clean and treat Lady Star's eyes. This was the only solution that I had to protect Lady Star's eyes from getting worse. I felt very guilty about Lady Star every time I held her in my arms and looked at her. I felt sorry for her that she had to deal with dried blind left eye for the rest of her life. Because the allergies and sickness that we got from my neighbor's birch tree were getting worse, Shaun asked my permission to hire somebody to take care of the front lawn for me. I agreed with him, and he hired people to take care of our front lawn.

In late spring 2007, when I went to my backyard to clean all the dried birch leaves and flowers that blew in from my neighbor's birch tree, I found the cherry floral tree on my left side was not growing properly. I decided to dig out the hard ground soil and replace it with new soft soil. I asked Shaun to help me to get pot soil from the Home Depot store. I dug out a lot of hard ground soil little by little from the ground and replaced it with new soft pot soil. One day when I had worked more than three hours in my backyard, I suddenly could not breathe well and felt dizzy. I stopped working right away and went inside my house. I took two Advil pain-reliever pills and laid down on my bed to rest. I felt that my chest bones on the right side were pushing down to my stomach and causing me great pain. I could not breathe well the whole night. I had to sit up to breathe. After my breathing started getting harder and harder, I stopped working in my backyard. Then I called Pleasanton KPMC adult medicine clinic in early June to set up my three months' checkup appointment on July 25, 2007, with Dr. Ma. Then I went in Pleasanton KPMC adult medicine clinic on July 25, 2007, to checkup with Dr. Ma. When I was in Dr. Ma's clinic, I told her I could not breathe well after I had worked in my backyard. She tested on my breathing level with a tube and prescribed me Albuterol-90 mcg of which two puffs were to be taken in by inhalation every four hours when required for shortness of breathing and QVAR-80 mcg inhalers of which two puffs to be taken in orally two times a day as directed. She referred me to go to the radiology department to take a chest X-ray and the laboratory department to take a blood test right away. I went down to the radiology department and took a chest X-ray after which she discharged me. Then I went to the laboratory department for my blood sample test. After I was done in the laboratory, I went to South Two pharmacy store to pick up two different kinds of inhalers and went home. As soon as I arrived home, I used the inhalers as directed by the doctor to help me breathe well every day. It seemed like I was getting asthma because when I laid down on my bed I heard a "ku-ku" sound from my lungs. I stopped going out to work in my backyard. After I used the inhalers for a certain period of time, I started hating to keep using the inhalers. I told myself I needed to find a better solution to solve this problem. I started to look for a better solution to solve my breathing problem. Then I received Dr. Ma's letter from July 26, 2007, to inform me that my chest X-ray was normal. I also received another letter from Dr. Ma to inform me about my blood test result. She indicated my triglyceride was high, but I had a good control on my diabetes (HGBA1c 6.1 percent). After a few months, I felt much better after I had rested at home, but I still could not breathe well. I called Pleasanton KPMC adult medicine clinic in August to set up my three months' follow-up appointment with Dr. Ma on September 11, 2007.

On September 11, 2007, I went to checkup with Dr. Ma in Pleasanton KPMC adult medicine clinic. But Dr. Ma was on vacation. Dr. Muniza M. replaced Dr. Ma to check up on me and asked me about my condition of breathing. I told her that I could not breathe well and I had bad allergy. She told me to keep using inhalers. Then she asked me to go to the laboratory department to have my blood sample test done without fasting. After she released me, I went down to the laboratory department to take my blood sample test. Then I went home. I received the letter with the results of my blood sample test from Dr. Muniza on September 15, 2007, to inform me that I had a good control on my diabetes (HGBA1c was 6 percent). I could even control my diabetes within the required data range, but I was still getting a bad itch and bad allergies from my neighbor's birch trees and I felt dizzy and threw up.

On January 15, 2008, I went down to Chinatown, Oakland, with Sirena to buy groceries. When we were there, I saw that a lot of American ginseng roots were displayed in Chinese groceries store. I decided to try using American ginseng roots to help my asthma and hard breathing that I had got lately. I bought home four pounds of American ginseng roots from Chinese groceries store. After I was home, I put ten pieces of American ginseng roots in a two-quart slow cooker and cooked for twenty-four hours minimum. Then I drank the American ginseng soup. I felt much better after I drank the American ginseng juice. I cooked American ginseng roots every day, and I kept drinking the American ginseng soup. After three months, my hard breathing was getting better. I did not have to get up to breathe again when I was on my bed. But I still could hear "ku-ku" sounds coming out from my lung. When I sat on my sofa and watched television, I still could not breathe well all the way, and I coughed a lot. I called Holly and talked to her about my bad asthma. I told her I could breathe better after I took American ginseng roots, but I still heard the "ku-ku" sound every night when I laid down on my bed. She asked me whether the "ku-ku" sound came from my throat or from my lung. I told her the sound was from my lung. Then I told her I was constantly drinking American ginseng juice. I knew my hearts and lungs were getting stronger. I could do deep breathing quite well lately. The only problem I had was I coughed a lot after I tried to do deep breathing. Sometimes when I drank hot tea or I smoked, I would choke and my throat would itch badly and make me to cough a lot.

On February 15, 2008, I checked up with Dr. Ma again. I told her I was still having problems with my breathing and I was unable to breathe with full strength. Sometimes I could not even drink a sip of hot tea and I coughed badly. After she heard I coughed badly, she prescribed me one bottle of Guaifen/Codein 100–10 g/5 ml liquid medicine for my cough. Then she referred me to take a blood sample test while fasting. I told her I had not eaten anything that morning before I checked in with her, and I would go down to the laboratory department to take a blood sample test after she released me. She said OK, and she released me. Then I went to the KPMC pharmacy store to get Guaifen/Codein 100–10 g/5 ml liquid medicine and went to the laboratory department to draw my blood for the sample test. After my blood sample was drawn, I went home. After I was home, I took two teaspoons of Guaifen/Codein liquid medicine orally every four hours. After I took Guaifen/Codein liquid medicine for a couple of days, my nose started to bleed. I stopped using Guaifen/Codein liquid medicine. I did not call Dr. Ma to let her know my nose was bleeding after I took Guaifen/Codein liquid medicine. After a few weeks, I received Dr. Ma's letter to inform me that my diabetic HGBA1c was 6.1 percent, but my triglyceride was high (247 mg/dl) and my potassium data was slightly high (5.5 meq/L). She asked me to repeat my blood sample test within one week. Before I went to take my blood test, I called Susong to let her know that I had high potassium data range in my blood sample test. She told me bananas contained high potassium and my potassium data range would be high if I ate a lot of banana. I told her that I had been eating a lot of bananas almost every day to help me in my bowel movement and that I will stop eating bananas to bring down my potassium data range to the required normal data range. After my sister reminded me bananas contained potassium, I stopped eating bananas. I went to the KPMC laboratory department on April 30, 2008, to take the blood sample test again. I received Dr. Ma's letter on May 2, 2008, to inform me that my potassium data range had dropped back down to the required normal data range of 5.0 meq/l.

On June 11, 2008, I checked up with Dr. Ma again. I told Dr. Ma that I was taking American ginseng juice every day and that I felt I was getting better with my hard breathing after I drank American ginseng juice. I was taking American ginseng juice every day and my mouth was getting bitter. In the last couple of months, because my mouth was getting bitter, I tried to reduce Metformin Hydrochloride 500 mg tablet to once a day instead of twice a day. She asked me how I knew when to reduce the medicine. I told her I checked on my urination daily whether I could go easily or not. If I could urinate easily after I reduced Metformin Hydrochloride 500 mg pill to once a day, then I took one tablet of Metformin Hydrochloride pill permanently once a day. Sometimes I tried to test eating some coffee ice cream and it seemed like I was OK. She checked my diabetic HGBA1c data for the past six months. They were 6 percent and 6.1 percent. All my total cholesterol, triglyceride, HDL cholesterol, LDL cholesterol were within the normal data range, and my glucose fasting data were 136 mg/dl and 139 mg/dl. They were above the normal data range. Then she told me that I was not diabetic anymore. I did not need to see her every three or four months anymore. She asked me twice a year to call in to check up with her. If I needed any medicine, she asked me to just call her. I said OK and that I would try to test myself for my diabetes and slowly stop the Metformin Hydrochloride pill. I said I would let her know the situation after I tested my urination. Before I left her clinic and went home, she reminded me not to eat too much sweet stuff. I was so happy to get the permission to reduce the Metformin Hydrochloride pill slowly, and I only had to take them when I needed to take. I called Holly to let her know about my allergy and that I was allowed to reduce the diabetic medicine. I also told her that the itch on my left foot toe had disappeared. Usually I complained to her a lot about the itching in my left leg all the way to my left foot toe. She always liked to tell me my toe itching was because of smoking. I disagreed with her, as I knew my allergy was not from the smoking. After a year, I continuously took the allergy medicines and stayed inside the house. My left leg and my left foot were getting cooler and cooler each day. My left foot toe was not itching anymore. Because of my cold feet, I had to wear socks all the time at home. After one and a half year, I was still taking the allergy medicines every day. My left foot was getting warmer and warmer. Finally, I did not need to wear socks on my feet again. My allergies were getting better and better every day after I closed all my windows and stayed inside my house. I was so happy to tell her; my doctor allowed me to reduce my diabetic medicines from twice a day to once a day. I felt like I was a new healthy person. I believed I could go outside to take care of the plants in my backyard again. So I went outside and worked in my backyard in the morning as usual and transplanted all the small trees from the small pots to the big pots. Then I moved all the pots to the right side of my side yard to block all the bad allergic leaves and flower pieces from my neighbor's white birch trees. I left the heavy pots to one side, which my children would move when they came home. Shaun hired the new gardener to take care of our front yard after my complaints about the allergy from the birch tree. When the gardener and his crew first came, I had to go outside to guide them as to what I wanted them to do in my front yard. I had to spend an hour standing outside to guide them. After I came back inside my house, I was getting quite sick. My ears, lips, and whole body were itching again and a lot of white pale spots had formed on my knees and legs. I tried not to work on my front yard as much as I could. I just let the gardener take care of the lawn and the bushes in my front yard.

On June 15, 2008, I went out to my front yard to check on my front lawn early in the morning around 8:30 a.m. I ran into a spot of weeds on the corner edge of my front yard lawn. The gardener had not pulled the weeds out from the lawn. When I saw the weeds, I tried to pull them out with my right hand. After I pulled out most of the weeds, accidentally, the soil in the lawn flew all over my right hand and body. Suddenly, I felt my right hand start to itch badly. I tried to clean the dirt soil on my right hand with my left hand. Then my body started itching badly. I ran into my house to wash my hands with soap and water, but the itch on my right hand did not go away. I kept on scratching my right hand until the skin on my right hand opened and peeled badly. After a while, my knees and legs started to itch, and I kept scratching them. I found my right hand was swelling really bad and there were small and big rashes. Then when I checked both my itchy knees and legs, I found a lot of different sizes of hives and rashes on them. Pale spots had formed on the bottom parts of both my legs. I put Calamine lotion on my hands and legs. But I was still struggling with the bad itch on my right hand and legs. I kept scratching on them. The more I scratched, the more the pimple rashes on my right hand spread to the nearby areas. Some pimple rashes were getting bigger and bigger and formed blisters. I decided to call my doctor to show her the rashes and hives on my body and my swollen right hand. I called Pleasanton KPMC adult medicine clinic at 1:45 p.m. The operator answered my phone. I asked the operator for my doctor, Dr. Ma, to inform her I had got a bad allergy accident in my front yard. I told the operator that I'd like to see Dr. Ma right away to show her the bad blister rashes and hives that I had got all over my hands and legs that morning while I was working in my front yard. But the operator told me Dr. Ma was on vacation. He referred me to talk to the emergency nurse. I told the emergency nurse about my allergy accident in my front yard. The emergency nurse told me to take Benadryl pills right away if I had them at home. I told her I had Benadryl pills at home. Then she instructed me to take two Benadryl pills and asked me to wait for her to call me back. I said OK to her and hung up the phone. While I was waiting for the nurse to call me back, I took two Benadryl pills right away. Then I used my cellular telephone camera to take pictures of my swollen hands, knees, and legs that had full of big and small hives and pimple rashes as shown in the pictures. The biggest hive that had formed on my right leg was two square inches.

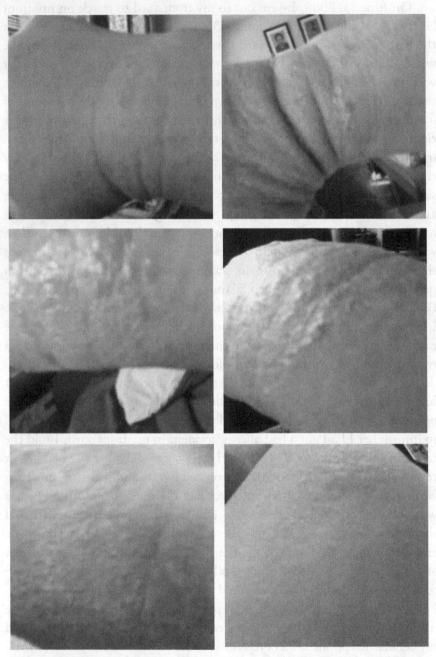

Blister rashes and hives were all over my swollen hands and legs.

I called Renee from the city of Pleasanton at 2:45 p.m. to set up an appointment with her to let her look at my blister rashes and hives on my swollen hand and legs that I had got from an allergy accident in front of my yard. The office secretary from the city of Pleasanton set up an appointment for me on June 17, 2008. Then the nurse from Dr. Ma's office called me back to set up an appointment the next day with Dr. Tobin at 3:00 p.m. I requested the nurse to give me five minutes' time to go in to show Dr. Tobin so that he would have a look at the blister rashes on my swollen hands and legs. But she refused to let me in and said Dr. Tobin's patient visiting schedule was full today. I requested her again. Then the nurse said she would check and call me back again. After 5:00 p.m., I did not get any return call from the nurse. I called my doctor's office again. The operator referred me to talk to the nurse again. I told her I was already in touch with the nurse from my doctor's office and I was waiting for them to call me back. I wanted to make sure whether they would let me go into the doctor's clinic today. I told her I would wait for the nurse to call me back and hung up the phone. I took two Benadryl medicine pills again before I went to bed. The whole night I struggled with my bad allergy, and it made me very uncomfortably sick.

On June 16, 2008, Dr. Tobin's nurse called me back in the morning and asked me to go to Pleasanton KPMC adult medicine clinic to see Dr. Tobin at 3:00 p.m. I told the nurse OK. But after I hung up my phone, I was very upset at the nurse, because they did not let me go in right away to see the doctor. I did not feel like going to see the doctor again after I had suffered from the bad allergy the whole night. Then I called Pleasanton KPMC adult medicine clinic to cancel my appointment with Dr. Tobin, and I let them know I was very upset at them. I refused to checkup with Dr. Tobin at 3:00 p.m. I told the nurse I had already suffered the whole night with the bad allergy and I was very sick. Then I hung up the phone. I was not aware that I should go to the minor injury clinic that day, but the nurse did not refer me to go to the minor injury clinic. I just had to wait at home for the doctor to call me back and tell me to go in. Next day, I used soap and water to wash my itching hands. When I washed my hands with water, my hands started to itch badly. I scratched my hands and a lot of blister rashes formed on my hands. The blister rashes spread all over my right hand and made my right hand swell badly.

On June 17, 2008, I took my two dogs with me to go to the city of Pleasanton to meet Renee. I met Renee in her office. I showed her all the blister rashes on my big swollen right hand, big and small hives on my legs, and pale allergy spots on both my knees and legs. I also showed her Lady Star's eyes. I told her we kept getting this kind of rashes and hive allergies from my neighbor's white birch trees, and we could not even enjoy our lives in our own home because of the bad allergy that we got from my neighbor's white birch trees. She looked at my hands and legs and the pictures that I had taken on the day of my accident. Then she suggested that I should let my doctor look at my swollen hands and legs. I told her I tried to contact my doctor, Dr. Ma, on the day that I got this accident, but Dr. Ma was not in the clinic. She was on vacation. The Pleasanton KPMC emergency nurse referred me to another doctor and would not let me in on the day when I got a bad allergy to show them what they looked like. She was also very upset with this case. She took notes and advised me to go to court again. Then I pointed my finger at Lady Star and told her to look at her left eye which was filled with thick dried layer of discharge. She tried to look at Lady Star's eyes. My two dogs were very friendly. As they had been running around, they had a strong body odor. I had not cleaned Lady Star's eye before I had gone to see her. I wanted Renee to look at how Lady Star's left eye looked like. I wanted her to feel how a healthy dog could get blind because of the substance from the birch acid. I told her to look at Lady Star's eyes and told her how she would feel to see somebody get hurt and had to go through the pain and the sickness caused by one bad tree. I asked her to tell my neighbor to cut down their bad allergy tree. Once my neighbor cut down their bad allergic white birch tree, it would create a very healthy environment in our neighborhood to save a lot of people's lives and get away from allergies and sickness. Otherwise people would get allergies and sickness just like the dogs' body odor and it would stay in the community, which would make people get sick and die forever. Then she told me she had a meeting to go and she would talk to Marlene, and she released me. I went home with my dogs.

I remembered I still had to take the blood sample test since the last time Dr. Ma had scheduled me to take a blood sample test in Pleasanton KPMC laboratory department. I went to Pleasanton KPMC laboratory department to check in at 2:18 p.m. I showed my right swollen hand to the front desk clerk. I told her that I wanted to find out myself what was in my blood when I got this bad allergy with red swollen blister rashes and hives on my hands and legs. Then I complained to her that Dr. Tobin had not accepted me to go in and see him on the day when I requested the nurse to let me go in to show the doctor the kind of allergy rashes and hives that I got on my hands and body in my yard. I refused to go in the next day to see Dr. Tobin when they called me to checkup with him the next day. Then the clerk looked at my hands and advised me to put cortisone lotion on my hands. But I said no and that just applying cortisone lotion would not be enough. I told her I needed the doctor to give me a cortisone shot for my bad allergy. Because the allergy rashes were not only on my hands and legs, but also I had breathed in a lot of poisonous birch substances from the air, pale spots had formed on my knees and legs. I also told that just like my hands and legs, my internal organs would also be swollen, forming blister rashes after I breathed in a lot of allergic powder. The clerk typed in all my information inside her computer and asked me to wait in front of the laboratory room. Then the technician called me in and drew my blood sample. After the technician drew my blood sample, one of the technicians came out and talked to me. She always liked to joke at me when she saw me. I showed her my swollen hands and my body which was full of blister rashes. I told her I had got a very bad allergy accident in my front yard while I was working outside my front yard. Then I told her I would like to review all my data from my blood sample tests after I got this accident and would compare all the data from different blood test results. Then I left and went home.

Next day, my allergies started getting worse. I was continuously taking Benadryl allergy medicines every four hours to get rid of the itching. Because I kept scratching my right hand, the blisters on my right hand broke and kept spreading to nearby areas. I used cotton to clean up the fluid from the broken blisters. I drank a lot of water to get rid of the poison from my body. But my whole body absorbed all the water that I drank. I could not urinate to take them out. No matter how much water I drank, only little water came out of my system when I urinated. I was getting scared, so I called Dr. Ma on July 26, 2008, in the morning to request her to let me in to see her, because I had got a bad allergy accident and I wanted to show her my swollen hands and legs with blister rashes and hives and pale spots on my knees and legs. She said OK and asked me to go in right away. She asked me to wash my right hand to get rid of the Calamine lotion first. I cleaned up the Calamine lotion from my right hand with soap and water. Then she checked my hand. She responded to me with surprise that she had never seen this kind of blister rashes on my hands and legs before. I showed her the pictures of my swollen right hand and my legs that I had taken when I had got a bad allergy a few weeks ago. She referred me again to see the allergy doctor to take the allergy skin test. I said I would talk to them if she referred me to see the allergy doctor. She said yes. Then she gave me the KPMC allergy department telephone number to call. She told me continuously to take the allergy medicines that she had prescribed me before. She prescribed me Fluocinonide USP 0.05 percent ointment to put on the blister rashes on my right hand. I told her I had already gone to the laboratory department to draw a blood sample last week to see what was in my blood. She said OK and asked me to take the blood sample test again after three months before I checked up with her. I said OK and left her clinic. I went to South Two pharmacy store to get Fluocinonide USP 0.05 percent ointment. I waited for a while in the pharmacy store. Then I bought my prescription Fluocinonide USP 0.05 percent ointment and I went home. After I was home, I called the KPMC allergy department from Pleasanton first with the telephone number that Dr. Ma had provided me to call. No one picked up the phone in Pleasanton allergy department. They left a message in the answering machine, asking the patient to call the KPMC allergy department in Livermore. I called the KPMC allergy department in Livermore with the number that they had provided in the answering machine for a patient to call. No one picked up the phone. So I left a message in the answering machine to have them call me back. Then I went out to my mailbox to get my mail. I received Dr. Ma's letter dated July 6, 2008, to inform me about my blood test result from June 17, 2008. She said my diabetic data was really high. She increased the strength of Metformin Hydrochloride tablet from 500 mg to 750 mg and indicated to me to take it twice a day as usual. After this accident, I continuously started taking Benadryl tablets that I had at home beside Fexofenadine allergy pill. Benadryl tablets made me very drowsy so that I had to lie down on my bed and sleep. I had to take the medicines for a couple weeks. Sometimes I could feel my heart beat fast at night once I laid down on my bed, but not the type of fast heart beat that we get after we exercise. I put the ointment that Dr. Ma had prescribed me every day until all the blister rashes disappeared from my right hand.

During the entire months of July and August 2008, the weather was terribly hot. The temperature was above ninety degrees. My house was heated up and very hot. I had to stay inside the house with the air conditioner on. I tried not to go outside as much as I could. But I still needed to go outside in the morning to water my plants; otherwise, all my plants would die if they did not get enough water. Once I went outside my yard, I felt very uncomfortable because of the itching after I came in; especially my lips were itching badly. I complained again and again to my children and to the city of Pleasanton. When Sirena came home on Sunday, we went to Bed Bath & Beyond store in Dublin shopping center to buy a vacuum cleaner for Sirena. I felt fresh and comfortable in the Dublin shopping center even when the weather was very hot. I showed Sirena that the management planner of that shopping center had planted all good and healthy trees in the Dublin shopping center. They did not contain the type of bad chemical acid like the acid from white birch trees. Even though the weather was hot, I still felt I got fresh air there. I did not feel any itching or dizziness. I stood in front of my car. I breathed in all the fresh air as much as I could get from that shopping center. Then we went inside Bed Bath & Beyond store. Sirena bought the vacuum cleaner, and we went home. After I arrived home, I felt itchy, and I complained about my allergy to Sirena again.

I remembered Charlene who had visited me so long before. I stopped her from visiting me after she complained that the turtles that I kept in my sink in the garage were very dirty. I had raised those two turtles since they were very little. I could not throw them away just like trash. I could only clean the dirty water for the turtles once a week. I did not have automatic air circulation system for my turtles in my garage. I did not want her to blame my turtles when she got sick. This was the reason I stopped her from visiting me at that moment. Then I started to look for people who would willingly keep my turtles. I also asked Sirena to find somebody who would take my turtles or find a place for putting the turtles away. Suddenly when I remembered Charlene, I called her to talk to her about my recent allergy incident, but she was not in her office. So I left a message to her to call me back. She called me back after she got my message. I told her about my allergy accident that I had got on my hands and body. I indicated to her that my doctor, Dr. Ma, had referred me to see the allergy doctor. She said it would be the best thing to do to see an allergy doctor if my doctor had referred me to checkup with the allergy doctor. I told her I had left a message to talk to the nurse from the KPMC allergy department to set up an appointment to checkup with the allergy doctor. I was waiting for them to call me back. She told me she was going to retire pretty soon, because her husband had gone through heart surgery not long ago and her husband wanted her to stay at home to take care of him. Then she mentioned Sara H. would replace her in Pleasanton Senior Supporting Group in Pleasanton Senior Center. She said Sara H. had the power to make my neighbor cut down his white birch tree. She also said that she would like to visit me before she retired. I said OK to her because she said she was going to retire. I told her that since she was a good friend of mine and I wanted her to call me and visit me any time when she had time to come out, but she was not allowed to come as long as my turtles were in my garage. Charlene offered to buy *The Scaring Birch Trees* book and gave me twenty-five dollars before. I refused to accept her money at that time. She mentioned to me again on the phone that Marlene would like to buy a book from me and she would pick up the book when she came. She said she would call me before she came to my house. I said OK to her and hung up my phone.

After a week, I did not get any return call from both Pleasanton and Livermore KPMC allergy department. I called Pleasanton KPMC allergy department again, but nobody answered the phone. I just left a message for them to call me back. Then I called the allergy department in Livermore. Nurse Ann F. picked up the phone and talked to me. I requested her to help me get the material charts that they used to test on the patients' skin in KPMC. Nurse Ann F. said they did not have fixed charts to test on patients' skin for allergy. Sometimes they had to make the decision from the skin test; sometimes they had to make the decision from the blood sample tests, depending on the type of allergy the patients were complaining about. If the kind of foods and things that they complained were available in the clinic, then the doctor would do the skin test for the patients to find the allergy to the foods that they mentioned. I told her on the phone that I had a very bad allergy to the white birch trees. I wanted to show her the pictures of the allergy blister rashes and hives that had formed on my hands and legs, which I had got from my front yard. She said OK. She set up an appointment for me to go in at 9:00 a.m. next day in Pleasanton KPMC allergy department to see her. I went in next day to Pleasanton KPMC allergy department to see Nurse Ann F. I met the front desk clerk Sue and told her I had come to see Nurse Ann F. Sue took me to Nurse Ann F. in her office. Nurse Ann F. invited me into her office. Then I showed her the pictures of my swollen right hand and legs with blister rashes and hives on my cellular telephone that I had taken when I got my bad allergy. I told her I had taken my neighbor to the court before. Because I did not have the doctor's letter to verify my allergies were from the white birch tree, the court had only asked my neighbor to cut two of his white birch trees. I could not make my brother write the letter for me. The court needed the verification letter from the doctor to order my neighbor to cut down all his birch trees. I requested her to refer me to see the allergy doctor that I could talk to. She advised me to set up an appointment with an allergy doctor to talk to them. She told me Dr. Teddy Young and Dr. Kate were the two doctors who were taking care of the allergy departments in Pleasanton and Livermore KPMC. She asked me to go back to my doctor if I knew what was causing me bad allergy. I told her I had told Dr. Ma that I was allergic to the white birch tree, but Dr. Ma kept referring me to see the allergy doctor to perform the allergy skin test. I did not understand what kind of allergy skin test she was referring me to take. I did not have any allergy to food and medicines. I never complained about any food that caused an allergy. Then I told her that because of the arguments we had out there I had some questions to ask the allergy doctor and that I would like to talk to one of them. Then she told me to set up an appointment with either Dr. Teddy Young or Dr. Kate. She gave me both doctors' business cards. I took the doctors' business cards and thanked her. I told her I would call her back. After we came out from her office, I gave her my book, *The Scaring Birch Trees,* to review, and I told her how the American Cancer Society had mistakenly stated the Red Indian people used birch leaves in their tea to treat diarrhea. I sent out somebody to check with Red Indians. They said they did not use birch leaves in their tea to treat diarrhea. I told her I was very familiar with the kind of plants and trees in Tri Valley area. All the trees and bushes were healthy plants. There were no allergic plants in the Tri Valley area except the white birch trees, which were the allergic bad trees. Most of the young teenagers in Tri Valley who helped their parents in taking care of the lawns at home were suffering from these kinds of bad allergies and had red blister rashes on their faces. I explained to her the reason that I wanted to talk to the allergy doctor. She suggested that I set up an appointment to checkup with one of the doctors. I told her I had to go to New York for a trip so as to stay away from this allergic house for a month, to check on how I felt in other places with no white birch trees again and I would call her back to set up an appointment with Dr. Young after I come back from New York. Then I left Pleasanton KPMC allergy department and went home.

Sirena called me to let me know that she had bought an air flight ticket for me on August 2, 2008, to go to New York. But next day when I called my sisters, I found that all my sisters would be on vacation and no one would be in the New York home in August 2008. So I decided to stay at home to get over this allergy case. I called the receptionist, Sue, in Pleasanton KPMC allergy department again to set up an appointment with Dr. Young, but no one was in the clinic to pick up the phone. So I left a message in the answering machine to have Sue from Pleasanton KPMC allergy department to call me to set up an appointment with Dr. Young for me. Then Charlene called me to inform me that she would come over to my house on August 30, 2008, before she retired from Pleasanton Senior Supporting Group at the end of this month.

On July 30, 2008, the receptionist, Sue, in the Pleasanton KPMC allergy department called me back to set up an appointment to see Dr. Young. While I was talking to Sue on the phone, I heard somebody ringing my front doorbell. So I asked Sue to hold on the telephone a few minutes so I could check who was at my front door. She said OK. Then I went to the front door and looked outside through the little door glass hole. I saw it was Charlene. I opened the front door for her to come in, and I told her I was on the phone with Sue of Pleasanton KPMC allergy department. She suggested I should go to talk to the allergy doctor. I said yes to her. I told her I was on the phone with the KPMC allergy department. I asked her to wait for a while. Charlene said OK, and she started playing with my dogs. I picked up the phone, and I talked to Sue again. I told Sue that the lady who had just come in my house was Charlene. She was the counselor from Pleasanton Senior Supporting Group. She had been visiting me every two weeks, for over three years now. I told Sue I wanted to set up an appointment with Dr. Young to talk to him about my bad allergies and sickness that I had got from my neighbor's birch tree. She said OK, and she set up an appointment on August 31, 2008, at 3:30 p.m. for me to see Dr. Young. I said thanks to her and hung up the phone.

I told Charlene I had already set up an appointment to see Dr. Young for my allergy on August 31, 2008. She said that it would be best for me to talk to the allergy doctor about my allergy from the birch tree. Then I told her about the accident that I had last time and how I got these bad allergies and blister rashes on my hands and legs. I showed her the allergy pictures that I had taken with my mobile camera. She was very upset after she heard about my accident. She offered to me to talk to my neighbor again. She went over to my right-side neighbor's house again to talk to John Clark for getting rid of his white birch tree. After a while, she came back with no good news. She told me John Clark had refused to cut his white birch tree again. She said she could not make him cut down his white birch tree, but one person could make him get rid of his bad tree. She said her name was Sara H. She was going to replace her in Pleasanton Senior Center after she left. Then I took her to my backyard to look at the fruit trees that I had grown for so many years. After we came back in from my backyard, she gave me twenty-five dollars for Marlene who had bought my book. I returned the money back to her and told her I wanted to add some more chapters in this book. After I had organized more proofs that the white birch trees were really allergic bad trees, I would print out the book and I would accept their money to buy my book. I said I would use the money that I had got from selling my book to build an analytical laboratory research center to find out more ingredients and chemical acids in the plants for the people. Then I went to my study room. I took out three more books from the box for her. She took the books and put twenty-five dollars back in her purse. Then she said she had to go home to her husband and left. Before she left, I gave her my cellular phone number for her to call and talk to me when she had time.

On August 31, 2008, I went to see Dr. Young in Pleasanton KPMC. I told him about my allergies and sickness due to my neighbor's birch tree. I showed him the allergy pictures that I got from the incident on my cellular phone. I explained to him about the type of foods that most Chinese people ate at home. I never complained that I got any allergy from any food and medicines. I knew my allergies were from the white birch trees after I tested directly on my skin with the fresh and dried birch flowers. I told him about the incident when I had transferred the dried white birch flowers from the paper envelope in which I had saved before into the new plastic bag: "Some of the powder from the birch flowers flew out from the paper envelope and landed on my face after I tapped the paper envelope and I got bad allergy rashes on my face. I got very itchy right away. I tried to clean my face with soap and warm water, but it was too late. I had already got the allergy rashes on my face and the itch would not go away. I kept scratching my face until my skin broke. A lot of small red blister rashes formed on my face. No matter how many times I washed my face, I still felt very itchy. After this incident, I did not keep dried white birch flowers in my house again. I did not have any dried birch flowers to show him at this moment." I told him that I turned in the dried birch flowers that I had before to the city of Pleasanton for them to review and that I requested them to take care of this case for me. But the city of Pleasanton did not take any action in this case to have my neighbor cut down their birch tree. I told him if he was interested to try out on his skin, he could get fresh flowers from the white birch trees. He shook his head. He listened to me carefully, and he looked at all my allergy pictures on my cellular phone. Then I showed him my pale allergy spots on my knees and legs. Then I mentioned to him about how the allergy doctors were using animal hair to test on human skin and that it was not an appropriate step to use animal hair to test on human skin since animal hair was not an allergic substance. I told him that they were just like human hair and they were not allergic to the people except when those animals carried allergic particles on their bodies inside the house. When they flicked their bodies after they came in from outside, the allergic particles would fly all over the place inside the house and possibly got into their uncovered food and caused them a bad allergy after they ate the uncovered food that contained bad allergic substances. When people complained about food allergy, we could prove the food that they complained about was allergic food or not, if we knew the ingredients of the food. The pets can never cause allergy to human beings. He agreed with me. I also mentioned to him that I had taken antibiotic medicine to protect myself when I got very sick all those years. I took American ginseng juice almost every day to protect myself from not getting sick. Then he reviewed my allergy symptoms and rashes from the pictures again. Then he said all my blister rashes and hives were called fixed maculopapular rashes with pustules. I asked him whether I still needed to get a skin test or not. He said they did not have anything from the birch tree to test on my skin. I asked him how to protect myself from getting an allergy from the white birch trees. He said I had to stay away from the birch tree. I told him this was my next-door neighbor's white birch tree, and it was impossible for me to stay away. I told him I had requested my neighbor to cut down his white birch tree before, but he had refused to cut it down for me. I also told him that I needed the doctor's letter to prove that I got bad allergies from his white birch tree, and only if I could show him my doctor's letter to prove that I am allergic to his white birch tree, I could make him cut down his bad white birch tree. I requested him to write a letter for me to show my neighbor. He said OK and wrote a statement: "This is a statement to certify that Ms. Chu's symptoms were fixed, maculopapular rash with pustules, which she states occur with exposure to birch tree and is not one that can be tested for with standard IgE-mediated allergy testing." (IgE stand for immunoglobulin E.) Then he told me again stay away from the white birch trees before I left. I told him I would. I needed to show his letter to my neighbor to let him know that my allergies were caused by his white birch tree. I took his letter and thanked him. Then I handed out my book *The Scaring Birch Trees* to him and requested him to read my book. If there was anything he would like to let me know, I requested him to call me. I thanked him again and left his clinic. I was so happy that finally I had got an allergy doctor's letter to prove my allergies were from the white birch trees. I kept telling the truth to every people whom I met in our neighborhood that the birch trees were allergic trees that could cause allergies and sickness. I kept asking people to be careful of the birch trees and to cut them down to prevent allergies and sickness.

Next day, I called Charlene to let her know that Dr. Young had issued me a letter and told me to stay away from the birch tree. She asked me to give a copy of my doctor's letter to my neighbor to indicate to him that my doctor had told me my allergies were from his white birch tree and requested him to cut down his white birch tree. I told her she knew that I had talked to him before, but he was very rude to me as he pointed his finger at me and yelled at me. He told me to do anything that I wanted to do with his tree, when I complained to him. I refused to talk to him again. I requested Charlene to talk to my neighbor to request him to cut down his white birch tree. She said she would help me talk to my neighbor, and we ended our conversation. Then I called Dr. Ma to let her know that I had checked in with the allergy doctor Dr. Young, and I let her know what Dr. Young told me. She said she would talk to Dr. Young to review my allergy symptoms caused by the birch trees. After a week, Dr. Ma called me back after she had talked to Dr. Young. She indicated to me that Dr. Young had told her to ask me to stay away from the birch trees. I told her I would try to stay away from the birch tree, but the white birch tree was my neighbor's white birch tree, which was just next to my house. It was impossible for me to stay away from the tree that was planted next to my house. I needed her to issue a letter for me to indicate that my allergies and sickness were from the birch tree. She asked me whether I could use her previous letter that she had written for me. I told her I could not use her previous letter because she did not indicate that my allergies were from the birch trees. I needed her to rewrite the letter to indicate that my allergies were from the birch trees. Then she promised to rewrite the letter for me and that she would call me back after she had finished her letter. I thanked her and hung up the phone.

I was so anxious to let Marlene know that I had finally got the letters from my doctors to indicate that my allergies were from the birch trees. So I called her to set up an appointment to show her the pictures of my allergy rashes that I had accidentally got when I pulled the weeds from my front yard recently and the letters from my two doctors, Dr. Ma and Dr. Young. She set up an appointment for me to meet her on September 11, 2008, at 8:30 a.m. in her office in Pleasanton Senior Center. Then I called Dr. Ma's office to find out whether she had already sent out her letter to me because it was very important to me. The nurse in Dr. Ma's office told me she would check with her and call me back. The nurse in Dr. Ma's office called me back on September 10, 2008, to let me know that Dr. Ma had already sent out her letter last week. She said I would receive Dr. Ma's letter in a few days by mail. If I did not receive Dr. Ma's letter through the mail, she wanted me to call her back. I said OK and hung up the phone.

On September 11, 2008, I had still not received Dr. Ma's letter through the mail yet. I went to see Marlene in Pleasanton Senior Center. I told her about my allergy accident in front of my house, how I had checked up with Dr. Ma, how Dr. Ma referred me to see the allergy doctor Dr. Young, and how I talked to Dr. Young about my allergy. I showed her Dr. Young's letter and the pictures that I had taken when I got the allergy rashes in my front yard. She reviewed the letter from Dr. Young and the pictures that I had taken and told me to give her a copy of Dr. Young's letter. She wanted to check with her friends to make sure the court and the city of Pleasanton would accept Dr. Young's letter to prove that my allergies were from the birch trees. Then I told her I had another letter from my primary doctor, Dr. Ma, and that I had not received Dr. Ma's letter yet through the mail, but as soon as I received the letter, I would fax it to her. She said OK. Then I asked for her advice about what I should do next. I wanted to know if they still wanted me to go to the court or just send out my doctor's letters to my neighbor. Marlene advised me to inform my neighbor first about my doctors' letters, indicating him to cut his birch tree. I requested her to send out a letter for me to inform my neighbor after her friends reviewed my doctors' letters. She said she would find out and let me know what would be the best thing for me to do. She mentioned to me about her daughter's allergy from her neighbor's cat. Then I asked Marlene who was Sara H. I told her that Charlene had told me Sara had replaced Charlene's position in Pleasanton Senior Supporting Group. She said she would take me to see Sara H. and let me talk to her. Then she asked me to go with her to Charlene's room. Sara H. was sitting on Charlene's desk. Marlene introduced Sara H. to me. I sat down on the chair in front of Sara's desk. I saw Sara H. had a red blister rash with a few small pieces of white skin meat on top of the blister rash near her mouth. It seemed like she had got burned with something on her lips. So I asked her what had happened to her mouth. Sara H. told me she got the allergy from the tooth stick that she had used for whitening her teeth. I was wondering what kind of tooth stick it was that she used to burn her mouth. So I asked her what kind of wood it was that made those tooth sticks burn her lip. She did not say anything to me and just shrugged her shoulders. Then I talked to her about my allergies from the birch trees. I described to her that my allergy was very bad and that sometimes when I stood up for longer than five to ten minutes my leg turned black and the black color would move up slowly all the way to my knee. I did not know how to show my doctor my symptoms that I had got at the time when my hands were swollen and my legs turned black. This time after I got my allergy incident, I called my doctor's office right away to inform them I had got a bad allergy incident in front of my house, but the nurse did not accept my request to go in and show my symptoms to the doctor. Then she advised me to just go to a minor injury clinic right away if I get any bad allergy or blisters on my body. The minor injury clinic or hospital emergency clinic had to accept me no matter what happened to me. I told her I did not know I could go in without the permission of the emergency nurse. I thought I could go in only when the nurse instructed me to go in. She said no to me. Then I said to her that if I was allowed to go to the emergency clinic anytime when I got the bad allergies, then I could get over one thousand dollars from my insurance company each time I went in the emergency clinic. I told her when I got allergies the next time I would go to the emergency clinic. Then I asked her about her replacement of Charlene's position in Pleasanton Senior Supporting Group and that Charlene told me she had the power to make my neighbor cut down his birch tree. She said no to me. She indicated that Charlene was still working in Pleasanton Senior Center. I did not know what to say to her because I did not know how they were arranging the staff inside their organization in Pleasanton Senior Center. Marlene took me back to her office. She made a copy of Dr. Young's letter and told me she would check with her friends. I reminded her again that I would fax her Dr. Ma's letter as soon as I received it. I asked her to give me her fax number. She wrote down her fax number on a piece of paper and gave it to me. Then I asked her what I should do next. She told me to let her talk to her friend and show her and discuss about Dr. Ma's letter whether this was the right way to express my allergies caused by the birch trees. I told Marlene OK and left her room.

After I talked to Marlene, I remembered the conversation that I had with Sara H. I tried to figure out what Sara H. had described to me when she said she was using a tooth stick to clean her mouth. I was thinking what kind of wood the tooth stick was made of. Then I figured out Sara H. must have said "paste" instead of "stick" to clean her mouth. After I left Marlene's room, I ran back to Sara's room to ask her again about her allergy on the tooth stick that she had been using for whitening her teeth. When I saw Sara H. in her room, I asked her again about the toothpaste that she was using and spelled out the word "P-A-S-T-E." She said yes to me. I realized I misunderstood her with regards the word of stick instead of paste. I said to her that the toothpaste companies were using hydrogen peroxide in the whitening toothpaste to whiten the teeth. Hydrogen peroxide was a chemical that had the strength to burn the skin and form a white skin on top of the blister rashes. I asked her whether she had changed back to the type of toothpaste with no hydrogen peroxide. She said yes to me and then I left. I went home on that day and tried to think why Sara H. had called that burn as an allergy. She must have been confused about the meanings of "allergy" and "burn." I thought it was necessary for me to call her to clear out the meaning of "allergy" and "burn." So the next day, I called Pleasanton Senior Center to talk to Sara H. about her burn that she had described as allergy. Sara H. was the one who picked up the phone. I told her she was using the wrong word to describe the burn as an allergy. She burned her lip with concentrated hydrogen peroxide from the toothpaste. I explained to her that I also used a lot of hydrogen peroxide liquid to whiten my teeth every day and I got burned inside my mouth when I used hydrogen peroxide. White meat showed up on top of the white swollen lines inside my mouth. Once I frequently started using hydrogen peroxide to clean my teeth, I did not have any more problems using it. She said yea. Then I told her that my sister's dentist had told my sister she had a lot of diseases inside her mouth because of the formation of white meat skin lines inside her mouth after the dentist cleaned her teeth with hydrogen peroxide. Actually, the white meat skin lines inside my sister's mouth were not diseases. They were the burn lines of hydrogen peroxide after the dentist applied hydrogen peroxide on my sister's teeth inside her mouth. The dentists were using the terminology "disease" instead of "burn," mixing up the meaning of the symptoms. I was sure a lot of people did not understand the meaning of allergy, burn, and disease. Then she said yea and we ended our conversation.

In the evening, I walked to my mailbox in front of my left neighbor's house to get my mails. I took out all my mails from my mailbox and walked back home. I sat in my family room and sorted all my mails. I found Dr. Ma's letter among the mails. I opened Dr. Ma's letter. She indicated that I was suffering with bad allergies that were related to the white birch trees. I took her letter and went into my room and checked my answering machine. I found a small red light was on in my telephone answering machine. Someone had left a message for me. I turned on my telephone answering machine. I found the message was from Cara Houck from Pleasanton Senior Supporting Group to inform me that she had replaced Charlene's position in Pleasanton Senior Supporting Group. She would be my new counselor.

Next day, I wrote a short note to inform Marlene that I had faxed Dr. Ma's letter to her. Then I faxed my short note and Dr. Ma's letter to her. Then I called her to let her know that I had already faxed Dr. Ma's letter to her and I wanted to make sure she had got it. Marlene answered the phone and said she had got Dr. Ma's letter and she would check with her friends about my doctors' letters and would call me back to let me know whether they would accept my doctors' letters that indicated my allergies and sickness were from my neighbor's white birch tree. I said OK to her and hung up the phone.

After a few days, I called Marlene again. She told me about my doctors' letters. She indicated that this was the right way for my doctors to describe that my allergies were from the birch tree. Since I had already turned in my doctors' letters to them, I requested her again to write a letter for me to inform my neighbor to cut down his white birch tree. I told her if she was unable to help me, I would hire a lawyer to send out a letter to inform him. Marlene said she would check whether I needed a lawyer. After one week, I called Marlene. She indicated that she would not write a letter to my neighbor to inform him to cut down his tree. She insisted that I did not need to hire a lawyer in this case and it would be very costly for me. She advised me to write a letter, enclosing my doctors' letters, to inform my neighbor about my allergies from the birch tree and request my neighbor to cut down his white birch tree. I said OK to her and hung up the phone. Then I wrote a letter to my neighbor, John Clark, to let him know that my doctors had already indicated that my allergies were related to his white birch trees and I wanted him to take responsibility for cutting his white birch tree. I enclosed my letter and a copy of Dr. Young's and Dr. Ma's letters inside the envelope, and I was ready to send my letter to my neighbor John Clark.

On September 22, 2008, I went to check up with Dr. Ma for my allergy problems. After she checked up on me, she advised me to set up an appointment with an eye specialist to check up my eyes, because of my high diabetic data that showed in my blood test result. I told her I would set up an appointment with the eye specialist doctor later. She advised me to take a mammogram X-ray. I said OK to her. She asked me to take the flu shots. I said OK. She asked the nurse to give me two different kinds of flu shots. Then I told her that my right toenail was causing a lot of pain lately. No matter how I tried to cut and fix my right toenail, it poked my toe meat and caused a lot of pain. She advised me to see the foot doctor and helped me set up an appointment with Dr. Randall on October 2, 2008. After I was done with my checkup with her, I thanked her for her letter that I had received through the mail. I told her I gave the copies of her letters to Renee of the city of Pleasanton and Marlene of Pleasanton Senior Center. She reviewed some of my background over with me. She asked me about the counselor from Pleasanton Senior Supporting Group. I told her Charlene had retired, Cara Houck was my new counselor, and she had replaced Charlene's position in Pleasanton Senior Supporting Group. Then I left the clinic and went to the KPMC laboratory department to get my blood drawn for my blood sample test. I saw a lot of people inside the laboratory department, waiting for their turns for their blood samples to be drawn. I went in and took the number slip from the machine. I asked the front desk clerk permission to go to the business office instead of waiting there for my turn to get my blood sample be drawn. The front desk clerk said OK to me. I went to the business office in South Two building to request them to fill up American International Group (AIG) insurance company's physician visiting claim form for me. The financial counselor Dee from the business office suggested that I use my yellow physician visiting payment receipt slip to claim for my physician visiting claims with my insurance company. She stamped the KPMC business office name and address on my yellow physician visited payment receipt slip and my credit card payment slip. She asked me to send out all the receipts that she had stamped to AIG insurance company to claim for my physician visit. She gave her business card to me to call her back if my insurance company denied accepting the yellow payment receipt copy. I said OK and thanked her. I went back to the laboratory department.

I went over to the front desk clerk to inform her I was back. She advised me to stay at the entrance of the laboratory room to wait for the next technician to call me. I stood in front of the entrance of the laboratory room. After a while, the technician called me in and settled me inside the laboratory room. The technician used a rubber strip to tie it strongly on my right arm. She searched for the different veins in my right arm. She switched to the cephalic vein on my right arm. She rubbed the alcohol on my arm and pushed the needle into my vein. Very little blood came out; it seemed like she did not get enough blood for my blood sample test. Then she pulled out the needle from my hand and used cotton to stop my blood and put a tape on my right arm. I told her I was getting scared the way she was searching my blood veins, because I had never seen any technician or doctor using that vein to take any blood out from my body in my life. After I said that, she referred me to another technician to draw my blood sample. The second technician came and released the rubber strap from my right arm and tied it to my left hand. Then she asked me to flip my left hand. She started to push the needle in one of the small veins branching out from the radical vein. Blood came out very slowly. She got less than half the test tube. Then she switched to another test tube. She got only 1/10 of the test tube of my blood. She lifted up the test tube and looked at it. Then she told another technician that she could not get enough blood from me for my blood sample test. She pulled out the needle from my hand. She pressed my vein with cotton and put a piece of tape on my left hand again. Then she threw away the previous two small test tubes that she had drawn from my hand and asked the third technician to draw my blood sample. After I heard the second technician tell the third technician that I did not have enough blood in my system, I requested the second technician to give me a cup of water to drink. The third technician came and released the rubber strap on my left hand and switched to my right hand again, tying my right arm with a rubber strap. The second technician came and gave me a small paper cup of water. I took the cup and drank the water. Then I asked the third technician to wait for a while. Then I let her start drawing the blood sample from my hand. She pushed a needle in one of the veins branching out from the radical vein on my right hand. This time the third technician successfully filled up half a test tube of my blood sample. Then she helped me to massage my right hand. I was very unhappy the way they had drawn my blood sample three times on both my hands. I joked around with them and said to them how come they could not remember the things that I had said before. She continuously massaged my right hand and responded to me that she remembered what I had said last time about the birch trees when I was there. Then she suddenly pressed my right hand very hard. I cried out loudly. She released my hand, untied the rubber string, and put cotton and a piece of tape on my hand. Then she wrote "Grace" on a piece of paper and stuck the paper on her right chest. I told her it was not nice for her to press my hand like this and hurt me. I told her I was not pleased the way she did that to me. Then I left the laboratory room with cotton and tape on my right arm and both hands. I knew all of my blood was very concentrated and it was hard for them to draw the blood sample from my blood system, even though I had drunk a big cup of water before I left my house. This was the worst day for me in Pleasanton KPMC laboratory department for drawing my blood sample. After I was done, I went to the KPMC head and neck surgery clinic to set up an appointment for my infectious ear. The front desk clerk set up an appointment for me on October 20, 2008, at 10:00 a.m. with Dr. Cornelius. Then I went to Pleasanton post office to mail out my registered letter, along with Dr. Ma's letter enclosed in it, to my neighbor John Clark and went home. I received the green return slip from the post office, indicating that John Clark had already received my letter after a week.

Since Dr. Ma was pushing me very hard to set up an appointment with the gynecologist doctor because of my allergy incident, I called to set up an appointment with Dr. Kevin S. W. of the gynecology clinic (OB/GYN) for my pap and HPV screening tests for cervical cancer on October 10, 2008, at 1:50 p.m. Next day, I called Pleasanton KPMC radiology department to set up an appointment for my mammogram X-rays on October 10, 2008, at 2:45 p.m. I had not called my eye doctor to set up any appointment yet, because I wanted to wait until my diabetic data went down. I knew I had a problem with my eyesight, and it was hard to urinate after I got the bad allergy accident. I drank a lot of water and kept taking the medicines until I could urinate easily, and my eyesight was also getting better. Usually if I lifted or carried heavy objects at home, it would cause my brain, right eye, and body a lot of pain. My right leg would swell really big, and I could not see well. Sometimes it would cause numbness of my brain. I had to take pain-reliever pills and rest for minimum one week to get rid of the pain. After the pain was gone, my eyesight would get back to normal. I received Dr. Ma's letter to inform me about my blood test's result dated September 23, 2008. She indicated to me to increase Metformin Hydrochloride tablet from 750 mg to 1,000 mg because my diabetic HGBA1c data was 6.6 percent and not much different from the previous diabetic data 6.7 percent and was almost still in the same data range. On the same day, I also received a telephone message from Cara. She asked me to call her back to set up an appointment for her to come to my house to visit me or to set up an appointment to go to her office in Pleasanton Senior Center to meet with her and talk. I called her back and set up an appointment to meet with her in her Pleasanton Senior Center office on September 26, 2008, at 11:00 a.m.

I went in Pleasanton Senior Center on September 26, 2008, to meet with Cara at 11:00 a.m. Cara was not in the office yet. I was half an hour early, so I talked to the lady in the front desk room and asked her about the class inside Pleasanton Senior Supporting Group room. She told me it was the psychology class for the elderly. She asked me to wait in the main Pleasanton Senior Center. So I came to the main lobby of Pleasanton Senior Center. I met the lady who was sorting the newspapers in the main lobby of Pleasanton Senior Center. I asked her about the class in Pleasanton Senior Supporting Group room. She told me she did not know anything about the class in Pleasanton Senior Supporting Group room.

Then I pulled a chair near her and sat down and talked to her. While I was talking to her, I found she had fair and smooth skin on her face. I asked her whether she had any skin cancer on her face before. She said she did not have any skin cancer on her face. Then I asked her whether she had any white birch tree in her house or in her neighborhood. She said no to me. Then I told her about an elderly that I had met in the Pleasanton KPMC main building lobby. This elderly had ½ × ½ square inch size of a red rash spot area on her face. She told me her doctor had indicated the red rash spot on her face was skin cancer after he diagnosed her skin. When I asked her whether she had any white birch tree in her house, she said she had a lot in her area. From the information I got from her, I presumed the skin rash on her face was due to the burn by the powder or the broken pieces of the white birch trees that caused itching. I told her all the doctors must get up and do something about the birch trees by telling people to get rid of them now. She asked me who would tell the doctors to do it. I told her I was the one who would prove to the doctors and tell all the people to get rid of the bad birch trees in order to protect the skin and various other kinds of cancers. I told her I was waiting for Cara to come in to have a meeting with me, but there was a class inside the Pleasanton Senior Supporting Group room and I was unable to wait there. She shook her head and got up from her seat to go into one of the offices to turn in the newspapers after she finished solving them. Then a guy came over to me and said he was working in Pleasanton Senior Center and he was the one who had arranged this psychology class in the Pleasanton Senior Supporting Group room because they did not have any spare room for this class. I did not say anything to him. I was sitting there alone until five minutes before eleven o'clock.

I went back to the Pleasanton Senior Supporting Group room to meet with Cara. When I was in the Pleasanton Senior Supporting Group room, one of the front desk ladies told me Cara was in her room. She asked me to wait for her to go in to inform Cara. I sat on a chair near the entrance door, waiting for Cara. She went in to inform Cara that I was here. Then Cara came out and took me inside her office. We sat down face-to-face to start our conversations. She asked me about the deal that I had made with the city of Pleasanton. Why did the city have to take responsibility for other people's allergy to pay me? I told her I had set up a deal and an agreement with the city of Pleasanton that they would agree to pay me five million dollars if I could find the chemical acid from the birch tree to prove to them that the birch trees were the allergic trees and harmful to all the people. I did the research and experiments and organized getting all the information about the white birch family trees to prove that they were the allergic trees which contained bad betulinic acid. I had already turned in my doctors' letters and all my allergy pictures to the city of Pleasanton to prove that birch trees are the worst allergic trees. The city of Pleasanton should organize the information to inform all the people who live in this city that birch trees are bad allergic trees, causing allergies and sickness. They should ask the people from the city of Pleasanton to get rid of the allergic white birch trees from their yards to provide good and healthy environment for all the people who live in this city. I told her I wrote so many letters to Renee and the city of Pleasanton earlier to ask them to take action by informing the people to cut down the white birch trees, and I did not receive any return action from the city of Pleasanton to take care of this case. I tried to persuade all the people again and again to cut down the white birch trees to avoid all kind of allergies and sickness. "Only if we are healthy, we can live happily with our family and friends. Otherwise, we will be very sick and we cannot enjoy our lives if we have an unhealthy environment." No matter how I tried to persuade the city to inform the people to cut down the birch trees, no one took action to inform the people to cut down the allergic white birch trees in their communities. Then I had to set a deal with the city of Pleasanton to pay me five million dollars if I could find out the type of chemical acids in the birch trees to prove the birch family trees were the allergic trees. I did a lot of searching and got into so many accidents. Even my female dog Lady Star got into an accident when I was researching the birch trees and her left eye got blind. After I organized all the information about the birch trees to indicate that the birch trees were the allergic trees, I turned in all the information and the doctors' letters to the city of Pleasanton. No one took action to do anything, except I heard Cara keep telling me that the city of Pleasanton did not have the money to pay me when she came to visit me. I told her I had set the agreement deal with Charlene to sell my twenty-nine-page book, *The Scaring Birch Trees,* for twenty-five dollars if all the people agreed to buy my book. If I could get enough money by selling this book, I would use that money to open an analytical laboratory research center in Tri Valley to search out the chemical ingredients from the plants that we had not analyzed yet. Charlene told me everyone had agreed to my idea of buying my book if

I published and sold my book. So I registered in the city of Pleasanton to get my business license and tried to print the book *The Scaring Birch Trees*. But unfortunately, I did not get a chance to sell my book. I told Cara I was trained by my parents to be the person who would keep the promise to get things done if I promised to do something. I kept my promise to search and prove that birch trees are allergic trees. All the people had to keep their promise to buy my book to pay me.

I'd like to share with my readers how my parents trained me to be an honest person. I grew up in my mom's lap when I was a child. My mom always guided me what kind of things I should say and what I should not say when she made me sit on her lap every day. She would be very angry if I lied to her or did the things that I was not allowed to do. She always guided me not to lie and took good care of myself and all my belongings. They were worried about me a lot as I was the youngest child in the family. I learned a lot of lessons from my parents. If I did not do things right when they asked me to do, they would ask me to do it again, until I did it right. They always advised me to remember the mistake that I had made as a lesson. My parents loved me dearly and bought a lot of toys for me wherever they went. My parents even let me have the safety key to open the safety box in their room. I kept all my money that I got from my father in the safety box. Every night, I helped him to count the money from the pawn shop. After he finished checking all the money and the account from the pawn shop, most of the times he let me keep all the changes from the pawn shop. I collected all the money in my metal box and kept it in the safe. I was allowed to open the safe anytime I wanted. I just had to go inside their room to open it. Then I checked how much money I had in my metal box every night, after my father let me keep the change from the pawn shop. I usually put my safety key in my little school bag. I was allowed to take my school bag to school with the safety key in it. They never inquired from me where I had kept my safety key. One day, my parents went to their friend's child's wedding. They locked their room before they left. They left their four youngest children at home. My father's car driver came to our house after they left, asking my sister Ivy to give him four hundred kyats (Burmese currency) as my father had not get a chance to pay him. Ivy knew I had money in my safe. She asked me to climb up over the divider wall of my parents' room and open the safe to take out four hundred kyats from my metal box to give to the driver. I listened to her, and I climbed up the divider wall of my parents' room and went inside the room. Then I opened the safe and took out the money from my metal box. I locked the safe and climbed back over the divider wall of my parents' room and gave the money to her. Then she gave it to the car driver. I put the safety key back in my school bag. When my parents came home at night, I told my mom I had taken out four hundred kyats from my metal safety box to help my father pay his car driver. I asked her to pay the money back to me. As soon as she found out I had climbed up over the divider wall to take the money out from the safe in her room, she got very upset and angry. She asked me to give the safety key back to her. She said I was not allowed to take out any money from my safety box while they were not at home. I went to my desk to take out my school bag. I tried to get the safety key from the front pocket of my school bag. But I could not find the safety key in my school bag. So I told my mom I had lost my key. She was very angry and upset. She took the duster stick to hit my body. I cried after she hit me with the duster stick and ran to the kitchen because it was paining a lot when she hit me so hard. She followed me to the kitchen and kept hitting me and telling me that I was not allowed to take out any money from my safety box. I cried and cried. When I ran to the living room, she followed me to the living room and kept hitting me. All my sisters were standing in the middle room with my father, just looking at me and did nothing to help me. When I ran into the middle of the room near my sisters, Ivy stepped in and stood in front of my mom, trying to block my mom with her body so as to not let her follow me. My mom asked her to move away, but she refused to do so, so my mom turned to her and used the duster stick and hit her. The duster stick broke. She stopped following me. Then I stopped running and hid myself in the kitchen corner near the bathroom, and I cried for a couple of hours. When it was time for us to go upstairs and sleep, my father came in the kitchen and took me upstairs. I had a lot of red strike scars all over my body. Next day, after I woke up in the morning, I went to my desk to take out my school bag and look for my safety key again, but I could not find it, so I dumped out all the books from my school bag to search for the safety key. I found my safety key was in the small front pocket of my school bag. I took the safety key out from my school bag and showed it to my father. When my father saw the safety key, he told me he was happy for me to have found my safety key. He allowed me to keep the safety key and advised me not to lose it again. I promised him I would be very careful next time in taking care of my safety key. I learned a big lesson after I got struck so hard by my mom. I was very careful and made sure I put the safety key in my front school bag pocket. But I did not get a chance to tell my mom that it was not my idea to get the money out from the safe. I was told to go in to get it. My parents never allowed us to lie, they always kept an eye on us, no matter where we are, what we do. In my life I never dared to lie to say things to hurt anyone if it was not the truth. This was the way I had been trained since I was a baby.

I told Cara I never dared to lie to people, and I just tried to find and dig out the cause of the allergies and sickness from the birch family trees to save the people's lives. I mentioned to her about the elderly with skin cancer whom I had met in KPMC. I told her I had advised the elderly to tell their doctors who treated their itching spots on their faces as skin cancers to match the itching area by measuring the size of the red rashes on the patients' faces to indicate where and how did the patients get the itching and how did they diagnose the itching areas as skin cancer. Then we talked about other poison plants such as poison ivy, poison oak, and poison sumac. I told her the people kept saying they were affected by poison, rashes, and blisters on their hands or bodies from these poisonous plants. But no one knew what kind of chemicals made their skin burn and form blisters and rashes on their skins. Cara said she had also got the poison from poison oak plants. Then I asked Cara how she had got poison from poisonous oak plants. She did not say anything. Then I explained to her that I could describe how she had got the poison from those poisonous oak plants. I told her when she passed these poisonous plants she would not get any pimple rashes or blisters unless she touched or came in contact with freshly broken poisonous oak leaves and flowers. Then she would get burns and blister rashes on the areas that had come in contact with the poisonous fluid from the oak plants. If the blisters on her skin broke, the fluid from the blisters would spread to the nearby area on her body. When all those poisonous plants died because of any reason, the fluid from these poisonous plants vaporized in the air. The plants and their leaves and flowers dried out and formed different-sized dried particles or powder on the ground and flew all over the places if there were strong winds in the areas. If the people came in contact or breathed in these dried poisonous particles or powder or moisture or gas from the air, it would cause burning inside their body and lead to allergies and sickness.

I mentioned to Cara about Marlene's daughter's allergy which she had told me last time. Then I told her that Marlene had said that her daughter was allergic to her neighbor's cat. When her daughter went over to her neighbor's house and asked them whether they had let their cat out or not, her neighbor told her they had never let their cat out. Then Marlene said her daughter's allergy was gone after she drank honey juice. I told her that the allergy of Marlene's daughter was not the type of the allergy that I was complaining of.

Then I mentioned to her about my next-door neighbor family in Pennsylvania. There were five members in the family and had a couple of big white birch trees in front of their house. John went to work and left home in the morning before 8:00 a.m. and came back home at night after 8:00 p.m. He never helped out in the yard even on Saturdays and Sundays when he was at home. Maryann was the one who took care of the kids, the lawn, the yard, and the house. She told us all her kids had eye problems just like her, except John who did not have any eye problem. After both their daughters grew up and moved out from their house to live with their families in their own apartments, Maryann said both her daughters' eyes did not have any diseases. But her son was still living with them. The doctor told them their son had eye cancer, and his eye cancer got worse. The doctor said her son had genetically inherited the eye cancer from his maternal side. When I went back to King of Prussia, I heard their son's eye cancer disease had got worse and spread to his brain, and he died because of his eye cancer disease. Then I heard that their two daughters had moved out from their house and were living in their own apartments. Maryann told me their daughters' eyes were fine. In this case, we could make an assumption that genetically any side of the parents did not have any eye cancer diseases, but accidentally, her son's eyes must have got burned by the strong acid from the birch trees that they had planted in front of their house. His eyes got infected, causing cancer and death.

Cara mentioned to me that doctors and researchers were repeatedly telling the people that the allergies that the people were getting were from the pollens of the flowers from the weed plants, but they did not mention the type of pollens from the flowers and plants and what kind of ingredients and chemicals from the plants were causing the people to get bad allergies. The doctors were just guessing that the allergies that the people were getting were from the pollens of the flowers. They did not even know what kind of pollens of the flowers of the plants was causing the allergies. They should not keep telling the people all these allergies were caused by the pollens from the weeds, if they did not know the kinds of weeds that they were talking about. They should know the types of weeds and pollens of the flowers that were causing the allergies. How did the weed plants look like? Then I stopped for a while, because I suddenly could not remember the name of the type of plants that the doctors used to call "weeds." I told her I had forgotten the name of the weeds that the doctors mentioned when they talked about the allergy. I asked her if she knew the name of the plants that caused allergy. She said no and shook her head. I told her in the future, if I got a chance, I would continuously research about more plants that had the capability to cause bad allergies and sickness. We concluded our conversation after 12:30 p.m. I left Pleasanton Senior Center and went home.

On October 2, 2008, I went for checkup with Dr. Randall K. T. in the podiatry clinic at 10:30 a.m. I showed Dr. Randall my right leg's toenail and told him I had a lot of pain in it. Once he looked at my toenail, he said he would perform surgery on it for me to right away get rid of the pain. Then he asked his assistant to settle me in his clinic. After his assistant prepared all the materials that were needed to perform the surgery, he started to work on my right toenail by injecting an anesthetic agent into the peripheral nerves to kill both side nerves of my right toenail, to get rid of the pain. While he was operating on my toenail, I told him that no matter how I fixed and cut my right toenail, it seemed like my toenail kept growing and poking my fat toe meat, causing a lot of pain. Even when I slept, I could feel the fluid in my fat toe meat being pushed in by my growing toenail and causing a lot of pain. Finally, I had to give up fixing my toenail and checkup with him. He laughed and told me that I had taken the right decision to come to him. The only way to solve this problem was to perform surgery and destroy the nerves on the side of the toenail. Then he said the surgery was called matricectomy. He said a lot of people were having this kind of toenail problem and he had to perform four to five cases of this kind of surgery a day. I covered my face with my yellow payment receipt paper and listened to what he was telling me. I was afraid to look at how he was operating my toenail, but I could feel how he was working on my toenail. It took more than an hour to get the surgery done. He used cotton and a bandage to tie my right toe. He wrote instructions on his release statement paper, telling me how to treat my foot in hot salty water every day for one month. Then he gave me his release statement paper and released me from his clinic. I took his release statement and went home. I followed his instruction on the release statement to treat my surgery toe in hot salty water every night until all the pain was gone.

On October 10, 2008, I went to Pleasanton KPMC gynecology (OB/GYN) department to checkup with Dr. Kevin at 1:35 p.m. The front desk clerk handed out one form for me to fill in. I took the form and filled in all the information that I knew. For some of the questions which I did not understand, I left the columns blank. I turned in the form to the front desk clerk and told her I did not know how to fill in some of the questions on the paper. She said this was OK and I did not need to fill in the information that I did not know. Then I went back to my seat and waited for a medical assistant to come out and get me. After a few minutes, a medical assistant came out and took me inside Dr. Kevin's clinic. She asked me to sit on a chair on the hallway. Then she asked me to put my right hand on the table. She tied my right arm with the wrapper of the blood pressure monitor machine. She pumped air into the blood pressure monitor machine's wrapper several times and released it. The blood pressure monitor machine could not read my blood pressure on my right arm. She untied the monitor machine's wrapper from my right arm and said the blood pressure monitor machine could not read my blood pressure on it, so she said she would use my left arm to read my blood pressure. She asked me to put my left hand on the table and tied my left arm with the monitor machine's wrapper. She pumped air into the monitor machine's wrapper. While she was pumping in air, I told her I did not have any blood in my system, and this was the reason the monitor machine could not read my blood pressure. She stopped pumping the air in the monitor machine wrapper and let the monitor machine read my blood pressure. The machine could not read my blood pressure again. She pumped the air in and tried again. This time the monitor machine successfully read my blood pressure. She wrote down the information on the sheet and took me inside the patient room and settled me there to wait for Dr. Kevin. After half an hour, Dr. Kevin walked inside the room and asked me to lie down on the patient bed. His medical assistant stayed with him in the room. He asked me when I had gone for my last visit to the gynecologist for a checkup. I told him I had never gone to see any gynecologist for over thirty years after my son was born. This was my fourth time I had checked up with a gynecologist. I told him that every time I received his letters before I threw them away in the trash can. He laughed. Then he checked up on me and took the tissues from my body for my pap and HPV laboratory test for cervical cancer. After he was done, he told me to get dressed and he left the room with his assistant. After I was ready, I went out of the patient's room and was just about to go to the main exit door to leave the clinic when Dr. Kevin came out of his office and handed out his release statement papers to me. Then he said he would like me to read his release statement papers. I took the release statement papers from him and told him I would read them and thanked him. Then he said he knew I had to go to the radiology department to take a mammogram X-ray and he would walk out with me to the exit door. He walked out with me to the exit door and opened the exit door for me. I came out from his clinic.

I went to the KPMC radiology department in South One building to take a mammogram X-ray. I checked in with the front desk clerk in the radiology department. After I checked in with the front desk clerk, I had to wait in the waiting room for fifteen minutes. The technician, Lisa, came out and took me inside the radiology clinic hallway. She handed out the form to me and asked me to fill in my breasts' history. I filled in all the information about my breasts in the form. When I saw Lisa come out, I gave the form to her. She took my form, and ushered me inside the mammogram X-ray room, asking me to change into the patient clothing. Then she asked me to stand in front of the mammogram X-ray machine. Then she took the mammogram X-rays of both my breasts. After she was done, she asked me to change back into my clothing. Then she asked me whether I had taken mammogram X-rays before. I told her I had taken mammogram X-rays before, but I did not remember the year when I had taken them. After a while, I remembered the year I had taken mammogram X-rays in New York was in 2001. I told her the year when I had taken my last mammogram X-rays. Then I told her when I had first checked up with Dr. Ma in the KPMC adult medicine clinic, I had filled up the form in the VCMC radiology department, requesting them to transfer all my old mammogram films to Pleasanton KPMC radiology department. When I checked with Pleasanton KPMC radiology department, they told me they did not have my old mammogram films from VCMC. I told her to check with Pleasanton KPMC radiology department to look for my old mammogram films. If Pleasanton KPMC radiology department did not have my old mammogram films, she could locate my mammogram films in VCMC in Pleasanton. She wrote down all my information on the sheet. Then I told her I had left breast surgery done before in Pennsylvania, because I had two plain areas on both my breasts, and I had to take the mammogram X-rays twice in the New York radiology department in 2001 to match the two films to make sure they had not been caused by X-ray machine error. I told her she would be very surprised to see my old mammogram films of two plain areas on both my breasts. She said she would locate all my mammogram films in Pleasanton KPMC radiology department to make sure they had all my old mammogram films. Then she released me and I went home.

On October 20, 2008, at 10:00 p.m., I went to Pleasanton KPMC head and neck surgery clinic for my appointment with Dr. Cornelius. When Dr. Cornelius saw me, he said he still remembered me that I had checked in to see him two years ago. I told him I remembered him too. Then I asked him whether he still wanted to refer me to the doctor from Fremont KPMC. He quickly responded to me with "no, no, no." Then he checked my right ear. He said my right ear was in good shape and Dr. Glenn had done a good surgery job on my right ear. Then he checked my left ear and said there was a lot of fluid inside my left ear. He drained out the fluid from my left infectious ear with a machine. Then he looked inside my left ear and said my left ear was infected badly, and he prescribed me Avelox/Moxifloxacin 400 mg antibiotic pill and Ciprodex otic suspension ear drops for my left infectious ear. He said he would not perform the repeat procedure for the ear surgery. He referred me to Dr. Sara S. C. and said she had already practiced in this field for two years. She had been doing a good job and had a lot of experience for repeat procedure in ear surgery. He would leave her to take the decision for my left ear as to what she wanted to do for me. I said OK. Then he left. I went out to the front desk clerk to set up two appointments on September 20, 2008. One appointment was with Cara T. for my hearing test at 9:30 a.m., and another appointment was with Dr. Sara at 10:00 a.m. Then I went to South Two pharmacy store to get Avelox/Moxifloxacin 400 mg (10 tablets) pills and one bottle of Ciprodex otic suspension ear drops. But when I saw the label of Ciprodex otic suspension ear drops, I remembered I had it at home, so I told the pharmacist that I had Ciprodex otic suspension ear drops at home and I did not want to purchase Ciprodex otic suspension ear drops. I just bought Avelox/Moxifloxacin 400 mg pills from the pharmacy store and then I went to 99 Ranch supermarket to buy lunch for myself. Then I went home.

I received a telephone call from Cara Houck on October 3, 2008. She informed me that Marlene had left a message for her to call me to find out what I wanted her to talk to my neighbor. I told her it was Marlene's idea to ask her to talk to my neighbor to get rid of their white birch trees. I told her I wanted her to study the environment in my neighborhood and take out time to come to my house to talk to my neighbor. She said OK and that she would call me back. But I called her back in the afternoon to set up an appointment for her to come to my house on October 6, 2008. She set up an appointment at 11:00 a.m. to come to see me before she talked to my neighbor. She came at 11:00 a.m. on October 6, 2008. She told me she had driven around my neighborhood before she came to my house and found there were so many white birch trees in my neighborhood. I suggested asking my neighbor why he did not want to cut his tree down. She said my neighbor did not have to tell her the reason why he did not want to cut down his white birch tree. I told her she had to get an answer from my neighbor regarding their cutting down their birch tree. My neighbor had to cut down his white birch tree to get rid of the allergies and sickness. That would be good for all of our neighborhood. Then she asked me what the use was of just asking only my neighbor's white birch tree to be cut. What about the rest of the white birch trees in our neighborhood? Didn't they expose the allergies and sickness to the people in those neighborhoods? I said the rest of the white birch trees from this neighborhood did not affect me much at this moment, because they were far away from my house, and if my neighbor cut down his white birch tree, it would get rid of my allergy that I had got from his birch tree. Once the people learned that my neighbor had cut down his birch tree, all the people from our neighborhood would follow him in cutting down their allergic birch trees. I told her that before when I told all my neighbors who owned the birch trees to cut down their birch trees, the owner of the right-end corner house across the street cut down all his big white birch trees as soon as he heard from me that the white birch trees were bad allergic trees. She asked me why all the people in my neighborhood hadn't complained. I said to her my neighbors in the left corner house complained a lot that they had been getting bad allergies before and they could not even lay their hands on their lawn and touch the grasses. When I told them about my neighbor's allergic birch trees, they said they had no right to complain about my neighbor's white birch trees, which were three houses away from them. I was the only one who had the right to complain about my neighbor's allergic birch trees that were growing next to my house and causing me bad allergy. I told her my neighbor's birch tree was getting so big and even the trunk was turning to a black color, and the poison from the tree was getting stronger and making our allergies getting worse. I told her I could not even leave my garage door open. Once I opened my garage door, air flew into my garage and all the dried birch flowers and leaves flew in and filled up my garage. The bad allergic particles from the birch tree were all over inside my garage. I could not even lay my hands on the food cans in my garage. Once I picked up the food cans in my garage, I got a bad itch and red rashes formed on my hands. When I opened the inner door to go inside my house, all the bad air from the garage flew inside my house. I had to breathe in all the bad chemicals from the air every day, because of the bad itch on my lips and pale spots on my knees and legs. I felt very sick. I requested her to tell my neighbor to cut down his white birch tree instead of forcing me to go to the court again, which Marlene never recommended me. If I had to go to the court, he had to pay me for my injury. The city of Pleasanton wanted her to take care of this case for me. This was the reason she got hired to replace Charlene's position; she was to visit me to help me solve my case. I showed her the letter that I had written to my neighbor. I urged her again to tell my neighbor to cut down his bad white tree. If he refused, I would have to take him to the small claim court again. The court would find him to pay me for my injury that I had got due to the bad allergy from his bad tree. She said OK and went over to my neighbor's house to talk to him, but she came back and told me no one was in his house. She said she would call my neighbor to talk to him on the phone. Then she left my house. Next day, I felt that I should prepare the documentation to take my neighbor to the court. I called the city of Pleasanton again to let them know I was going to the courthouse to pick up the form. Then I went to the courthouse to pick up the form again. I told the front desk clerk at the courthouse that I had got my doctors' letters indicating that the birch trees were allergic to me and that they had told me to stay away from the birch trees. All these years, my sister Holly and my brother Harvey provided me antibiotic medicines and eye medicines for Lady Star and Sir Space. I had told the truth before when I was in the court that the birch tree was the allergic tree, and if I had not had my sister and brother to help me in providing the medicines to me, I would have to spend a bundle of money to keep seeing the doctors for my allergy. If I had to add in all the cost of the medicines that my sister and brother had provided to me all these years, he would have to pay me a lot. Then I called Renee to set up an appointment on Monday to see her to get some advice from her about the claim of the payment if I took my neighbor to the court. Renee's secretary told me she was not in her office and she would have Renee call me back. Then I called Cara again on Monday to make sure she had talked to my neighbor to remove his white birch tree.

On November 4, 2008, in the morning, the technician Lisa from Pleasanton KPMC radiology department called me back to let me know that I needed to take a new ultrasound screening test in the Walnut Creek KPMC radiology department to review my breasts' condition. Then she said she had set up an appointment on November 13, 2008, for me to take a new ultrasound screening test in Walnut Creek KPMC. I asked her whether there was anything wrong with my mammogram films. She said nothing was wrong in my mammogram films and the doctor just wanted me to check my breasts by an ultrasound screening test to review my breasts just to make sure everything was OK. Then I asked her why I had to go to the Walnut Creek KPMC radiology department to take the ultrasound screening test. She said there was no ultrasound doctor to read the ultrasound screening test in Pleasanton KPMC radiology department. I thanked her and hung up the telephone. I did not feel right that they suddenly scheduled me to go to another KPMC facility in other city. Because of my car accident, I was scared to drive myself to another city, which was far away from Pleasanton. So I called Pleasanton KPMC in the night to check with the operator whether Pleasanton KPMC radiology department had an ultrasound machine in the radiology department. I told her I had taken an ultrasound screening test on my right leg before in Pleasanton KPMC radiology department. She indicated that Pleasanton KPMC radiology department had the ultrasound machine, but she did not know the reason the technician had set up the appointment for me in the Walnut Creek KPMC radiology department. She referred me to talk to one of the managers from the KPMC main office to check the reason Pleasanton KPMC radiology department did not have a doctor to read the ultrasound screening test. I said OK. She switched the telephone line to the KPMC main office to let me talk to the office manager. The manager in the KPMC main office picked up the phone. I asked the manager why Lisa from the radiology department had referred me to the Walnut Creek KPMC radiology department to take the ultrasound screening test. She explained to me that Walnut Creek KPMC had all kinds of computer machines to detect the diseases. If they found anything wrong on my breasts after the doctor read the ultrasound screening test, they could use other computer machines to detect my problem right away. She asked me whether I would like to file a complaint against the mammogram X-ray technician who had referred me to Walnut Creek KPMC radiology department. I said no to her and hung up the phone. I sent out text messages to both my children to ask them to take me to the Walnut Creek KPMC radiology department to take an ultrasound screening test. Shaun called me after he received my message and told me he would drive me to Walnut Creek KPMC to take an ultrasound screening test.

On November 13, 2008, Shaun came home early in the morning and took me to Walnut Creek KPMC to take the ultrasound screening test for my breasts in the radiology department at 10:45 a.m. We arrived at Walnut Creek KPMC at 10:00 a.m. and parked our car in the KPMC garage parking lots. Then we went up to the fourth floor to check in the radiology department. After I checked in with the front desk clerk, it was still an hour early. I suggested that Shaun and I went to the coffee shop to have a cup of coffee instead of waiting here. Shaun said OK. I went to the front desk clerk to ask permission to go downstairs to have a cup of coffee. The front desk clerk said no and asked us to wait here. We waited there for half an hour. The nurse T. Quenedo called me to take me to the ultrasound room. After I was inside the ultrasound room, she asked me to change into patient clothing. Then she left. After a while, she came in and asked me to lie down on the patient bed to screen both my breasts with an ultrasound machine. She checked my right breast a couple of times on the computer screen. Dr. L. S. Cheng came in to perform the ultrasound screening test on me. Dr. Cheng carefully checked my breasts on the computer screen and told me everything was good. I asked him whether he had reviewed my old mammogram films that I had taken in New York. He said he did not know anything about my old mammogram films. Then he released me. Then I asked him to check whether I should wait for any release statement to take home. He said he did not have any release statement for me at that moment. He said the doctor would send out the screening test result through the mail to me after the doctor had reviewed it, and he discharged me. I left the Walnut Creek KPMC building with Shaun and went home. Shaun took me to a Chinese buffet restaurant in Dublin to have luncheon on the way back home. We enjoyed very much our luncheon in the restaurant. We went home after we finished our lunch. I was a little tired and went to asleep as soon as I arrived home. When I woke up in the evening, I saw Shaun cutting the lawn. I prepared some food for him to take back to Davis. After he was done with the lawn work, he took the food that I had prepared for him and went back to Davis at 4:30 p.m. Before he left, he went to the mailbox to pick up all the mails for me. I was happy to receive a card from Dr. Kevin, informing me that my pap and HPV screening test for cervical cancer were normal.

On November 20, 2008, at 9:30 a.m., I checked in with Cara T. Cara T. tried to perform the hearing test for me, but she was unable to perform it on my left ear. I could not hear well when she asked me to repeat the words that she mentioned to me because I had a lot of black fluid blocking my left ear. She requested Dr. Sara to drain the fluid out of my left ear with the draining machine. Dr. Sara drained all the fluid out of my left ear and then Cara T. performed a hearing test on me. After she was done, she told me I had hearing loss in my left ear. Perhaps I needed to wear hearing aid. Then she took me to another patient room to wait for Dr. Sara. Dr. Sara came in at 10:00 p.m. and checked in both my ears. She told me my right ear looked fine after my ear surgery done by Dr. Glenn. She asked me about Dr. Cornelius and the medicines that Dr. Cornelius had prescribed to me. I told her Dr. Cornelius had prescribed me Avelox/Moxifloxacin 400 mg antibiotic tablets and Ciprodex otic suspension ear drops. She asked me whether the medicines that Dr. Cornelius had prescribed me worked for me. I said no. Then I told her about Dr. Glenn who had told me earlier I needed to operate my left infectious ear. She looked at my left ear and said I had a lot of bad fluid inside my left infectious ear. She used a cotton swab to clean up the fluid in my left ear and said my left ear was infected badly. She explained to me how she was going to perform the surgery by cutting the back of my left ear and then opening my left ear to clean the infectious area and replace a new eardrum for me. Then she said that I needed to take a CAT scan X-ray of my left ear first and that the CAT scan X-ray technician would call me to set up an appointment after one week. I requested her to perform my left ear surgery as soon as possible. Because my left ear had been infected for over six years now, she said she would take care of everything for me to perform the surgery as soon as possible. I said OK to her. Then she wrote the "masterdectomy" word down on her business card and gave it to me. I took her business card and left her office. On my way back home, my heart was very heavy and I was very upset at my neighbor. Because of their bad white birch tree, I had to cut my left ear from the back to perform another ear surgery again.

As soon as I arrived home, I gave Marlene a call to let her know that my left ear was infected badly and that the doctor had told me I had to perform another surgery on my left ear for infection and have my infectious eardrum replaced again. I told Marlene this was not a good sign for me to keep getting ear infection from my neighbor's birch tree and keep replacing my eardrum. I needed to get a definite answer from her as to when my neighbor would remove their bad allergic white birch tree. I requested her to talk to my neighbor again. She said Cara would call me to set up an appointment to come to my house and talk to my neighbor. I said OK and hung up my phone. The technician from Pleasanton KPMC radiology department called me in the afternoon and asked me to go to the radiology department the next day to take a CAT scan X-ray at 1:30 p.m. I said OK to the technician. Then Cara called to inform me at 3:00 p.m. that she would come with Marlene to my house on Monday, November 24, 2008, at 3:00 p.m. to visit me and talk to my neighbor.

On November 21, 2008, I went to Pleasanton KPMC radiology department for my CAT scan X-ray. I arrived at the KPMC radiology department at 1:00 p.m. and was half an hour early. I asked the front desk clerk whether the technician could take the CAT scan X-ray for me now. She said all the technicians were having luncheon in the upstairs cafeteria. She did not think they would do it for me now. She advised me to go to the upstairs cafeteria to have a cup of hot coffee and come back down at 1:30 p.m. I said OK. I went to the upstairs cafeteria. I bought a cup of hot clam chowder soup for myself. The lady cashier in the cafeteria charged me $2.89 for a cup of clam chowder soup. Then she said I had to pay extra twenty-five cents if the total food price was less than four dollars. She asked me whether I wanted to get other things. I said no, I did not want any other things. Then she told me I had to pay extra twenty-five cents. I said OK and handed out my credit card to her to let her charge twenty-five cents more. She entered the food cost in the computer and handed out the receipt slip to me to sign it. I signed the receipt slip and gave it back to her. I took my clam chowder soup and went to a corner table. I sat down on the chair and started having my clam chowder soup. A lady employee brought her luncheon to my table and sat next to me. She was eating her lunch. I talked to her about the KPMC cafeteria system and that I was very surprised with this system. She said she did not know anything about it. I told her the lady cashier at the cafeteria had charged me extra twenty-five cents, since the total food cost was less than four dollars. She said she did not know anything about this. While I was having my soup, I looked around the whole cafeteria room. I saw a lot of patients and employees were inside the cafeteria, enjoying their lunches. I saw two disabled patients on wheelchairs in the cafeteria room, eating their lunches with their friends. When I saw them, I felt bad for them. I wanted them to be perfect just like any other healthy people. I was very afraid of becoming disabled just like them. I had learned to protect myself since I was four years old, after I got into a bad accident that broke my lip and left a deep scar on my lip. I still remember that when I was four years old I was very naughty. Every day after dinner, my mom would settle all my three elder sisters at the round table in the living room to make them complete their homework. My mom would be busy in the kitchen all the time. I played in the living room myself. Sometimes I rode my small bike inside the house; sometimes I jumped from one chair to another chair behind my sisters' seats, and all my sisters never complained about me when I jumped around the table from one chair to another chair behind their seats until I was tired. Sometimes if I was too active, they would force me to sit in the middle of the table to watch them studying. One day while I was jumping from one chair to another chair behind my sisters' seats, I accidentally slipped and hit the back corner edge of one of my sisters' chairs and fell on the floor. My mouth was bleeding heavily. I cried and cried. As soon as my mom heard me crying, she ran to me and helped me up. She saw my mouth was bleeding very heavily. She and my father tried to find the wounded area in my mouth to stop the bleeding, but the blood would not stop flowing and it kept bleeding from my left upper lip. It took a while for my father to stop the blood to flow from the wounded area on my left upper lip. Then they cleaned my mouth with warm water, using cotton. They found out the left side of my upper lip was cut and broken, over a half an inch big cut. They put medicine on my wounded upper lip. I cried and cried, because I had a lot of pain. My mom put some sugar in my mouth to stop me from crying. After a while, I stopped crying. This accident made my parents so scared that my mom put me on her lap and kept telling me day and night not to jump around the chairs again as I would hurt myself. Then she pointed at my broken lip and kept saying it would look very ugly if the wounded area left a big scar on my lip when I grew up. She wanted me to be careful no matter what I did to protect myself. After that accident, I was so scared to hurt myself because I would get big pain and a big scar on my lip. So I stopped jumping from one chair to another chair. This was the only accident I had in my life in which I hurt myself. I did not like to have any scar left in my body. I did not like to be a disabled person. No matter where I went, no matter what I did, I watched out carefully my surroundings and took good care of myself not to get hurt. But unfortunately, I got hurt by the other people who set up the car accident against me. I did not know why they wanted to hurt and kill me. Whenever I saw handicapped people around, I did not feel comfortable with them. I was scared to become a disabled person just like them. We all should learn to take good care of ourselves and others by looking at the handicapped people and seeing how hard it is for them to sit on wheelchairs and how much they need the people to take care of them. We should behave well and be considerate enough to take good care of ourselves and others. I felt bad for them. I got very upset with those people who made other people become handicapped, because of their careless mistakes.

After I finished my soup in cafeteria, I went back to the radiology department at 1:30 p.m. CAT scan X-ray technician Mrs. Bunn came out and took me inside the CAT scan X-ray room. She asked me to take out all my jewelries and eyeglasses from my body. I took out all of them from my body. She asked me to lie down on the CAT scan X-ray patient bed and started to take X-rays of my ears. After she was done, she asked me to put back my jewelries and eyeglasses. I did the way she said. Then she said my doctor would call me after she had reviewed the CAT scan X-ray films. I shook my head, and she showed me the exit door to go out from the CAT scan X-ray room. She was a very nice and polite lady. I liked her a lot. I stopped in the laboratory department on the way out from KPMC South One building. I saw a man and a woman cleaning the floor in the laboratory room. I stopped and asked them where Grace was. They said they did not know. Then I joked at them by shaking my right hand and crying, "ah-ah-ah . . ." just like last time, when I had cried as Grace pressed and hurt my hand. They all laughed, and I left KPMC South One building and went home.

After I arrived home, I went to my mailbox to pick up my mails. I found a letter from California Franchise Tax Board, indicating that they had not received my income tax returns from 2006. They also indicated that the city of Pleasanton had informed them about my earnings from my Peak Farm Company and my Lincoln Life Insurance. I called California Franchise Tax Board as soon as I read in their letter that I needed to explain to them why I had to close down Peak Farm Company. Then I explained to them I did not get a chance to print and sell my book, before California Franchise Tax Board sent out a letter to me and asked me to close down the Peak Farm Company business license from the city of Pleasanton if I did not get any sales tax from my company. California Franchise Tax Board suggested that I not waste any money on paying business license tax, postal stamp fees, and postal mailbox, so I cancelled my business license from the city of Pleasanton and my postal mailbox. California Franchise Tax Board also inquired from me about my Lincoln Life Insurance. I explained to them that I did not receive any dividend from Lincoln Insurance Company. I did not know why they kept sending out the 1099 tax form to me each year, to make me keep paying the income tax. I did not claim my disability from them at the time I was in a bad car accident and got hurt badly. Earlier, when I had talked to Lincoln Life Insurance Company about my disability insurance, the company had promised to reimburse the amount of money back to me for the time I was disabled. They sent out the claim form to me. I had the claim form, but I did not get a chance to fill up the form to send it back to them to claim. The lady from the California Franchise Tax Board called me and left a note, asking me to fill up the form and send it back to them. She also advised me to call the city of Pleasanton to find out the date when I had closed my business license. I said OK. We finished our phone conversation. I called Pleasanton business license department to request the manager Karen to find out the date that I had closed my business license for my Peak Farm Company. Karen found out my business license closing date for me. It was on March 17, 2007, that I had closed my business license from the city of Pleasanton. I gave Sirena the Franchise Tax Board form. I told her I did have a big loss on my Peak

Farm Company by selling my books. I did not get any money from my friends after I sent out the books to them. She took the form from me and put it in her bag. Then she said she would let her CPA take care of my income tax. Then she suggested that I went to Best Buy store to shop for a new television because my television was broken. When we were in Best Buy store, we found they had a Samsung television for sale with the right price. Sirena bought the Samsung television and had the Best Buy store deliver the new television to my house on December 2, 2008. After we bought the television from the store, we went home. When we reached home, Sirena prepared food for both of us. After we ate, she went home.

On November 24, 2008, Monday, at 3:00 p.m., Cara called me to let me know that she and Marlene were just about to leave Pleasanton Senior Center to come to my house. They arrived at my house at 3:45 p.m. I took them to the family room. Marlene told me that she had seen my neighbor hiring painters for painting his house, and it seemed like they were going to move out. After I heard that my neighbor was going to move out, I told her I did not want him to move out before he cut down his tree. I did not like to deal with another new owner again about this tree. Marlene mentioned about the cypress trees and that the cypress trees had big roots and they were also very messy. I told her cypress trees were just like any other trees. They had big roots and a lot of small roots branched out from the big roots in the ground, but cypress trees were just like pine trees. They were not allergic trees. We could call cypress trees as medicine trees. I told Marlene that I heard the news on a Chinese television channel reporting that Chinese researchers were using the hair lotion made from cypress tree oil to help smooth the skin and regrow the people's hairs on their heads. I told Marlene that I was very tired that I had to keep bringing them up and complaining about my neighbor's birch tree again and again. I explained to her another secret as to why people's lips were so itchy without touching the white birch trees and their discharge. I explained to her that the trees were just like human beings. The moisture and the odor from their trunk, branches, leaves, and flowers spread into the air in hot weather. When you walked and passed by somebody in hot weather, you could smell the bad odor from the person that you passed by, if that person was sweating and had a bad odor. The same concept we could apply to the trees with regards to them having odor or being odorless. You would smell the tree's odor if it had an odor when you passed it, but not all the odors from the trees would be the same, because each type of tree contained a different kind of chemical acid. The white birch tree was an odorless tree, but the moisture from the white birch trunk, birch branches, birch leaves, and birch flowers contained the same kind of acid from the white birch tree. They were in the air all the year round, making people get itching after they breathed in the bad acid of the white birch tree from the air every day. Then I picked up the perfume machine to spray on them in the family room, and I explained to them the acid moisture from the birch trees was in the air just like the perfume stayed in the air after I sprayed it from the perfume machine into the air. The perfume smell stayed all over my family room. Marlene said she did not smell any odor from the perfume machine. I stopped spraying the perfume in the family room and I looked at her amazedly. I told Marlene that I hated the big maple tree in my left neighbor's yard and I had to keep cleaning their big maple leaves and big round fruits that kept falling on to my left front yard, but I never went to them to complain about the messy maple trees and their discharges. I only went to my right-side neighbor to keep complaining about their white birch tree. I insisted them to cut down their white birch tree, but my neighbor kept refusing to cut down his bad allergic white birch tree. I did not know how to make him cut down his white birch tree. I did not want to bring up this problem and this case repeatedly to keep complaining. I did not want to go through another ear surgery again and again. I did not like to suffer from bad allergies and sickness caused by my neighbor's bad birch tree. I wanted my neighbor to cut down his white birch tree so that I would come out of this allergy. Then I asked Marlene how she wanted me to solve this problem—whether she wanted me to take my neighbor to the court to have it order my neighbor to cut down their birch trees or I wanted to move out from this house. She said she would like me to wait, but if I liked to move out, she would not stop me, but she did not want me to move out from this house where I had been living for so long. She did not want me to go to the court either. I told her I liked to clear out this problem before I moved out from this house. No matter who moved into my house, I would like to give them the best of the best luck and the best of health to stay in this house. I did not want them to go through what I had to go through. I told them I had proofs in the form of my two doctors' letters, which indicated that I was very allergic to the birch trees. Then I took out my two doctors' letters and made copies of them for Marlene again. Then Marlene said they would go and talk to my neighbor now and left my house. I went outside with them. Marlene told me not to worry about it and that she would get my neighbor's telephone number to talk to him and make him cut down his white birch tree. She said if he did not agree to cut down his birch tree after she talked to him in person, then she would advise me to take him to the court. When we were outside, we saw three big trucks were parked in front of my neighbor's driveway. A few people were standing near the trucks in front of my right-side neighbor's garage. After Marlene and Cara saw the people at my neighbor's house, they decided not to go in and talk to my neighbor; instead, they told me they had another meeting and they left my house. After they left, I came back inside my house with a heavy heart. I was very upset about this case. I called Renee again after they left. The receptionist, Marylou, picked up the phone, and I asked for Renee. She said Renee was not in her office. I left a message for Renee, informing her that Marlene and Cara had come to my house to help me talk to my neighbor and persuade them to cut down their big white birch tree. But they left instead of talking to my neighbor. Then I hung up my phone. Then I called Cara, leaving a message on her answering machine to call me back.

On November 25, 2008, I called Renee again. Marylou picked up the phone. I told her I wanted to talk to Renee. She immediately transferred me to Renee's telephone line. Renee picked up the phone. I told Renee that Marlene and Cara had come to my house to talk to my neighbor and have them cut down their bad white birch tree. They came into my house and talked to me for a while. They told me they were going to talk to my neighbor. They took my two doctors' letters from me and left. But after they went outside, when they saw there were big trucks in front of my neighbor's garage, they did not go in and talk to my neighbor; instead, they left. I did not know what to do anymore. Renee tried to convince me not to worry about anything, saying that the weather was getting cooler. The weather would help the allergy to be a little bit better. I told her no; as long as the birch trees were around, they would spray their chemical substances into the air, causing all of us to get allergies and sickness all the year round. Renee said she would talk to Marlene about this case again, and we ended our conversation.

On Thursday, November 25, 2008, I baked turkey and chicken in the morning and waited for my children to come home for Thanksgiving dinner. Sirena arrived home at 11:30 a.m. She prepared mashed potatoes, bread stuffing, and gravy for Thanksgiving dinner. After she was done, we waited for Shaun to come home. As soon as Shaun arrived home, we started to have Thanksgiving dinner, and we enjoyed our food a lot; in particular, my two dogs were happy to get big pieces of turkey and they enjoyed their food so much. After Thanksgiving dinner, my two children rested for a while. Then they moved the old television to one corner to make place in the family room for the new television to arrive. They cleaned the house for me. After they were done cleaning, they both left and went home.

On December 1, 2008, I went to my garage to clean my garage cabinets. I got so sick after I came back inside my house from my car garage. My lips were itching badly. My whole legs and knees had big pale spots. I took two pills of Claritin allergy medicines to get rid of my allergy, besides the medicines that my doctor had prescribed to me. I stopped using Benadryl allergy medicine when I found out it made me so drowsy. Then I called Cara again after 4:00 p.m. She said she did not get my neighbor's telephone number to talk to them. She said she would talk to Marlene and call me back after she got my neighbor's telephone number from her. On December 2, 2008, Best Buy store called me in the morning to let me know that their delivery men would not be able to deliver the television on the time that they had stated they would do it. They said they would deliver the television in the morning. I said no problem to them. Two delivery men from Best Buy store arrived at my house at 10:00 a.m., assembled, and tested the new television for me. After they were done, they took my two old televisions and left. I opened my front screen door for them. Even in those few steps that I took, during which I helped the delivery men of Best Buy store by opening my front screen door for them to move the old television out from my house, my lips, legs, and knees were itching badly. On December 4, 2008, Cara called me back to let me know that she would talk to my neighbor about their birch tree and asked them to get rid of them.

On December 8, 2008, I called Pleasanton KPMC South Two pharmacy store to order my prescriptions. Then I called Pleasanton KPMC adult medicine clinic to set up an appointment for my three-month follow-up doctor visit with Dr. Ma. But Dr. Ma had been transferred to KPMC in Union City, which made it more convenient for her to commute from her house to her KPMC clinic in Union City. She left Pleasanton KPMC adult medicine clinic on November 1, 2008.

Pleasanton KPMC gave me a new list of doctors' names to replace Dr. Ma as my new adult medicine doctor after Dr. Ma left. I chose Dr. Jennifer, B. C., as my new adult medicine doctor. When I called to set up a follow-up appointment with my adult medicine doctor, the operator asked me the reason I called to set up an appointment to see the doctor. I told him I could not do anything about my allergy as my neighbor did not cut down his white birch tree and I had to call in for a follow-up appointment to checkup with my doctor. The schedule operator set up an appointment on December 31, 2008, at 3:30 p.m. for me to checkup with Dr. Jennifer. Then I went to Walmart store to get tuna fish can food after 11:00 a.m., but Walmart store had ran out of tuna fish can food, so I just bought some cookies from Walmart store. Then I went to the Indian supermarket to buy some vegetables and went to Dublin Chase bank to deposit my money.

While I was in the Chase bank, only two bank clerks were taking care of the customers. I was the only customer waiting for the bank clerk to call me to take care of my deposit money. When one of the bank clerks finished helping the customer, she called me to go to her. So I went to her and took out my deposit checks from my purse and put them on the counter desk. Then I told her I wanted to deposit my money in my checking account. When she picked up my checks from the counter desk, she started to sneeze a few times and then stopped. Then she pointed her finger accusingly at my jacket and said her sneezing was caused by the dog hair on my jacket. I said no. I told her that her sneezing was not caused by the dog hair on my jacket. After she heard me say no to her, she did not say anything back to me and just entered the data into the computer to deposit my checks for me. After she finished depositing my check in my checking account, I went over to one of the bankers and explained to them I was doing a lot of study on human allergies and sickness and I was also studying the types of things that caused the people to sneeze. Most of the people never thought of the right reasons that made them sneeze. They liked to blame on the things that they saw in front of them after they sneezed. I was not happy that the bank clerk had accused me that the dog hair on my jacket made her sneeze. The jacket that I was wearing had been washed and dried many times. There were still a few dog hair stuck on my jacket, but they were no longer having any particles that would make people sneeze. The actual reason the bank clerk sneezed was either the dirt on the counter desk flew into her nose when she picked up the checks from the counter or cold air blew in from outside when the customers opened the bank entrance door. If she got sick after this sneezing, I could presume that she did not have enough resistance to the cold air that blew in from outside when the customers opened the door to come in or go out. I was home all this year with my two dogs. Their hair and their bodies' odor were all over my house. Their hair and bodies' odor never disturbed me at home to make me to get sick or sneeze. I did not believe all those dogs and their hair could cause any allergy to mankind. Maybe they could make the people get a tickle-type of itch when their hair contacted with the people's noses, but they could never cause the people to be exposed to any allergy. But some animals were having a strong bad odor just like human beings were having a bad odor on their body in the hot weather. Maybe sometimes their odor would make you feel dizzy and throw up, but they would never make you sneeze. I studied very carefully about the type of things that would make me sneeze at home. Sometime I sneezed so badly when the cold air blew in from outside when I opened my windows. I had to close my windows right away, and then I stopped sneezing. Sometimes when I sat on my sofa, I suddenly felt cold. I sneezed for about fifteen minutes and then stopped. A lot of fluid came out from my nose. Sometimes tears came out from my eyes after I sneezed a lot when I came in from my garage in winter time. Sometimes when I poured red pepper powder in my food, I sneezed when I smelled the pepper scent. It did not make any sense to accuse the object that did not even have the ability to make the people sneeze. I like to advise all people to learn to find out the truth what is really causing them to sneeze before they accuse anything. I hated it so much when I heard the allergy doctors accusing the dog's hair for causing the bad allergies after the dog owners had the allergy skin test. Then the doctor would recommend the dog owners to get rid of their beloved pets. It was a very unprofessional technique for the doctors to ask the pet owners to get rid of their beloved pets. If there are objects that could really make us sneeze or get a bad allergy, we would not be able to stop sneezing, as long as those objects were around us in our environment. We should get rid of those objects from our environment. I was getting very frustrated because every time when I asked my neighbor to get rid of their bad allergic birch tree, they refused to get rid of it. If they do not get rid of it, then the allergies and sickness would stay in our environment forever. I could not do anything, except to move out from this house or take my neighbor to court, so that the court would order them to cut their bad white birch tree.

Dr. Sara called me on December 17, 2008, after she reviewed my CAT scan X-ray film to inform me that my left ear was infected badly. My surrounding ear bone and eardrum were infected badly. She said I had to have surgery performed on my left ear to clean all of the infectious area inside my left ear and get the eardrum replaced. I requested her to do the surgery as soon as possible. She said she had no control of scheduling the ear surgery, but she would let the surgery scheduler to schedule my ear surgery as soon as possible. She said that the surgery scheduler would call me to inform me the date for my ear surgery. I said OK and hung up the phone. Then I remembered every time my father went to the salon shop, he took me with him to cut my hair when I was very young. I had seen the barber in the salon shop put a few drops of liquid from a small bottle inside my father's ears and allowed it to stay inside his ears for a few minutes. Then the barber would cut my father's hair. After he finished cutting my father's hair, he would clean my father's ear discharge. I believed the liquid that the barber used in my father's ears was hydrogen peroxide. I decided to try and use 3 percent hydrogen peroxide liquid to clean my left infectious ear daily, while I waited for my ear surgery. When I used 3 percent hydrogen peroxide liquid to clean my left infectious ear, it seemed like I had got a good result. The infection in my left ear was getting better. The black and yellow fluid from my left ear reduced. I felt very comfortable and I could hear well after I used hydrogen peroxide to clean my left infectious ear. I continuously used 3 percent hydrogen peroxide liquid to clean my left infectious ear during the time I was waiting for my ear surgery.

On December 31, 2008, I went to Pleasanton KPMC adult medicine clinic at 3:30 p.m. for my first checkup with Dr. Jennifer. After I checked in with the front desk clerk, I went across the clinic hallway and knocked on the clinic door. The nurse came out and I handed my payment receipt slip to her. She took it and told me Dr. Jennifer was with another patient. She asked me to wait in the waiting room. I said OK, and she closed the door. While I was waiting for my doctor, I decided to go to the restroom, so I went outside the hallway to the restroom. After I came back, one of the patients told me the nurse had been calling me to go in. So I knocked on the door again; the nurse came out and took me inside the clinic. She measured my blood pressure and my pulse. Then she took my weight. After she was done, she took me inside the small room to wait for Dr. Jennifer. After I stayed inside the room for a while, I did not feel like waiting inside the room, so I went out to the hallway. Then I saw a girl coming out from another patient room next to my room. When she saw me, she said she would be with me shortly. I said OK to her and went back to the patient room. I presumed she must be Dr. Jennifer. She was so little and very active. I stayed inside the room for a while. I felt I could not sit there waiting for my doctor, so I got up and went back out to the clinic hallway. I looked at all the plants' pictures hanging on the wall. I saw one of the plants' pictures on the wall was of the plant that I was looking for a long time ago, so I went to one of the nurses and asked her for the name of the plant on the wall picture. She said she did not know the plant's name. I told her I had a lot of that kind of plants in my house, but I did not know their name. Then I went back to the patient room to wait for my doctor. After a while, Dr. Jennifer came in the room and checked my medical records on the computer, and she asked me some questions that she needed to know from me and entered all the information in her computer. I told her about my allergies that I had got from my neighbor's white birch trees and that I had taken Claritin allergy medicine for my allergies. I also told her I had taken antibiotic medicines at home to protect myself, besides the medicines that the doctor had prescribed me to take when I got bad allergies and sickness from my neighbor's birch tree. I also told her I needed to get my left infectious ear operated, but Dr. Sara had told me I needed to wait for another four months to wait for my turn for my left infectious ear to be operated. I mentioned to her, while I was waiting for my ear surgery, that I had used hydrogen peroxide to clean my left infectious ear and it seemed like it was getting better. She told me to call Dr. Sara again to check for my surgery date. I told her that when I had requested Dr. Sara to operate my left infectious ear in a short period of time, she told me she could not control the scheduling of the surgery and the surgery scheduler would call me to inform me my ear surgery date. But Dr. Jennifer insisted to me to call Dr. Sara again to set up another appointment to see her. I said OK. After she finished reviewing my records and checked up on me, I told her I had a lot of pain in my right chin, the right side of my chest, my back, and my right stomach. The bottom part of my ribs seemed like it was being pulled down with the weight of my body every time I carried stuff over ten pounds. She asked me to lie down on the patient bed. She tried to press the right side of the ribs to locate the actual pain there. Then she referred me to take a blood sample test with fasting and to checkup with her after three months. I told her I had not eaten anything except water since last night and I could take a blood test after she released me. She asked me when I had eaten my last meal yesterday. I told her 8:00 p.m. She said I could go to the laboratory department to get my blood sample drawn. Then she released me.

I went to the laboratory department in South One KPMC building. When I reached there, I went inside the laboratory. I saw there were a few patients inside the laboratory. I took the number slip and waited for my turn to check in with the front desk clerk. I saw Grace was standing at the front desk. I went to her and asked her to draw my blood sample for me. She said yes to me. When the front desk clerk called my number, I checked in with the front desk clerk. Then I went to the blood withdrawal room, peaking inside; when Grace saw me standing in front of the blood withdrawal room entrance, she asked me to go inside the room and sit down on a chair while she took care of another patient. After a while she was done with the patient and was labeling blood sample tubes. I told her how she had hurt my hand last time when she pressed my hand with force and that I did not want her to hurt me again. She laughed. At that time, another technician came to me to draw my blood sample. I was so afraid to let that technician draw my blood sample, because I was afraid she would repeatedly inject the needle in my veins without getting any blood sample from my hand. My bad allergies were causing my blood to become very thick. It was very hard to draw the blood sample from my arm. I knew Grace was very good at drawing the blood sample from my hand, so I turned to her to ask her to do it for me. She said yes to me and asked me to wait for a while. After she finished labeling the patient's blood sample, she came to me and warmed up my hand with a small warmer plastic bag for a few minutes. Then she drew my blood sample from my hand. I remembered she was the one who had told me before that I would have to stick with them for a long time when I first came to this laboratory. After she was done drawing my blood sample, she showed me the picture that she had taken with two red-haired monkeys in Philippines. Both the monkeys were so cute. I told her about how African people kept killing big gorillas and elephants in Congo. They had almost killed all the beautiful gorillas, elephants, and other species in Congo, Africa. The African people were making the biggest mistake in kill all those animals in the jungles, because the safari in Africa was the only one left in the whole world. They should value their jungles, and this was a very good resource for them in attracting a lot of tourists to visit their country. Then I gave Grace back her pictures and left KPMC and went to 99 Ranch supermarket. The supermarket was very crowded and full of shoppers on that day. I bought some food from the restaurant to take home. After I was home, I prepared food for my New Year's Eve dinner. After midnight, I called my children and my sisters, wishing them the best in the coming New Year of 2009.

On January 1, 2009, I woke up at 7:30 a.m. I felt very fresh. I let the dogs out into my backyard. Then I made a cup of hot tea for myself. After I had drunk the tea, I prepared food for my children, who were coming home to have lunch. My children were home after 12:15 p.m. They asked me whether I would like to eat out to celebrate New Year in the restaurant. I said no because food was almost ready, as I had prepared all the food and had been waiting for them to come home and eat. All the dishes were done. I asked them to eat since they were hungry when they came home. They ate and enjoyed the food very much. Shaun helped me clean the kitchen after he was done with his lunch. Sirena had a sore throat and was sick. I gave her some antibiotic medicine and let her rest in the family room. Then I made pizza for dinner. After they ate their dinner, they went home. On January 2, 2009, Shaun called me in the morning. He offered to buy rice for me in Costco store when he came home the next time. I asked him not to go to Costco to buy rice himself, as I wanted to go with him when he came home. Then I called my ear doctor Dr. Sara's office on January 6, 2009, to leave a message with her assistant to call me back. Then I realized I had forgotten to check with Dr. Jennifer about my blood test result when I was in her office. So I called and left a message with Dr. Jennifer to call me back. Dr. Jennifer's assistant called me back at 2:00 p.m. and informed me that Dr. Jennifer had received my blood test result and she had already sent out a copy to me yesterday. Then I told her I wanted to know about my health, as I had forgotten to ask my doctor when I was there. She said she would check with Dr. Jennifer and call me back. After half an hour, she called me back and told me that Dr. Jennifer would let me know if there was anything wrong with me. I thanked her and hung up my phone.

I received my blood test result dated January 5, 2009, from Dr. Jennifer on January 10, 2009. My diabetic data had gone down from

6.6 percent to 6.3 percent. My glucose fasting data had gone down from 135 mg/dl to 101 mg/dl within three months. This was the first time my glucose fasting data showed 101 mg/dl after I got my allergy for so many years. When I reviewed and compared all my data of diabetic HGBA1c and LDL cholesterol from the blood test result data chart, the data from the chart indicated that my allergy from the birch trees had caused me to get diabetes. My diabetic data and LDL cholesterol data had gone up really high and made me sick at the time I had got the bad allergy in my house. I had to keep taking the allergy medicines and stay inside my house. When I did not get enough exercise inside my house, my triglyceride data went up really high. After I reviewed all my blood test results and compared all the data from the chart, I decided to check up my eyes' vision. I had not gone to check my eyes since last time when Dr. Ma referred me to check my eyes. It was too late for me to call Pleasanton KPMC optometry department to set up an appointment for my eyes' checkup. I called Holly to tell her about my blood test. She told me some people had diabetic data over 9 percent. I told her my diabetic data had gone up to 6.7 percent when I got the bad allergy on my hands. I took antibiotic pills as soon as I got a bad allergy and got sick. Last time I tried not to take antibiotic pills when I got the bad allergy. My body was heated up and it made me very sick. I had to take antibiotic pills to get rid of my sickness.

On January 12, 2009, I went to Safeway supermarket to buy groceries at 9:00 a.m. After I came back home and put away all my groceries, I felt pain in my back. So I sat down on my sofa and rested. Then I turned on my television. I could not see the television screen clearly. I felt my eye vision was lost. So I called Pleasanton KPMC optometry department to set up an appointment with Dr. Debra A. on January 20, 2009, at 1:50 p.m. I told the operator that Dr. Ma had referred me to set up the appointment to check my eyes, because of my high diabetic data. When the operator heard about my diabetes, she told me I should set up an appointment with Dr. Huang for my red eye ophthalmology test. I said OK; then she set up an appointment with Dr. Huang on February 9, 2009, at 2:50 p.m. for me. Because I did not know what kind of test was the red eye ophthalmology test, I called the optometry department many times to find out what it was. Finally, I understood what the red eye ophthalmology test was after the operator explained to me. The test was to check whether I had diseases in my eyes since I had high diabetes.

I went to checkup with Dr. Debra at 1:50 p.m. on January 20, 2009. Dr. Debra examined my eye pressure. She said my eye pressure was good. She used her eye checking machine to test my eyesight. I could see the alphabet letters very clearly on the first and second lines, but it was not bright enough to look at those alphabet letters. I felt my eyes were very uncomfortable and did not show brightness like before. The brightness changed when I looked at the projected alphabet letters on the wall. I could see the letters on the third line, but I could not distinguish what the letters were. Each time I went in to check up my eyes, I could understand the brightness of the letters when the doctor switched the rows of the letters, but this time, I felt the brightness was not changed. I told Dr. Debra that the brightness of the letters was no different. She said she would start all over again and ask me to read the projected letters on the wall. Then she asked me to read the alphabet letters again. After she was done checking my eyesight, she said my eyesight had increased only a little bit. She wrote down the measurements of my eyesight on the spectacle prescription paper and gave it to me. Then I asked her whether I should see Dr. Huang to check up my eyes. She recommended me to see Dr. Huang to take an ophthalmology test to make sure my eyes were OK. I thanked her and asked her whether I needed to change my eyeglasses with her spectacle prescription since my eyesight had not increased much at this time. She said my eyeglasses were still good, and I did not need to get a new pair of eyeglasses if I felt I could still use the eyeglasses that I had. After Dr. Debra was done with me, she released me. I left her clinic and went home.

I got a call from the Walnut Creek KPMC surgery scheduler on January 20, 2009, to ask me if I could come in for my left ear surgery the next day in Walnut Creek Kaiser Permanente Hospital, because one of Dr. Sara's patients had cancelled the surgery on January 21, 2009, and she wanted me to go in for surgery on my left infectious ear the next day. But I had not done any preparation for my ear surgery and I did not know how to go to Walnut Creek and Antioch KPMC, so I told the surgery scheduler I did not know how to go to Walnut Creek Kaiser Permanente Hospital. The surgery scheduler told me to go in Antioch Kaiser Permanente Hospital on January 29, 2009, to get my ear surgery done. I told her I did not know how to go to Antioch Kaiser Permanente Hospital either. I requested the surgery scheduler to let me see Dr. Sara before my ear surgery. The surgery scheduler asked me to go to Walnut Creek Kaiser Permanente Hospital to see Dr. Sara right away in the evening. But I refused to go in, because I did not know how to go to Walnut Creek Kaiser Permanente Hospital. I told the surgery scheduler that I did not know how to go to both hospitals. I told the surgery scheduler that if she had called me a few days earlier, I would have called my daughter Sirena to take me to the hospital. But I requested her to let me see Dr. Sara to check my left ear first before she performed ear surgery because I had been using hydrogen peroxide to clean my left ear every day and my left infectious ear was getting a little bit better. The fluid from my left ear had stopped flowing out. The surgery scheduler advised me to call Dr. Sara's clinic to set up an appointment for the day I could go in to see Dr. Sara. I said OK and hung up the phone. Then I left a text message to Sirena to, asking her whether she could take me to the Walnut Creek KPMC. Sirena did not call me back right away.

On February 4, 2009, the nurse from the KPMC optometry department called me to cancel Dr. Huang's appointment on February 7, 2009, and rescheduled my appointment with him on March 4, 2009. She said Dr. Huang had to go to a meeting on February 7, 2009, so he would not be able to see me. I said OK to her and hung up the phone. Then the nurse called me back to tell me I could just take pictures of my eyes without seeing the doctor. I did not know which was which. I just said OK to her to take pictures of my eyes and set up the appointment on February 17, 2009, at 1:30 p.m. Then she said if I accepted to take pictures of my eyes, I did not need to see Dr. Huang, and she would help me cancel the appointment on March 4, 2009, with Dr. Huang. Since I did not know the procedure of how they took the eyes' pictures and how they reviewed them, I requested the nurse to take a decision for me. The nurse advised me to go into the optometry department on February 17, 2009, to find out how they took the pictures of my eyes and asked me to keep the appointment date with Dr. Huang on March 4, 2009.

After I talked to the nurse from the ophthalmology department, I called the head and neck surgery clinic to leave a message to Dr. Sara for setting up an appointment to check up my left ear. But no one called me back from the head and neck surgery clinic to schedule my appointment to see Dr. Sara. I called Pleasanton KPMC head and neck surgery clinic on February 11, 2009, to set up an appointment again with Dr. Sara. The clerk at the head and neck surgery clinic picked up the phone. I told the clerk I wanted to set up an appointment with Dr. Sara to check up my ears. I also mentioned to her that I had heard my left eardrum making a flipping sound in my left ear last night, just like the flipping sound of my new eardrum after it was replaced fourteen years ago. If it was unnecessary to perform the ear surgery, I did not want to get it done. I wanted the doctor to look at my ear to make sure I really needed to operate my ear. So the clerk scheduled my appointment on March 19, 2009, to see Dr. Sara in Walnut Creek KPMC head and neck surgery clinic, but I requested her to schedule my appointment with Dr. Sara in Pleasanton KPMC. She told me Dr. Sara would not be in Pleasanton until June. If I wanted to see Dr. Sara, I had to go to Walnut Creek KPMC head and neck surgery clinic. Since I did not know how to go to Walnut Creek, I told the scheduling clerk that I would wait till she came back to Pleasanton. So I cancelled my March 19, 2009, appointment with Dr. Sara.

On February 17, 2009, at 1:30 p.m., I went to Pleasanton KPMC ophthalmology department. I met the medical assistant, Lydia. Lydia told me I had to choose whether I wanted the pictures of my eyes taken with the computerized camera machine or to checkup with Dr. Huang. I told her I did not know which would be the best for me to do. Then I asked her if taking pictures were better than seeing the doctor. She said it did not make any difference in taking pictures or seeing the doctor, but if I took my eyes' pictures, it would be kept in my medical record files, and these eyes' pictures could detect all the diseases in my eyes. Then she told me if I accepted pictures to be taken of my eyes, I had to cancel my appointment with Dr. Huang. I told her I had checked with my eye specialist Dr. Debra, and she had recommended me to see Dr. Huang to make sure my eyes were OK. Lydia said Dr. Debra would give me the same answer if I asked Dr. Debra now. She advised me to go into Dr. Debra's office to ask her whether I should choose to take my eyes' pictures or to see Dr. Huang. I said OK. She went into Dr. Debra's office to get her for me. Dr. Debra came out from her office with Lydia and told me if I accepted my eyes' pictures be taken I did not need to see Dr. Huang. I told her I accepted pictures being taken of my eyes. Then she asked me to sit in front of the computerized camera. After I sat in front of the camera, my eyeballs could be seen on the computer screen. I saw my eyeballs on the computer screen. I was scared to see my eyeballs moving around on the computer screen. Then she asked me again to make sure I would allow her take the pictures. She said if I allowed her to take pictures, I had to cancel my appointment with Dr. Huang. I said OK to her for canceling the appointment with Dr. Huang on March 4, 2009. She cancelled the appointment with Dr. Huang for me. Then she advised me not to move my eyes and just look at the camera. She carefully screened both my eyes and took pictures of my eyes at different positions. After she was done, she showed me both my eyeballs on the computer screen and said it did not show anything wrong with my eyes. Then she told me after the doctor reviewed my eyes' pictures on the computer, the doctor would send out the results to me within seven to fourteen days. I said OK and thanked her. Before I left, I asked her again to make sure I did not need to see Dr. Huang again. She said no and that if I needed to see the doctor they would let me know. Then I left. I met Dr. Debra in the hallway. She told me to make sure I understood the reason I did not need to see Dr. Huang anymore. I said yes to her. I told her I was very happy to hear nothing was wrong with my eyes. I said thanks and hugged both of them. Then I left the ophthalmology department and went home. After I reached home, I tried to call Sirena to let her know the good news about my eyes. After a couple of weeks, I received Dr. Wei Jiang's letter dated February 18, 2009, indicating that both my eyes had no sign of diabetic retinopathy at this time. He recommended me to repeat the screening test after two years. He reminded me to keep my diabetes low and to control my high blood pressure to minimize the chance of losing my eye vision due to diabetic retinopathy. After I got my eyes checked, I tried not to watch television all day long, because I did not want to ruin my eyesight. As usual, I went to my backyard to take care of my fruit plants in the morning. Sometimes I stayed outside in my backyard till noon to transfer my small plants to the big pots. Every day after I came in from outside, both my ears and lips would itch. I cleaned both my ears with 3 percent hydrogen peroxide liquid. I knew my left ear was infected badly again.

On February 26, 2009, after I worked outside my yard and came into my house, I went into my room and laid down on my bed. I felt both my ears were so itchy, and a lot of fluid was flowing out from my left ear. I turned my body to the left to move my right arm over my body to the left side to get the Q-tip cotton swab from the top of my CD player to clean my left ear. After I picked up the Q-tip cotton swab from the CD player, I tried to move my right arm back to the right side. Suddenly, I felt pain in my right shoulder. I could not move my right arm back to the right side. No matter how much I tried to move my right arm back to the right side, it did not work. My right shoulder had stiffened. So I pushed my right arm with my left hand back to the right side with force until my right arm was touching the surface of my bed. Then I tried to push away with my right hand the blanket out from my body to the right side. I could not lift up my right arm and my right hand. I had great pain in the nerves of my right shoulder, and my right shoulder had stiffened, causing great pain. I had push with my left hand the blanket out from my body to the right side. Then I flipped myself down from my bed to the floor until both my legs touched the ground. Then I got up from the floor. I went to the sink counter near my bathroom to get Advil 200 mg medicine bottle. I took out one tablet of Advil pill from the bottle and took it with water. Then I went back to lie down on my bed. I tried to test lifting up my right arm again and again, but I could not lift it. I gave up and just went to sleep. I could not sleep well. Next day, after I got up, I took Advil pain-reliever pills again and tried to adjust my right shoulder by rolling both my arms and exercising. After a few days, my right shoulder pain increased. I called Pleasanton KPMC adult medicine clinic to set up an appointment for my three-month follow-up appointment with Dr. Jennifer. The operator set up the appointment on April 13, 2009, for me. I told her I wanted to ask Dr. Jennifer whether I should take a blood sample test before or after I checked up with the doctor. The operator told me she would send the message to Dr. Jennifer and have her call me back and let me know. The medical assistant from Dr. Jennifer's clinic called me back the next day to tell me that Dr. Jennifer was not in the office and that she would check with her on Monday when she came back on Monday and that she would call me back after she talked to Dr. Jennifer. Then I told her I had got an accident on my right shoulder and I could not lift and move my right shoulder as it was very painful. She said she would call me back on Monday to instruct me what I should do with my shoulder after she talked to Dr. Jennifer. I said OK to her and hung up the phone.

On Sunday March 1, 2009, when Sirena came home, I told her I needed her to go with me to get some groceries from the supermarket because I had got an accident on my right shoulder and was in great pain and could not carry anything. She asked me whether I had called my doctor. I told her I had already called my doctor and the nurse told me she would call me back on Monday after she checked with Dr. Jennifer. Sirena took me to Safeway supermarket in Dublin and bought some groceries, and we came back home. She helped me to put away all the groceries and cooked dinner for both of us. After she was done cooking, we ate dinner together. Then she fed the dogs chicken and rice for me. Then she cleaned the kitchen. After she was done cleaning the kitchen, she went home at 7:00 p.m. I kept taking Advil pills every four hours to get rid of the pain in my right shoulder, but my pain did not go away. While I was waiting for my doctor to call me back, I applied low heat to my right shoulder with a heat pad, and slowly I moved around my right shoulder to exercise. As usual, I prepared food for myself. But on March 10, 2009, when I was cutting the chicken to prepare dinner for myself, my knife slipped and hurt my palm with the knife's holder. I had great pain in my palm, but I just ignored the accident. I finished cutting the chicken and put it away in my refrigerator. That night, I had great pain in my right palm. When I got up in the morning, I had severe pain in my right hand that I could not touch anything with my right hand.

On Wednesday, the nurse from Dr. Jennifer's clinic called me back in the evening to tell me that Dr. Jennifer wanted me to take a blood test first before I went in to see her. Then I asked her about the pain in my right shoulder and hand. She advised me to go to the minor injury clinic if I had a lot of pain, but it was too late for me to go to the minor injury clinic, so I decided to go in the next day if I did not get better. I took Advil pills again in the night. Next day after I woke up, I had great pain in the center of my right hand palm and I could not even touch or lift anything. With my left hand, I shifted the car gear and drove my car to Pleasanton KPMC minor injury clinic. Once I was in the minor injury clinic, I did not have to wait long to get to the front desk clerk that day, because there were only a few patients. I checked in with the front desk clerk. The front desk clerk asked me what had happened to me. I told her about my right shoulder and right palm injury. She asked me to checkup with the minor injury clinic head nurse first and asked me to go to the head nurse's room. I waited in front of the head nurse's room. After a while, the head nurse came and took me in her office. She asked me what had happened to me. I told her I had got an accidents and that I could not lift my right arm and also that I had a lot of pain in my right shoulder and right palm. She asked me how. I told her last Thursday night my right shoulder had stiffened when I tried to get a Q-tip cotton swab from the top of my CD player. I pushed my right hand with my left hand back to the right side with force. Then I stayed on my bed the whole night. Next day I exercised both my shoulders by rotating both my arms round and round to fix my right shoulder. I thought my right shoulder would be getting better and my pain would go away after I exercised my right shoulder. But the pain in my right shoulder and right middle palm did not go away. I could not lift or touch anything with my right hand. I explained to her that I had called my doctor and waited for her to call me back on Friday. The medical assistant from my doctor's office had not called me back until yesterday. The medical assistant instructed me to go to the minor injury clinic in Pleasanton KPMC, so I came here today. Then she asked me to lift up both my arms to check my right shoulder. I told her I had a lot of pain in my right shoulder when I lifted up both my arms. I also told her about the accident yesterday when I had used the knife to cut and chop the chicken. The knife slipped from my hand and hurt my right palm with the knife holder. After she checked my right shoulder and my right hand, she asked me to go to the front desk clerk to register first. Then she said she would have somebody take me to the radiology department to take an X-ray of my right shoulder and my right hand. I went to the front desk clerk to check in. After I checked in with the front desk clerk, the clerk asked me to go to the male employee that the head nurse had sent out, who would take me to the radiology department. I went to him. He asked me to sit on the wheelchair and took me to the radiology department to check in with the front desk clerk. After a while, the X-ray technician took me inside the X-ray room to take X-ray. After I was done taking X-ray, the nurse took me back to the minor injury department and settled me inside the clinic room, and she asked me to change into patient's clothes and wait for the doctor to come in and check up on me. After a while, Dr. Harold K. H. came inside the room and reviewed my right shoulder's X-ray on the computer screen. He told me my right shoulder joint was in place. Then he asked me how I had hurt myself. I told him about the incident of my stiff right shoulder that had happened on the night of February 26, 2009, and how I tried to fix myself at home after my shoulder was stiffened; instead of calling the ambulance to take me to the emergency clinic, I pushed my right arm all the way down to the bed with my left hand. I told him I could not lift anything with my right hand and my shoulder was in great pain. When I called Dr. Jennifer to inform her about my right shoulder's accident, the medical assistant instructed me to come in here. Then I told him about the accident on the center of my right palm and how painful it was. I could not lift or touch anything with my right hand. He asked me what kind of things I did. I did not know what he meant. I did not know how to answer his question. So I just said I did a housewife's jobs. I said housewife's jobs meant cooking, cleaning, and taking care of my house. Then I told him about my car accident and how my chiropractor had pushed my chest bone back in for me many times in the past when I had dislocated the bone on my chest after the car accident. I told him how I had pain in my right brain, my right chest, and my right swollen leg after my car accident; then I showed him my right chest bone and my right swollen leg.

Dr. Harold examined my right chest bone and my swollen leg; he advised me to see an orthopedic surgeon for my chest bone. He said he did not think an orthopedic surgeon would do any surgery on me. Then he asked me to stand in front of him and lift up both my arms and stretch my both arms horizontally, and he asked me to put up my thumbs. I did the way he instructed me to do. I told him I had great pain in my right thumb when he asked me to put my thumb up. I told him I felt just like a fat string pulling my thumb from my right arm. He told me there were two different kinds of injuries that I had got at this moment. He wanted me to call Dr. Jennifer to set up an appointment to see her within the next week. Then he told me to come back to the minor injury clinic after five days. He set up an appointment for me with the orthopedic doctor, Dr. Jodi R., on March 17, 2009, at 1:30 p.m. Then he asked me what type of pain-reliever pills that I was taking after the accident. I told him I was taking Advil pills. He said he would prescribe me three 200 mg of Advil pills, to be taken three times a day for three days at home. Then he asked me to change back into my regular clothing, and he went back to his office to prepare for the release statement. After he was done, he came back out and gave his release statement to me. I took the release statement from him and thanked him. The nurse from the minor injury clinic helped me to set up an appointment on March 23, 2009, at 9:45 a.m. with Dr. Jennifer. Then she released me. I could not use my right hand to shift my car gear because of the pain in my right hand palm. I used my left hand to shift my car gear and drove home slowly. After I was home, I stopped doing all my housework and yard work. I took 600 mg of Advil pills three times a day for three days as instructed by Dr. Harold. After three days, the pain in my right palm was reduced and I could touch and pick up small things with my right hand.

On March 17, 2009, at 1:30 p.m., I went back to Pleasanton KPMC minor injury clinic to checkup with the orthopedic doctor, Dr. Jodi. After I was in Dr. Jodi's clinic, he asked me about my shoulder's accident and how I had hurt myself. I told her the same things that I had told Dr. Harold. She checked and tested the movements in both my shoulders and my neck. Then she said she recommended me to checkup with the physical therapist a couple of times. She reminded me not to call her, and she wanted me to checkup with Dr. Jennifer first. If Dr. Jennifer would not recommend me to see a physical therapist, she would call me to set up an appointment for me to see the physical therapist. Then she prescribed me thirty tablets of Cyclobenzaprine Hydrochloride 10 mg pill to take one pill a day, and on her release statement, she asked me to take continuously 600 mg of Advil pills until all my pain was gone. Then she released me. I took the release statement paper from her. I thanked her and came out from the minor injury clinic. I went to Pleasanton KPMC South One pharmacy store to purchase thirty tablets of Cyclobenzaprine Hydrochloride 10 mg pill, and I went home. I took one tablet of Cyclobenzaprine Hydrochloride 10 mg pill a day and three Advil pills for three times a day as instructed by Dr. Jodi at home.

On March 23, 2009, I checked up with Dr. Jennifer in the adult medicine clinic. After Dr. Jennifer's medical assistant took me inside the patient room, he asked me how I had got the accident on my shoulder and right hand. I told her how my right shoulder had stiffened when I turned my body to the left to pick up the Q-tip from the top of my CD player and how I had fixed my right shoulder after I got up in the morning. After she was done reviewing my accident, she told me to wait for Dr. Jennifer. After a while, Dr. Jennifer came in and asked me to lift up both my arms to check my shoulders and to test my body positions. I told her I had pain in my right shoulder and my right palm. After she checked on me, she said my right arm and neck position was not right. She advised me to see a physical therapist. Then she mentioned about my appointment on April 13, 2009. I just said I'd keep it. Then she gave me the release statement and the physical therapy clinic telephone number for me to call and set up an appointment to see the physical therapist. After I arrived home, I called the physical therapy clinic to set up an appointment with Dr. Amy C. on April 6, 2009, at 2:00 p.m.

On April 6, 2009, I went to Pleasanton KPMC laboratory department at 12:30 p.m. to draw my blood sample. There were a lot of patients waiting inside the laboratory to draw blood for blood tests. I went inside the laboratory to take the number slip to check in for my turn. I waited for a while in the waiting room. The front desk clerk called me. I went to the front desk clerk to check in. I saw Grace was in the laboratory. I requested the clerk to let Grace draw my blood sample. The clerk said OK. After I checked in for my blood sample test, I waited in front of the laboratory entrance for Grace to call me in. After Grace finished helping the patient, she called me in to sit on the chair and helped me draw my blood sample. After she was done, I left Pleasanton KPMC South One building.

I went to KPMC physical therapy clinic. I had never been to KPMC physical therapy clinic. It took a while for me to drive around to locate the KPMC physical therapy clinic building. Finally, I found the physical therapy clinic building near Stonebridge mall. I parked my car in front of the physical therapy clinic building. I went inside the building. I saw the KPMC pharmacy store was in the first floor. I was still early to check in with my physical therapist's clinic. I went in the KPMC pharmacy store to look around. Then I saw potato chips on the shelf. I picked up a potato chip bag and went to the cashier to pay. The pharmacist Karen came out to the cashier register. I gave her my credit card to charge the potato chips. She refused to accept the credit card. I asked her why. She said the store had to pay the credit card company $0.60 for each transition for the customer's credit card. I was very surprised to hear what Karen told me. Then I remembered why the girl in the cafeteria of South One building charged me $0.25 more when I bought clam chowder soup from her. I told her I did not have any cash in my wallet. I put back the potato chips on the shelf. Then I went up to the third floor on the elevator to the physical therapy clinic. I checked in with the front desk clerk. She said I was an hour early and I could fill up the form to check in with her. I said OK and took the form from her. I filled in all the information in the form and turned in the form to the clerk. I sat in the waiting room for a while. I did not feel like waiting in the physical therapy clinic. I went back down to the first floor. I went to my car to get the change to buy potato chips in the pharmacy store. After I took the change from my car, I went back into the KPMC pharmacy store and bought the potato chips. I sat outside the clinic building and ate my potato chips. After a while, I did not feel like sitting outside the building to wait for my physical therapy appointment. I went back up to the third floor and waited in the waiting room for my physical therapist Dr. Amy to call me in. One of Dr. Amy's patients was supposed to be in the clinic at 1.30 p.m., but the patient had not shown up in the clinic yet. The front desk clerk told me the patient was supposed to be here at 1.30 p.m., and it was already fifteen minutes late. If the patient did not show up in another fifteen minutes, Dr. Amy would take me in. I said OK to her. But the lady patient showed up and checked in with her. Then the front desk clerk asked the lady patient to wait in the hallway. She went inside to inform Dr. Amy in her office. Dr. Amy came out and took the lady patient to the patient room. After she was done taking care of the lady patient, she came back out and took me inside the patient room. She reviewed the history of my accident with me. Then she took out one bundle of rubber strings in different colors and the instruction guideline paper folder. She took the first page out from the folder and guided me on how to follow the instructions starting from the first page for exercising my arms, shoulders, and hands. Then she took the bundle of rubber strings and asked me to go to the clinic door with her. She chose a green rubber string from the string bundle to hang on the door knob. She showed me the first step on how to use both my hands to pull and release the string from the door knob to exercise my hands and my shoulders. She suggested that I use the technique that she showed me to exercise my hands and my shoulders every day. Then she advised me to go down to the KPMC pharmacy store on the first floor to get a red rubber string for myself to exercise at home. She gave me all the guideline instruction papers and told me to follow the instruction step by step to exercise my hands and my shoulders. After she was done with me, she told me to come back after three weeks, but I suggested that she set up an appointment for four weeks, because I wanted to learn and slowly make my body to adopt the exercises that she had taught me. She said OK and discharged me. I went to the front desk clerk to set up my next appointment with Dr. Amy on May 13, 2009, at 1:30 p.m. Then I went down to the first floor and bought the red rubber string in the KPMC pharmacy store and went home.

After I reached home, I tied the red rubber string on the door knob in the hallway. Then I followed the technique given in the instruction papers that Dr. Amy had instructed me to use for exercising. I did the exercises with the rubber string twice a day, in the morning and in the evening. The first day I started with ten times each of pulling and releasing the rubber string with each of my hand in both directions first.

Then I used both my hands as showed in the guideline instruction papers to exercise back and forth for my arms and shoulders. I felt tired at first when I used the rubber string to exercise both my arms and shoulders. After a week, my body and both my arms and shoulders started getting ice-cold. I had to wear a long-sleeved sweatshirt every day to get rid of the coldness in my body, arms, and shoulders after I exercised. I slowly increased the number of times to pull and release the rubber string each week to build up both my arm muscles. I increased it to four times each week for pulling or releasing the rubber string, depending on how my arms and shoulders could adopt the exercises. These exercises helped me to adjust and balance my neck nerves, shoulders, and arms. After two weeks, pain in my right chin, neck, and shoulder were gone. I felt very comfortable in continue doing these exercises every day. When I exercised with the rubber string, I needed to be careful while pulling and releasing the rubber string; otherwise, I could hurt myself. I learned carefully to use these exercises to adjust my shoulders and body. I was very impressed with the doctor who had invented this technique to adjust and balance my neck nerves and tendons, arm muscles, and shoulders.

On April 13, 2009, I went to KPMC adult medicine clinic to checkup with Dr. Jennifer for my three-month follow-up checkup. She told me my blood test result was improving. She had already sent out a copy of my blood test result to my house. I told her that I had not received it yet. Then she recommended me to take fish oil 1,000 mg tablets to improve the joint movements in my body. Earlier, Dr. Ma had recommended me to take fish oil tablets, but I had refused to take them because I did not like the smell of fish in the fish oil tablets. After I got my joint accident, Dr. Jennifer insisted me that I should take fish oil tablets. She told me I should go to the pharmacy store to get 1,000 mg of fish oil tablets and take it every day. Then she advised me to come back after four weeks to check with the nurse and turn in the list of all the medications that I was taking till date and to get my body temperature, blood pressure, pulse, and weight taken, and then she released me. Her medical assistant helped me to set up the appointment on May 13, 2009, at 2:30 p.m. to come back to the clinic for doing the procedures as instructed by Dr. Jennifer. After I was done with Dr. Jennifer, I went to KPMC South Two pharmacy store to get one bottle of 1,000 mg fish oil tablets and went home. Once I reached home, I called KPMC adult medicine clinic to leave a message for Dr. Jennifer to check with her how many fish oil tablets I had to take each day. After I left a message for Dr. Jennifer, her assistant called me back in the evening and instructed me to take two fish oil tablets twice a day every day. I said OK to her and hung up the phone. I started to take two 1,000 mg fish oil tablets twice a day every day. Then I organized all the medicines that the doctors had prescribed me to take every day and listed them on a sheet of paper as follows:

Metformin Hydrochloride (1,000 mg)	2 tablets twice a day
Fexofenadine (60 mg)	2 tablets twice a day
Lovastatin (40 mg)	1 tablet once a day
Fish oil (1,000 mg)	4 tablets twice a day
Cyclobenzaprine Hydrochloride (10 mg)	1 tablet once a day
Advil (200 mg)*	*Take when needed
Tetracycline (250 mg)*	

- Since I had not received my blood test result from Dr. Jennifer through the mail, I called Pleasanton KPMC adult medicine clinic to leave a message for Dr. Jennifer, indicating that I had not received my blood test result through the mail as yet on April 28, 2009. I requested her to allow me to pick up my blood test result in her clinic. Next day, her assistant called me back and told me to go and pick up my blood test result in the clinic. I said OK. I told her I would come over that day to pick up my blood test result. After an hour, I prepared myself to go to Dr. Jennifer's clinic to pick up my blood test result. I went to Pleasanton KPMC adult medicine clinic. Once I was in Dr. Jennifer's clinic, I knocked on her clinic door. The nurse opened the door, and I told the nurse the reason I had come to the clinic. The nurse told me to check in with the front desk clerk to get a check-in statement first. So I went to the front desk clerk to get the check-in statement to pick up my blood test result from Dr. Jennifer. The clerk issued me the paperwork to check in with her clinic. I took the check-in paper to Dr. Jennifer's clinic and knocked on the door. The nurse opened the door. I gave my check-in paper to her. She took the check-in paper from me and took me inside the clinic. She helped me print out my recent blood test result from the computer and gave it to me. I took the blood test result, thanked her, and left the clinic and went home.

On May 6, 2009, Dave and Neal, two outside contractors, came to my house to audit and rate my house, telling me they would help me save my energy bill. When they called me, they mentioned the company name of PG&E. I thought they were the employees from PG&E and that PG&E had sent them out for auditing and rating their customer's energy bill to prevent leaking energy, so I responded to them and left my name and my telephone number on their answering machine to call me back. Next day, Dave called me back after I left a message on his answering machine. He informed me that he would come to my house next day and asked me to give him my home address. But when he asked me to give him my home address, I felt a little bit strange. If he was a PG&E employee, then why did he still need to ask me to give him my home address? I became suspicious of him. I refused to give my home address to him. Dave was very unhappy that I refused to give him my home address. He forced me to give my home address to him and asked me why I had left a message on his answering machine if I did not want him to come to my house. I told him I thought he was an employee from PG&E. Then he said he had just wanted to come to my house to look at my house and help me save my energy bill. Because he gave me enough reason for me to give out my home address to him, I gave him my home address. Dave called me the next morning again to ask me the directions to my house. He said he had tried to find my street on the Pleasanton map, but he could not find it. I gave them directions on how to come to my house. Dave then told me he had found my street on the map after I gave him the directions on how to come to my house. Then I hung up my phone, and I went outside to my front yard to water my plants while I waited for them to come. After half an hour, I saw a van stopping in front of my house. The driver got down from his van and told me his name was Dave, introducing himself to me. Then I took him in my house. I still believed he was the employee of PG&E. After he came into my house, I took him to my heater section to let him check out my heater, just like the last time when the employee from PG&E had come to my house five years ago to check on my heater. But he did not even look at my heater. It seemed like he was not interested to check on my heater like the employee from PG&E who had come to my house to check on my heater. I became very uncomfortable with him. At that time, another guy came and rang the doorbell. Dave opened the door for him to come into my house. He introduced him to me that he was his partner, Neal. Then Dave took out a small computer machine from his bag and looked around at the ventilation hooks in my house and tried to measure the data points from the ventilation hooks to the small computer machine. He said the data points of all my ventilation hooks that showed in the computer machine were really good. I did not know what he meant and what kind of results he wanted from my house. Then he asked me to show him the attic door to go up to the attic. I told him the attic door was in my room. He said he needed to get the ladder out from his car to go up to the attic. So he went outside to his car and took out the ladder from his car and brought it into my house. I took him to my room to show him the attic door. Neal also came in with us to my room. Then Dave climbed up the ladder and removed the attic door's cover. He used his flashlight to look at the attic. After a while, he came back down and put his ladder back in his car. Then he came back in. He took out a paper from his bag and wrote something on his paper. I did not know what he wrote on that paper. I was just looking at him, waiting for him to finish his writing. After he was done, he told me the total rating points of my house on his paper was forty points out of hundred points. I did not know what categories were in his paper and how he was rating to give out such points to my house, making the judgment on my house to tell me I had only got forty points out of hundred points. I asked him what kind of total rating points he was talking about. Dave did not give any answer or explanation to me. Then he asked me my monthly PG&E bill. I told them it was between eighty and hundred dollars during winter and forty and fifty dollars during summer. Then he told me he would help me save my PG&E bill and he wanted me to look at his experiment. Then he asked me to wait for a while. He went outside to his van and took out the insulation fabrics box, which had two divided sections and two electric lights. He brought them inside my house. He asked me where the electric wall outlet was that he could use for his experiment. I showed him the closest electric wall outlet in my living room. He put the insulation fabrics box and two electric lights near the wall outlet that I had showed him. He took out the box cover of the insulation fabrics box, which had two section holes, and assembled two electric lights on the box cover holes of the insulation fabrics box, and he put the box cover with the lights back on the insulation fabrics box. Then he attached two thermometers to each section of the walls outside the insulation fabrics box. He took out the electric wire hooker from the box. Then he connected the electric wire with the living room wall outlet. Then he told me to listen to his experiment. He started his conversation by telling me that both sections of the box had the same kind of insulation fabrics. But he covered the insulation fabrics in one section with an aluminum foil sheet and the insulation fabrics in another section without an aluminum foil sheet. He turned on the lights in both sections of the box. He asked me to concentrate on the temperatures of both thermometers after ten to fifteen minutes. He asked me to read the temperatures on the thermometers after fifteen minutes to compare the temperatures on both of them. He explained to me the temperature in the section with the insulation fabrics covered with an aluminum foil sheet was thirty degrees less than the temperature in the section in which insulation fabrics was not covered with an aluminum foil sheet. He said there was a thirty degrees difference in temperature in both thermometers of the box. I told him that I understood what he was trying to tell me, and this was just like we used the aluminum foil sheet to wrap the meat to protect it from getting burned when we baked the meat in the oven or when we barbecued the meat on the grill. Then Dave told me Neal was his boss. He asked Neal to give out his business card to me and asked him to talk to me about the aluminum foil sheet. Then Dave unassembled the lights from the insulation fabrics box and put all the accessories inside the tool bag. Then he took the insulation fabrics box and his tool bag from my house and put them in his van.

Neal talked to me to persuade me to put an aluminum foil sheet on my attic to save the energy bill. He said it would cost me around thirty-five hundred dollars if I put the aluminum foil sheet in my attic, and I would also get back one thousand dollars tax credit from the federal government for assembling the energy saver aluminum foil sheet in my attic. I told him I had to ask my son about it. Then he asked me to give him my son's name and telephone number so that he could talk to my son. But I gave him my son's name. I refused to let him have my son's telephone number. I told him my children were not living with me. But I would contact them and talk it over with them, and after we took a decision, if we wanted to put the aluminum foil sheet in my attic, I would have my son contact them. Neal said OK to me and told me they had to leave; he wanted me to call them after we had decided to put the aluminum foil sheet in my attic. I said OK. Then I stopped them and asked them to give me their rate sheet to review my energy bill. Dave said they never gave out their rate sheet to any customer. I insisted on him giving me a copy of the rate paper of my house so that I knew what kind of rating points he was talking about and what kind of things we needed to improve our home in order to save our energy bill. He said he did not have an extra sheet to give me. I told him I had a copy machine in my house to make a copy of his rate paper. Then he gave me his paper. I made a copy of their rate paper on my copy machine and gave it back to him. Dave took back their rate paper and left. I was afraid at first when Dave had called me to push me on the phone to give out my address to him. I felt much better after I saw him and his partner. They did not look like bad people. I had some confidence on them, and I was even joking with them. I studied their energy rate paper in the night and tried to understand how they were rating to give out the points on the rated paper to rate my house. Since I did not have any pool or computerized thermometer to read the temperatures inside my house, I did not get any point on that. I was not happy the way they were rating my house. I was very happy to have been living in this house for many decades as I had a roof to cover myself and my family, so I felt deep appreciation for the house that we lived in. I did not have any complaints about this house. I was very satisfied with the insulation that I had in my attic. If I put the aluminum foil sheet in my attic, the black moss would grow in my attic if water came in accidentally from the small open window in the attic. Then it would create more work for me and I would have to spend a bundle of money to replace the insulation fabrics in my attic. The aluminum foil sheet had the ability to absorb more coolness from outside and make my attic cooler in winter time. Then I would have to spend more money on my electricity bill in winter time. I realized Dave and Neal only wanted business to make money from me without giving any consideration of the cost of electricity bill for the whole year. I decided to find out more about them and why they had come out to my house to give out that kind of rating, making me very unhappy.

After a few days, I called PG&E to let them know about Dave and Neal and asked them who they were. PG&E told me they were not employees of PG&E and they were only outside contractors who were trying to get business from PG&E customers. I told PG&E that I was really amazed that they were using the PG&E name to sell their business to come to my house. I was displeased with the way they were rating my house. I also told them it was not a good idea to put aluminum foil sheets in the attic, because I did not want to spend more money later to replace the new insulation fabrics if a lot of black moss grew in the attic insulation fabrics. After I called PG&E, I called Dave and Neal back, but no one picked up the phone. I just had to leave a message on their answering machine to say thanks to them for coming by to rate my house. I let them know the reason I did not want to assemble the aluminum foil sheet in my attic.

On Sunday, May 10, 2009, I was very upset at my children when they came home after noon time, because one of the toilet pipes in my room was leaking, and I was not feeling good about fix the leaking toilet pipe in my room myself. I needed Shaun to help me fix the leaking toilet pipe. When I saw both of them come into the house, I screamed at both of them. Then I asked Shaun to fix the toilet pipe for me. Shaun went to Home Depot store to buy a new valve to replace the old one for my leaking toilet pipe. After he bought the valve, he came home and replaced the old valve with a new valve, fixing the leaking toilet pipe in my bathroom. After he changed the new valve, it was still leaking. He told me to keep an eye on the pipe until he came home the next time. He said if the pipe was still leaking, he would have to call the plumber to fix the toilet pipe. Then he went home after dinner in the evening.

On May 13, 2009, before I went to checkup with Dr. Amy, I went to Orchard Supply Hardware store first to find a valve for the leaking toilet pipe in my bathroom. I asked the employee at Orchard Supply Hardware store help me to get the right size of the valve for the leaking toilet pipe. He guided me to get the right size of the valve to fix the toilet leaking pipe in my house. I bought the regular size of valve that the employee at Orchard Supply Hardware store recommended me to buy. After I bought the valves for my toilet from Orchard Supply Hardware store, I went to Chase bank to deposit my check. After I was done depositing my money in the bank, I went to Dr. Amy's clinic at 1:15 p.m.

After I was in Dr. Army's clinic, I checked in with the front desk clerk. Then I waited in the waiting room for my doctor to call me in. While I was waiting, I got to know a lady who had fallen and got hurt badly six months ago. She asked me what was wrong with me. I told her about my car accident and my shoulder accident that I had got recently. I showed her my swollen legs. She asked me whether I had gone to see an acupuncture doctor to fix my swollen legs and body. I told her my brother was a doctor and he never recommended me to check with an acupuncture doctor to fix my body. He only recommended me to see a physical therapist to fix my body. Then she was telling me about her daughter and the pain that her daughter got in her neck after her car accident. Her daughter went to see an acupuncture doctor several times to get rid of the pain from her neck. I told her that her daughter must have got the minor pain in her neck after her car accident. I told her my lawyer had recommended me to checkup with a chiropractor to fix my body when I had my car accident, but my chiropractor and his associate doctors screwed up my body, making my right side of the body swell after one of his associate doctors pressed my back hard to level my spinal cord. When he could not fix my body, he told me he could not fix my body and he released me. I told her I did not know how and who could fix my swollen body. After she heard the story about my car accident, she just shook her head and said nothing to me.

Dr. Amy came out to take me into her office at 1:30 p.m. Then she asked me how I was doing. I told her I felt much better after I had used her technique to exercise my arms. I told her my body and both my arms had become very ice-cold after I did the exercises under her instruction after the first two weeks. I had to use a heat pad to get rid of the coldness that I got from my exercises. Then I felt very comfortable after the coldness was gone, and my muscles started getting stronger. But unfortunately I could not get rid of the pain in my right palm. The pain kept coming back in my right palm when I used my right hand to dig the ground with the digger. I also had a lot of pain in my neck after I worked outside in my yard again. She reminded me not to do any digging or lifting at home until I was totally getting better. She said that would hurt me more. I told her I did not have anybody to help me to do the jobs at home. If I needed to do it, I had to do it. Then she checked both my shoulders and asked me to put both my hands on my back. She asked me whether I had pain. I told her I did not have any pain at this moment. She asked me to take out the instruction papers that she had given me last time. I opened my folder to take out the instruction papers that she had given me last time. When she saw the list of the medicine papers that I prepared for Dr. Jennifer, she took the paper and read it. Then she told me to stop taking Cyclobenzaprine Hydrochloride 10 mg pill after I had finished all the tablets that I had. I said OK to her. Then she looked at my other medicines and asked me about my allergies. I told her I was getting bad allergies from my neighbor's white birch trees and

I was sick all the time. I also told her my allergies would be gone if my neighbor cut down his allergic birch tree and I did not need to take any more of these allergy medicines. But she said I needed to take Metformin Hydrochloride 1,000 mg pills continuously because my allergies had already damaged my body and the diabetes would always be there. I told her that I had got my diabetes when I tried to taste the birch flower fluid without knowing their chemical ingredients. I also told her how the diabetic medicine Metformin Hydrochloride 1,000 mg pills dried out my shoulders' joints and made them stiff. She shook her head, and she started using her yellow pen to highlight the techniques on the instruction paper for me to exercise. She indicated to me that she wanted me to do the exercises every day. Then she told me I was done with her and I did not need to make another appointment to see her again. I was happy to hear she had discharged me and thanked her. Then I left Dr. Amy's clinic.

I went to Pleasanton KPMC adult medicine clinic to checkup with Dr. Jennifer. I went to the front desk clerk to get the check-in statement. After I got the check-in statement from the front desk clerk, I went to Dr. Jennifer's clinic and knocked at the clinic door. The nurse opened the clinic door. I gave her my check-in statement and my medicine list paper that I was preparing for Dr. Jennifer. The nurse took my check-in statement and told me to hold on to my medicine list paper, asking me to wait for fifteen minutes in the waiting room. After fifteen minutes, the nurse came back out to take me inside the clinic, to measure my blood pressure and my pulse. My blood pressures were 130 and 84. My pulse was 115. The nurse told me my pulse was too high. She was not pleased to see my pulse above 100. She said the normal pulse should be below 100. I did not know what to tell her. I just said to her not to worry about me. I had been meditating to control my anger and frustration all these years. I told her, "When I get angry, I just cry out loud. I meditate myself at night to forget the anger and frustration that I have and leave them in the past. When I get up next day, I smile again." She said this was good for me and recommended me to keep doing my meditation. Then she advised me to set up an appointment to checkup with Dr. Jennifer after three months. Then she released me. I went to 99 Ranch supermarket in Dublin to buy groceries and went home. After I was home, I went to pick up my mails from my mailbox. I answered all my mails. I cooked and ate my dinner at 5:00 p.m. Then I went outside to my backyard to water my plants. After I came in from my backyard, I did not feel good, so I went to bed. Unfortunately, I woke up in the middle of the night and threw up badly. I was so sick. I took one antibiotic tablet and Advil pills, and then I went back to sleep. I remembered the nurse told me she was not happy with the pulse count that I had after she had measured my pulse count, which was above hundred when I was in Dr. Jennifer's clinic. I realized that the nurse already knew I would be getting very sick. But I did not call the doctor. I took an antibiotic medicine and Advil pills to overcome my sickness. I felt better after I woke up next day.

On May 15, 2009, I called Pleasanton KPMC head and neck surgery clinic to set up an appointment to see Dr. Sara for my left infectious ear. The scheduling clerk told me I had to go to Walnut Creek KPMC head and neck surgery clinic to checkup with Dr. Sara if I wanted to set up an appointment to see her. I asked the scheduling clerk when Dr. Sara would come back to Pleasanton KPMC head and neck surgery clinic. The scheduling clerk told me she would be back in July, but her appointment schedule was not open yet. The scheduling clerk asked me to call back the next week. I requested the scheduling clerk to leave a note for me to let Dr. Sara know that I would be the first patient to see her when she come back to Pleasanton KPMC head and neck surgery clinic. She said she would leave a note for me. I called back Pleasanton KPMC head and neck surgery clinic the following week. The scheduling clerk told me she was not sure whether Dr. Sara would come back to Pleasanton KPMC head and neck surgery clinic. She insisted on me seeing Dr. Sara at Walnut Creek facility. Since no one could drive me to Walnut Creek KPMC, I asked her whether there would be other doctors available for me in Pleasanton KPMC to check my left infectious ear. The clerk told me if I chose another doctor I could never go back to Dr. Sara again. I said OK. Then she gave me the names of Dr. Cornelius and Dr. Chin to me. I told her Dr. Cornelius did not take care of repeat ear surgery, so I chose Dr. Chin to set up an appointment on July 9, 2009, at 10:30 p.m. After I hung up the telephone, I felt very unhappy the way the scheduling clerk told me I could never go back to see Dr. Sara again. I was not happy the whole night. The more I thought about it, the more I got upset. So I called Holly to ask her why I could not see my doctor again if I switched to another doctor. She said all the doctors understood the patient's situation, and they would never get mad if the patients switched to another doctor because of the distance of the clinics. I still did not feel good. So I called back to the head and neck surgery clinic to cancel my appointment with Dr. Chin and rescheduled the appointment date on July 1, 2009, with Dr. Sara. Then the scheduling clerk asked me why I had not set up the date with Dr. Sara in June. I did not say anything to her. My reason for not seeing Dr. Sara in June was I continuously wanted to treat my left infectious ear with hydrogen peroxide. My left ear infection dried out after I treated the ear with hydrogen peroxide, but I felt that my ear was still swelling with the infection behind my eardrum. I wanted to continuously treat my left ear for one more month with hydrogen peroxide to clean the infection, and then I put a few drops more of hydrogen peroxide liquid in my left infectious ear and kept it inside my ear for more than four hours a day to treat it. I used a Q-tip cotton swab to clean all of the hydrogen peroxide liquid out from my left ear. Then I put Ciprodex otic suspension ear drops in my left ear and kept the medicine inside it for the whole night and let it drain out itself. It seemed like my ear infection was getting better. No black fluid was flowing out. When I used a Q-tip cotton swab to clean my ear, I found a lot of yellow thick fluid on the cotton swab. So I was a bit afraid my ear infection was not totally gone. This was the reason I requested Dr. Sara to look at my left ear. Hopefully I did not have to go through ear surgery. Since I had gone through so many accidents in the past, I was afraid to drive my car out from the city of Pleasanton. I called Sirena and Shaun and asked them to take me to Walnut Creek KPMC head and neck surgery clinic to checkup with Dr. Sara. Both my children came home on Sunday, May 24, 2009. Sirena told me she would take me to see Dr. Sara on July 1, 2009. I said OK to her. Sirena's and Shaun's birthdays were only nine days apart. I usually celebrated their birthdays together every year. When they were young, I usually invited a lot of their friends to our house to celebrate their birthdays together. After they both graduated from the universities, I did not arrange any more birthday parties for them. I took both of them out to the restaurant to celebrate their birthdays together with me this year.

On June 15, 2009, I called Pleasanton KPMC adult medicine clinic to set up an appointment with Dr. Jennifer for my three-month checkup on July 15, 2009. On July 1, 2009, Sirena came home at 10:00 a.m. to take me to Walnut Creek KPMC to see Dr. Sara in the head and neck surgery clinic. She was very busy. She had been talking on the phone since she had arrived home. Even when we arrived in the KPMC head and neck surgery clinic's waiting room, she was still on the phone, talking to her clients. Dr. Sara's assistant came out at 11:20 a.m. and took me inside the patient room, asking me to wait for Dr. Sara. After a while, Dr. Sara came in and checked both my ears. She tested my hearing in both my ears with a tuning fork. She said my hearing in my left ear was not much different from my right ear. Then she checked my left ear. She pulled out small pieces of hard shell from my left ear. Then she said she still recommended me to do the surgery in my left ear. She said this was the best way for me to get rid of the infection totally from my left ear and it would make my hearing get better. I agreed with her and said OK. I told her that my glucose fasting data had dropped to 115 mg/dl, but was still above the normal data range. I told her if I had to do the surgery on my left ear, I'd like to do the surgery in the second week of August after I came back from Philadelphia. I told her in the first week of August I would be in Philadelphia and would be back on August 9. Then she checked on my left ear again and asked me whether I wanted to wait for another six months. I said OK, I'd wait for another six months, since I wanted to make sure my glucose fasting data went down to the normal data range before my surgery took place. She wrote a note on her business card, asking me to call her back in December to set up for a January 2010 appointment. I took her business card from her and thanked her. I came out from her clinic. I met Sirena outside the hallway, and then I remembered I did not have any Ciprodex otic suspension ear drops at home, so I went back to Dr. Sara's clinic. But her assistant stopped me in the hallway. I told her assistant that I wanted to ask Dr. Sara to prescribe the ear drop medicine for me. She told me to wait in the hallway and went inside the clinic to let Dr. Sara know that I wanted to talk to her. After a few minutes, Dr. Sara came out to see me. I requested her to prescribe Ciprodex otic suspension ear drops medicine that Dr. Cornelius had prescribed for me before. She said OK and left. Sirena dropped me home and went back to work. Next day, I called Pleasanton KPMC South Two pharmacy store to mail Ciprodex otic suspension ear drop medicine to my house. After a week, I received the ear drop medicine from KPMC pharmacy store in the mail. I started continuously using it every morning and night. I tried to clean my left ear with hydrogen peroxide in the morning, and at night, before I went to sleep, I applied a few drops of Ciprodex otic suspension ear drops in my left ear after I cleaned it with hydrogen peroxide. I left Ciprodex otic suspension ear drop liquid in my left ear and let the liquid flow out itself. Early in the morning, I found a lot of yellow fluid flowing out from my left ear. I used the Q-tip cotton swab to clean out all the yellow fluid from my left ear. I applied hydrogen peroxide solution and Ciprodex otic suspension ear drop inside my left ear alternately to control my left infectious ear so that it wouldn't get worse.

On July 7, 2009, I went to Pleasanton KPMC laboratory department at 12:30 p.m. I checked in with the front desk clerk. I asked the clerk where Grace was. The front desk clerk told me Grace was off and he would draw the blood sample for me. I had not seen him before in that laboratory. I asked him whether he was a new technician. He said he was not a new technician here. I was not sure he could draw my blood sample smoothly. So I told him he was not allowed to draw my blood sample more than once. He said he could do it and asked me to wait for a while for him to finish what he was doing. After he was done, he went inside the laboratory. A few minutes later, a black lady clerk came out to take care of me. After she was done, she asked me to wait in front of the laboratory room. I did not have to wait very long. The technician called me and took me inside the laboratory room and asked me to sit down on a chair. After a while, the technician that I had met in the front desk came out and drew a blood sample for me. I told the technician to take my blood sample from my right hand instead of the right arm because no technician had successfully drawn blood from my right arm before. So he shifted to my right hand and tied my right hand with a rubber string. I asked him again whether he could really draw my blood sample. He said yes to me. I told him to make sure he would do it one time only and he was not allowed to repeat it again because I did not have any confidence in him. I told him if he repeatedly did it, I would use my finger to hit his head. I bent my first finger to show him with action of hitting his head. He said he would try his best to help me and left. Then another technician came to me and released the rubber string from my hand, and I told him the same thing. He said he would try to draw my blood sample, and then he left again. I sat there and waited for them to come out to draw my blood sample. After a while, another old female technician came to me. This female technician seemed like a very experienced senior technician. I advised her to draw blood sample from my left hand. She said OK. She flattened my left hand and then pushed the needle into my left hand without any hesitation. I saw a lot of blood coming out from the small plastic pipe into the test tube. After she collected the first test tube, she changed to another test tube to collect another bottle of my blood sample. I could tell she was a very experienced technician. She drew two small test tubes of my blood samples from my left hand successfully. I did not feel any pain in my left hand. She put cotton and a tape on my left hand and told me I was done. I left the laboratory department happily as I did not have to repeatedly draw my blood sample and went home.

On July 15, 2009, I went to Pleasanton KPMC adult medicine clinic for my appointment with Dr. Jennifer at 11:15 a.m. After I was in Pleasanton KPMC, I checked in with the front desk clerk, and then I went to the patients' waiting room, waiting for Dr. Jennifer's medical assistant to call me in. After half an hour, Dr. Jennifer's assistant came out and took me inside the clinic to measure my pulse, my blood pressure, and my weight as usual. Then she took me into the patient's room to wait for Dr. Jennifer. After a while, Dr. Jennifer came inside the room. She told me she had already sent out my blood test result to my house as usual. She said my blood test result was good, and all the data were within the normal data range. Then she asked me how I was doing. I told her I was still getting bad allergies from my neighbor's birch tree as usual. My ears and my lips were itching all the time and I had swelling in my legs. I was just recovering from my shoulder accident. She looked at my legs and said it did not look that bad. She insisted to me that I had to take the colorectal cancer screening test in Walnut Creek KPMC Gastroenterology department, and she set up an appointment for me with Nurse Joan Stanley on September 17, 2009, at 3:00 p.m. Then she told me I needed to get my blood sample test done in the laboratory department before my next visit with her. She set up an open date for me to go to the laboratory department to draw my blood sample. Then she asked me to come back for my follow-up checkup after three months. I said OK. I requested her to give me a copy of my blood sample test result again. The nurse helped me to print out the blood test result and gave it to me. I took my blood test result from the nurse and went home.

Chapter Four

Review Blood Test Results

After I received the wedding invitation card from my sister Susong for her daughter Sabrina's wedding in August 2009, I asked my children whether they would like to go to Sabrina's wedding in King of Prussia. Shaun suggested that all of us should go to Sabrina's wedding. After we discussed and we all agreed to go, Sirena told Shaun to buy the airline tickets for the three of us to go to Philadelphia for Sabrina's wedding. Sirena came home on Sunday to go to Stonebridge mall in Pleasanton with me to shop for our dresses that we were going to wear for my niece's wedding. We found the dresses that we liked to wear for the wedding in Macy's store; we bought them and went home. Sirena told me Shaun had already booked red-eye air tickets from United Airlines to go to Philadelphia from San Francisco airport on July 31, 2009. She told me Shaun would go to San Francisco airport and meet us there; she would pick me up at 7:00 p.m. to go to the airport. She asked me to get ready and pack all my clothing and presents that I needed to take to Philadelphia. I said OK to her. Then she told me she had already asked her friend to come and take care of the dogs twice a day for me when we were not home. I reminded her to tell her friend that it was very important to clean Lady Star's eyes every day, because her eyes would be covered with a hard layer of discharge. She needed somebody to clean her eyes every day for her, otherwise she could not see well. She said she would tell her friend to take care of Lady Star's eyes and asked me not to worry about them. I started to organize all my clothing and things that I needed for my daily use in King of Prussia. Then I took out my small CD player to replace the old batteries with the new ones, and then

I selected a couple of CDs that I would like to take with me. I kept them in my CD bag. Then I wrapped the green gemstone bracelet that I had bought for my niece Sabrina as her wedding present in wrapping paper. After I organized all my stuff to get ready for my trip to King of Prussia, I prepared fresh chicken and hamburgers for the dogs to be kept in the refrigerator for Sirena's friend to come and feed the dogs when I was away from home.

On July 31, 2009, Friday morning, I cleaned Lady Star's both eyes with wet tissues and applied antibiotic eyedrops in her eyes. I filled up water in the dog water bowl and put dried snack food in the special bowl that I usually kept in the kitchen for them to eat when they were hungry; even if no one would be home to feed them, they had enough dried snack food to eat for one week. Then I went outside to my backyard to water all my plants to make sure they got enough water while I was gone. Sirena came home at 6:00 p.m. from her work to take me to the airport. She told me Shaun would go to San Francisco airport by himself and would meet us at the United Airlines departure entrance in San Francisco airport. She had already informed her friend to come over to my house to take care of the dogs for me. I reminded Sirena to tell her friend to make sure she remembered to feed my three turtles in the garage water sink. Sirena asked me to put enough green vegetables in the water sink for three days for my turtles. After two days, she would come back home to take care of the turtles. Then she went in my room and checked my stuff, and when she saw my luggage bag was too small to put all my clothing in, she suggested that I take her bigger luggage bag to put all my clothing in; she said I would have more room to put more things in when I came back from King of Prussia, if I bought a lot of stuff there. I said OK to her. She took out all her clothing, books, and other stuff from her luggage bag, and she helped me to put all my stuff in her luggage bag. After she was done, she put all her stuff in my smaller luggage bag. After we were done arranging our luggage bags, Sirena took the luggage bags to my car and loaded them inside my car trunk. When my two dogs saw us moving around in and out the house, they became very excited; they both started crying loudly, making a lot of noises in the kitchen, and pushing the kitchen gate door to indicate that they wanted to go with us. Unfortunately, we were unable to take them with us to travel three thousand miles away to the East Coast. When I heard them crying, it was really very hard for me to leave them at home for nine days. Because they had been with me since Sirena had brought them home when they were four weeks old, I would miss them a lot. Then I came back in my house to check and make sure all my windows and doors were locked. I went to my garage to check on my three turtles to make sure they had enough food to eat while I was gone. I went back to the kitchen to say good-bye to my dogs and told them to behave. I heard Sirena calling me from outside and telling me that we had to go. I went outside to my garage and got inside the car. Then we went to San Francisco airport.

Sirena was using Bay Bridge to go to San Francisco airport, and it took more than an hour to arrive there. When we arrived in San Francisco airport, Sirena lost her way in the airport parking lot, and she had to drive a couple of times in and out from San Francisco airport to look for the airport parking lot. Finally she found the way to go into the airport parking lot; she drove into the parking lot and parked our car. Sirena unloaded our luggage bags from my car trunk; then we went to the entrance of the United Airlines departure section to meet with Shaun. Shaun was already waiting for us at the entrance of the departure section of United Airlines; as soon as he saw us, he came to us, asking us to get in line with other people. There were a lot of passengers already lining up for security check to get in the departure gate. I asked him while we were lining up for our security check where he had parked his car; he told me he had parked his car in his friend's house in San Francisco city. His friend had driven him to the airport and had dropped him in front of the United Airlines entrance.

Since the terror attacks in our country on September 11, 2001, United States federal government had set the rules and regulations for all the airports to provide security check on the passengers and their luggage bags before they were allowed to get in the departure gates. The security guards were standing at the gates, checking the passengers and their identification cards to make sure they were the right persons to travel before they allowed the passengers to go inside the departure gate. After they checked the passengers' identification cards, they allowed them to go in the luggage bags checking machine section for checking the passengers' luggage bags to make sure they did not carry any explosive fluids or devices on to the airplane. All the passengers moved slowly toward the security guards for their turns. Finally it was my turn. I approached one of the security guards; the security guard asked me to give him my driving license. I took out my driving license from my small purse and gave it to him. He took my driving license; then he looked at me, and matching the picture from my driving license, he asked me why I looked a lot younger than the picture on my driving license. I told him I was sixty-one years old and it was my picture on my driving license. It seemed like he did not believe me I was sixty-one years old, and he asked me which year I was born. I told him my birthday; he tried to match my birthday that I had told him to my driving license. Then he said OK and allowed me to go in the luggage bag checking section.

I went in, put my small CD bag on the counter, and waited for my children to help me load my luggage bag on the counter. After a while, I saw Sirena and Shaun come in, load their luggage bags on the counter, and take out all their jackets and their shoes from their bodies and put them in the airport buckets. Then they came to me to help me load my luggage bag on the counter; they asked me to take out my jacket and shoes and put them in the airport bucket. After I took out my jacket and shoes to put them in the airport bucket, they pushed all our luggage bags and the airport buckets from the rolling counter machines to the security guards to let them check. After the security guards checked our luggage, they asked us to go through the security gate to make sure we did not carry in any weapons or explosive materials on our bodies to the airplane. After we passed the security check, we went to the departure gate of United Airlines and waited for our flight to take off. We had to wait for half an hour in the departure gate. Shaun bought three bottles of drinking water for all of us inside the departure gate. I took one bottle of water from Shaun. I went to the restaurants near the departure gate to look around to see what kind of foods they were selling inside the airport. After I looked around, I came back and told Sirena that they only had ham sandwiches in the store. Then Sirena went out to the front section of the airport to get fried shrimps and fried vegetables in the Japanese restaurant and she came back. We waited patiently at the departure gate for more than half an hour for the flight attendant to announce that we would be allowed to go inside the airplane. At 10:15 p.m., the flight attendant finally announced that the passengers should get ready to go inside the airplane. We lined up with the other passengers to approach the flight attendant to check our air tickets.

We went inside the hallway after the flight attendant checked our air tickets and allowed us to go in. We passed the long hallway to get inside the airplane. There were not so many people ahead of us inside the airplane; this made it easy to find our seats. Shaun put all our luggage bags in the luggage cabinet shelves above our seats. Sirena asked me to get in first to sit on the seat that was next to the airplane window. After I was seated, Sirena got in the seat next to me. Shaun sat on the seat in front of us next to the window. The passengers got inside the airplane, put their luggage bags away in the luggage cabinet shelves above their seats, and sat on their seats. After all the passengers were seated and settled inside the airplane, a United Airlines flight attendant announced that the airplane was ready to take off exactly at 10:30 p.m. from San Francisco airport to Philadelphia airport. The airplane moved slowly out from the departure gate and took off. The weather was clear that night, and we felt asleep in the airplane. We woke up when we heard the flight attendant announce that the airplane would arrive in the Philadelphia airport soon, asking us to fasten our seat belts. We fastened our seat belts to get ready for the airplane to land in Philadelphia airport. After fifteen minutes, our airplane landed in the Philadelphia airport smoothly. It was a direct flight from San Francisco to Philadelphia, and we arrived in the airport in the morning.

We got out from the airplane and walked out from the arrival gate to pick up our luggage bags in the luggage pickup section; then we went out from the building to the outside sidewalk of the airport. We stood on the sidewalk for a few minutes, waiting for the airport bus to take us to the car rental section near the airport. There were many different rental companies in the airport; their buses moved in and out from their rental companies to the airport and from the airport to their rental companies. When Sirena saw the bus from Enterprise Car Rental drive in, she stopped the bus. As soon as the bus driver saw her, he stopped the bus in front of us, and we got inside the bus. The driver took us to Enterprise Car Rental. We got out from the bus and went inside the Enterprise Car Rental building. It was early in the morning, so there were only a few customers inside the building. Shaun asked us to sit down on the chairs in the waiting room, as both my legs were swollen quite a lot after I had been in the airplane for more than six hours. I sat down on the chair with Sirena. Shaun went to the counter to rent a car. After Shaun rented a car, the clerk from the rental car company took us to the rental car parking section next to the company to show us our white compact rental car. Shaun opened the car trunk and loaded all our luggage bags inside the car trunk, asking us to get inside the car. Once we were inside the car,

Shaun checked the fuel tank indicator; he found the fuel tank was almost empty. So he got out from the car and went back to the building to talk to the clerk about the fuel in the car. The clerk came out with Shaun and took him to another blue compact car next to the white compact car; she got inside the blue compact car and checked the fuel tank indicator. After she checked the blue compact car's fuel tank was full, she gave Shaun the key of the blue compact car and let Shaun take it. Shaun took the blue compact car's key from the clerk, gave her back the white compact car's key, and then he asked me and Sirena to get inside the car. After we got inside the blue compact car, Shaun drove the car carefully to the exit gate of Enterprise Car Rental. Then he stopped the car next to the exit gate and asked the guard about how to go to King of Prussia. The guard guided him to use Pennsylvania Turnpike to go to King of Prussia. Shaun thanked the guard, and he went on Pennsylvania Turnpike and drove carefully all the way to King of Prussia.

It was Saturday morning. I did not see too many cars on Pennsylvania Turnpike. When I looked up the sky, it was not a pleasant day; the sky was filled with scattered dark clouds, and it seemed like it was going to rain. Shaun took the King of Prussia exit to go directly to Susong's house. He told me that Susong wanted him to drop me in her house first before they went to check in for their rooms in the Crown hotel next to King of Prussia Plaza. When we arrived in front of Susong's house, we all got out from the car. I saw my sister Ivy Chow had just arrived and parked her car behind us. Then she got out from her car. I had not seen her since I had left King of Prussia in August 2001. She looked great. She said she was very happy to see us. Then she went to the front door of Susong's house to ring the doorbell. I saw Susong as she opened her front door and came out of the house; when she saw us, she invited us to go inside the house. She must have been very busy; she looked a bit older than before. We all went inside the house together. Shaun and Sirena came inside the house with my luggage bag. Susong asked Shaun to drop my luggage bag in my room upstairs. She went upstairs with Shaun to show him the room that I was going to stay for a couple weeks. Shaun left my luggage bag in my room; then he came back down with Susong.

I went in the kitchen and saw Margaret in the kitchen, cooking Burmese fish noodle soup for everybody. As soon as she saw us, she invited us to eat the soup. She was generally a good cook and enjoyed cooking different kind of foods in the kitchen. I sat on the kitchen chair facing the front door. I put both my legs up on another chair next to me. Both Sirena and Shaun came in the kitchen and sat on the opposite side of the kitchen table. Margaret brought the soup to the table for all of us. After Shaun and Sirena ate their Burmese fish noodle soup, they went to the Crown hotel to check into their rooms for the night.

After my children left, I went upstairs to my room and rested for a while. I took out the picture of my great-great-grandmother Phoebe Apperson Hearst and the old *Valley Times* newspaper from my luggage bag and I went to Susong's room. I saw both Margaret and Susong were sleeping in Susong's room. Margaret was asleep in Susong's bed. Susong was lying on her floor mattress; it seemed like she was very tired. They said they had slept late last night, preparing for the wedding. I gave Susong the old *Valley Times* newspaper to look at my chicken; then I told her to read the *Valley Times* newspaper that was published in 1997 to prove that I had really designed the incubators and raised the chicken. I told her to look at the chicken picture in the newspaper that was taken in 1997. She took the newspaper from me and started reading it. Then I took out the picture of my great-great-grandmother Phoebe Apperson Hearst to show Margaret and Susong and said that that was our great-great-grandmother Phoebe Apperson Hearst. They both looked at the picture without saying anything to me. Then Susong continued reading the newspaper. I sat on the bed and moved the picture to let Margaret see the picture clearly. She took the picture and looked at it clearly; she gave it back to me and then closed her eyes again.

I took the picture and went back to my room and put it away in my luggage bag, because I did not want to ruin it. Then I took out my cellular phone and went back to Susong's room to show them the pictures that I had taken at home with it. I opened the graphic section of my cellular phone and asked Margaret to review all the allergy pictures on it. She took my phone and reviewed all my allergy pictures; she said they were terrible. While she was looking at the pictures, I climbed up on the bed and laid down next to Margaret. After she was done looking at my allergy pictures, she gave the cellular phone back to me. I asked her whether she would like to look at my great-great-grandmother's picture that was hanging in my family room. She said OK, so I opened the graphic section to access my great-great-grandmother's pictures, zooming in one by one on her pictures to show her, indicating to her to look at the straight yellow light on the pictures. I told her I saw this yellow light every night on my great-great-grandmother's picture that was hanging on the wall in my house. I did not know where this yellow light came from. I could not point out where this yellow light was coming from. After she looked at the zoomed picture of my great-great-grandmother, it seemed like she got scared; she slid down from the bed and went to the bathroom. I took back the newspaper from Susong after she had finished reading it.

I went back to my room and put away the newspaper in my luggage bag. I folded all the blankets on my bed to make it higher. Then I laid down on my bed and put my big swollen legs up on top of the blankets. I felt very tired and both my legs were swelling badly. After I rested for a while, Susong came into my room, asking me to get ready for Sabrina's wedding. I got up to change my dress and put makeup on my face. Susong came into my room and gave me a pair of new diamond earrings to wear for the wedding. I refused to accept her diamond earrings. I told her I did not want anything from her. I gave the diamond earrings back to her. She said that those diamond earrings were from my mom, and she insisted that I should take out the old earrings from my ears and wear the new ones; she helped me take out my old earrings, put on the new diamond earrings on my both ears, and then left. Ivy came in and told me she had slept in this room last night; she just wanted to take her luggage bag out from this room. She picked up all her clothing and luggage bag and left. After a while, she came back in with a red bag that had money in it and gave it to me; then she asked me to give that red bag of money to the groom when he offered me tea during the wedding ceremony. Then she mentioned the diamond earrings. I did not understand what she was telling me. I tried to finish my makeup to get ready for the wedding.

After I was dressed up and ready for the wedding, I heard a lot of noises coming from downstairs. So I went downstairs to check who were there. I saw my sister Daisy and her husband just about to come inside the house through the front door. I saw Daisy's husband was walking very slowly and looking very sick. I asked Daisy what was wrong with him; she said he had had a heart surgery not long ago. Then they went in the kitchen. I saw Harvey was sitting on the sofa alone in the living room. He looked older than he was before; a lot of old-age moles were growing on his face. I sat down with him on the sofa and talked to him for a while. Then I saw Rosie and her family come in. When Rosie saw me, she did not recognize me and kept looking at me strangely. Then I laughed at her and called her. She came to me and sat with me on the sofa; then she said that we had not seen each other for almost eight years since 2001 and that she did not recognize me anymore. She was looking great and healthy. We talked for a while in the living room. I saw all my other sisters and their family come in from the front door.

When all the invited guests arrived, Sabrina's wedding tea ceremony started. Sabrina and her groom Adam offered tea to all her aunts and uncles; in return all her aunts and uncles gave red bags of money and jewelry to the couple and wished the couple the best of luck. After it was done, Susong invited all the guests to have luncheon in her house. After luncheon, I rested for a while in my room. Sabrina and her groom had arranged a big wedding ceremony in Audubon Park. I went to Audubon Park with my sisters; a lot of guests were coming, and at the wedding ceremony, Sabrina and Adam arranged drinks, dinner, and desserts for the guests. We all enjoyed the dinner very much. After dinner, the dance party started; the couples danced with their guests until midnight inside the park. After the wedding ceremony was over, all the guests left, I went back to Susong's house with Ivy and her family.

I was tired after I was home. I went upstairs to my room to lie down on my bed. Susong's family came home and was very busy downstairs, taking care of their in-laws and guests. I did not join them. It was raining heavily accompanied by thunderstorms after midnight, so I could not sleep well that night. I heard somebody turning the hallway light on. I got up from my bed to check who had turned on the hallway light. I did not see anybody, so I went downstairs to check who was downstairs. I went to the living room, kitchen, and family room downstairs, but I did not see anyone in there. I came back upstairs and turned off the hallway light, and I went back to my room. After a while, I heard somebody turning on the hallway light again. This time I did not go out and check who had turned on the hallway light again. I believed Susong was the one who had turned on the hallway light to go downstairs and work in the kitchen.

Next day I woke up early; it was still raining on and off. I got up and looked outside at the backyard from the window in my room. I saw a lot of broken branches from her old big tree lying all over the backyard after last night's thunderstorm. After a while, Susong came and knocked on my room door. I got up from my bed and opened the door for her. She came into my room and told me to get ready to go to the Crown hotel to have breakfast. I told her I was very tired and that I would like to stay home, but she insisted that I should get ready to go to the Crown hotel; she said she had already ordered breakfast for all of us in the Crown hotel. So I changed my clothing and went down to the kitchen, waiting for Susong to go to the Crown hotel. I looked around her house; just like before, she had kept her house very clean. She had not made a lot of changes in her house, but her kitchen ceiling had been patched in with a small wooden board. I asked her what had happened to the ceiling, and she said her kitchen ceiling was leaking water, so they had just cut out the ceiling board to find out where the leaking water was coming from, and they had temporarily put a small wooden board to cover the leaking area in the ceiling after they found water was leaking from the upstairs bathtub; they were looking for somebody to fix the upstairs bathtub.

Then she went upstairs to change. I went outside to her backyard to look at the ants that used to travel to her upstairs bathroom earlier through the gutter pipe outside her house. A lot of ants were still there, still climbing up and down the outside corner gutter pipe just like before. I tried to find a trace of all these ants. I found all these ants were commuting back and forth from her neighbor's yard to her house. Then I looked up at the sky. The sky was dark and filled with heavy clouds; it seemed like it was going to rain soon. Then I looked at her siding walls. I saw with amazement that one section of her siding walls close to her upstairs window had greenish spots; it looked like tiny greenish plants were growing on the siding wall. When I heard Susong calling me to go to the Crown hotel from inside, I went inside the house. When I saw her, I asked her about the greenish plants growing on her outside siding wall; she said she knew about it, but she did not have time to fix it yet. Then she said that we had to go, so we got inside the car. Susong's husband Richard drove us to the Crown hotel.

When we arrived at the Crown hotel, I saw all my sisters, brothers, and their families were already in the breakfast room inside the Crown hotel; some of them were already having breakfast and some were still getting their breakfast from the food counters. I went to the food counters and picked all the food that I liked and I went to a table near the hallway next to my brother's table. I put my plate on the table. When I was just about to sit down, Shaun came to me and asked me to go with him to the inner breakfast room to have breakfast with him and Sirena. So I took my breakfast plate and followed him to the breakfast room. Sirena was already sitting at the table, waiting for me and Shaun. I went to Sirena's table and sat down with my children and had breakfast with them. Then Susong came and joined us to have breakfast with us. After we ate the breakfast, the waiters took all the plates from the table and cleaned the table for us. Margaret and Rosie came and joined us at our table. My other sisters, brothers, nephews, nieces, their spouses, and their children came to our table and talked to me. I had not seen them for over eight years. I was happy to see them again. Then some of my sisters with their family left the hotel early and went home to other states. Some were still staying in the hotel for a couple more hours and left to go back to their home.

After everyone left, I went back home with Susong and Richard. When I was sitting with Susong in the kitchen, Shaun, Sirena, and Sabrina came home. Shaun put a pizza box on the table and told us they had gone to the King of Prussia mall and walked around a little bit to shop, but they did not find anything they liked inside the mall, so they left the mall and went to the Italian pizza restaurant in Norristown, where we used to eat pizza when we lived in King of Prussia. He said he had ordered one whole pizza and they ate inside the restaurant. He brought home the leftover pizza after the three of them finished eating inside the restaurant. He told Susong that he liked the pizza at that restaurant. I opened the pizza box and had one small slice of pizza. Then Shaun told me they would stay here for a while and would go to the Philadelphia airport a bit earlier to get the earlier flight to go back to California. If they could not get the earlier flight, they would wait at the Philadelphia airport to take their regular flight to go back to California. They stayed in the living room with Richard for a while; then they came and said good-bye to Susong and me, then left to go to the Philadelphia airport with Richard. I was very tired, so I went upstairs to my room to take a nap. Susong was busy in her kitchen as usual.

On Sunday morning, August 2, 2009, Susong came upstairs to tell me Edward had just called her to let me know he was going to take me to visit my parents' grave in New York Manhattan Cemetery on Tuesday. Ivy came to Susong's house on Sunday evening and brought fried beef for our dinner. She did not use any ingredients for marinating the beef when she cooked. When I took one small piece of beef in my mouth, the beef tasted terrible, so I told Ivy that her beef tasted terrible. But I was hungry, so I just had to eat it. Then I went upstairs to my room and took a nap. I woke up at 8:00 p.m. I felt I was a little bit hungry, so I went downstairs to the kitchen to look for something to eat. I did not know when Sabrina and Adam had come home; I saw them in the family room, looking at the picture book and talking. The television was on. I opened the refrigerator and looked for something to eat. I saw two buns, leftover fried noodles box, and some fried chicken inside the refrigerator. I could not find rice to eat with chicken, so I took out the fried noodles box from the refrigerator and warmed up the noodles in the microwave oven. After the noodles were warmed up, I took the noodles box out and put it on the kitchen table. I sat down on the chair. I moved the noodles box in front of me, and I was just about to eat the noodles when I saw Richard come in from the garage. When he saw me eating the noodles from the noodles box, he asked me whether I was going to finish all the noodles. There was not much fried noodles left inside the box, so I told him yes. Then he went upstairs.

Then I heard arguing voices coming out from upstairs; it seemed like Richard and Susong were arguing upstairs. Listening to them made me very uncomfortable. So I ran upstairs to check what was happening to them. I kept calling Susong when I was upstairs; I did not see Susong. But I saw Richard was sitting in his room in front of God's statue and praying. When he saw me, he told me Susong was in the bathroom, taking a shower. I went to the bathroom inside Susong's room, looking for her; the bathroom door was closed. I went back down to the kitchen to eat my noodles. Then I heard the arguing voices from upstairs again. So I went to the family room and asked Sabrina whether she could hear the arguing voices. She said yes, she heard the arguing voices, which were coming from the television; the television was showing criminals arguing and fighting inside the jail. When I looked at the television, I saw pictures on the television, but I did not hear any sound from the television. So I told her to go upstairs to find out what was wrong upstairs. But she insisted the voices were from the television, so I did not say anything and finished my noodles.

After I finished my noodles, I left the empty noodle box in the kitchen sink and went upstairs to my room. I saw Susong coming out from the bathroom, holding her clean clothes in her hand. I believed she had not taken a shower yet. I did not say anything to her and went to my room. I laid down on my bed and tried to figure out where the arguing voices were coming from. I felt upset about the answer I had got from Sabrina. Then I heard my cellular phone ring. I picked it up; it was from Sirena. She told me they had got early air tickets to go back to California. Shaun had gone back to Davis, and she was already home with the dogs in her bedroom. I asked her about the dogs. She said the dogs were fine and very happy to see her home. She had fed them fresh chicken for dinner. When she left them in the kitchen and went to her room, both the dogs kept crying in the kitchen and would not stop scratching the kitchen gate; she had to go back out to the kitchen and take them into her room, but Lady Star refused to go into her room when she was in front of my room. She just sat in front of my room and kept scratching my room's door, looking for me. It seemed like Lady Star missed me a lot and she was looking for me, as she would be on the sofa with me day and night when I was home. Sir Space did not miss me that much, because he was used to staying on the carpet floor. Sirena put the telephone to Lady Star's ear, suggesting that I talk to Lady Star to get her to be quiet. I talked to Lady Star. I told her to stop scratching my room's door. Sirena told me she quietened after she heard my voice on the telephone. Then I asked Sirena to let me talk to Sir Space. Sirena put the telephone to Sir Space's ear. I talked to Sir Space. After I finished talking to my dogs, I told Sirena to take them back out to the kitchen and let them stay there, just like when I was home. She said OK and hung up the phone. Then I went to sleep.

On August 3, 2009, Monday, my telephone's alarm bell woke me up at 8:00 a.m. to remind me to take my medicines. I got up and went downstairs to the kitchen, looking for something to eat before I took the medicine. I saw Susong was very busy putting away all the clean cups and plates in the kitchen shelves, cleaning the kitchen. I just went to the refrigerator, looking for something to eat. I saw one pork bun inside the refrigerator. I took it out from the refrigerator and put it in the microwave oven to warm it up for one minute. Then I took the pork bun out from the microwave oven once it was warmed up. I put it on the kitchen table to let it cool down a little bit. I sat down on the chair. Susong gave me a big cup of bitter melon juice to drink. Then I saw Adam come down from upstairs, carrying one bucket of dirty clothing to wash. When he saw me, he said hello to me and asked Susong where the washing machine room was. Susong took him to the washing machine room, for him wash his dirty clothing. After a while, he came out of the washing machine room to the kitchen. I was sitting in the kitchen and waiting for the pork bun to cool down a little bit more. When I saw him, I offered him the pork bun to eat, and he said he would like to have one for himself. So I told him to get the pork bun himself from the refrigerator. He went to the refrigerator and opened it to look for the pork bun. He could not find it, so he asked me where the pork bun was. I told him that there was a bun wrap inside the refrigerator. He said he could not find it. When Susong heard that he could not find the pork bun inside the refrigerator, she went to the refrigerator to help him get the pork bun, but there was no pork bun left inside the refrigerator. Susong told him to eat a strawberry bun kept on the table. He said OK; then he took one strawberry bun out from the strawberry bun package and sat down in front of me. Susong gave him a cup of milk. I started eating my pork bun. I had finished eating my pork bun when Sabrina came in with a lunch bag of leftover ham and turkey sandwiches, and she sat down next to me. She took out all the sandwiches from the bag and offered me half of her ham sandwich. I took it and started eating with her. Adam was very surprised when he saw us eating ham and turkey sandwiches in the morning. I told him this was the way we ate our food to survive. We did not have fixed times for our breakfast, lunch, and dinner. We ate whatever we had in front of us whenever we were hungry.

After we finished eating, Susong told them to go upstairs to pack their stuff to get ready to go back to New York the next day. They went upstairs, and after a while, they came back down together with a bucket of dirty clothing, and they went to the laundry room to take care of their dirty clothing. After a while they came back out of the laundry room with a bucket of clean clothing and folded them in the family room. I went back to my room to take my medicine. On my way upstairs, I jokingly told Adam to help his mom fix the kitchen ceiling and the greenish plants on the outside siding wall. I went into my room and stayed there until Susong came and knocked at my door to tell me to come down to see Edward. I went downstairs. I met Edward at the front door. He handed out an envelope to me, asking me to buy whatever I needed for myself in King of Prussia. I opened the envelope in front of him. I saw hundred-dollar bills inside the envelope. I gave him back the envelope, telling him to keep the money for himself. But he insisted that I keep the money to buy anything I liked for myself in King of Prussia.

Then he told me he would take me to New York tomorrow to visit my parents' graves and asked me to get ready the next morning. I said OK and went upstairs to my room.

After a while, I came back down to the kitchen at lunchtime and sat down on the chair that I usually sat on. Susong put the food on the table for me and Edward to eat after she finished cooking. Then Adam brought in coconut juice cans from the garage; he gave one can to me and one can to Edward, and he put a couple of cans on the table and left. I joked with Edward, telling him all those coconut juice cans were for me, not for him. Edward stayed quiet. I told him I usually bought the coconut juices from 99 Ranch supermarket and that the prices were $1.38 for two cans when they were on sale. Adam must have heard the conversation between me and Edward, because he came back in from the garage and told us the regular sale price for this coconut juice can was one dollar each. They were not cheap. I told him I drank a lot of coconut juice in California, and I usually got $1.38 for two cans. When he heard that, he brought in more coconut juice cans and put them on the table. Then he brought in two bottles of peanut butter for us to try; he gave one bottle to me and said that was the best brand of peanut butter that his brother had given him from his grocery store in Chicago. He asked me to try this brand of peanut butter, and he gave one bottle to Edward. We did not use much peanut butter at home, so I just kept it on the kitchen table. After luncheon, Edward went home. I went back upstairs to my room.

After a while, Rosie and Edward came to Susong's house again. Susong came upstairs to tell me they were going to shop in the King of Prussia mall and asked me to go with them. I told them I did not want to go to the mall, because both my legs were swollen badly. I told them to go without me, but Rosie and Susong insisted I should go and walk around inside the mall to get some exercise. I went to the mall with them. First, I went with them to the cosmetic section in Macy's store; they were looking for branded cosmetics and said so to the saleslady. I just walked around in the women's clothing section in the store, waiting for them. After they were done, they went to Rite Aid store to look for cosmetics again. I was tired, so I just sat on the bench in front of Rite Aid store, waiting for them to finish shopping and go home. Rosie did not go in with them; she just sat with me on the bench. I told her the worst thing that had happened in California recently; a police officer had killed a man who sat on the bench outside a Starbucks coffee shop, smoking a cigarette. The police officer had gone to the man and accused him that the man was smoking cigarettes in the area where it was not allowed to smoke; the man had ignored the police officer and continued smoking his cigarette. The police officer got upset and shot the man and killed him. She said she had never heard of anyone killing somebody because they were smoking a cigarette; how could the police officer kill a man just because he was smoking a cigarette? She said it was legal to smoke as long as the stores were allowed to sell cigarettes; she could not believe the government would set this kind of law in this country of killing somebody just for smoking a cigarette. Then I told her other things were happening in California, which made people sick in the heart.

Susong and Edward came out from Rite Aid store after they bought the cosmetics that they were looking for, and then we walked to the parking lot to go home. On the way to the parking lot, Susong showed me a big red hive on her arm that she had just got in the store; she kept scratching her arm, blaming it on the perfume in the store. I was really amazed that she still blamed the things that were not even causing her to get allergy rash. I explained to her again that her allergy was from the allergy powder that somebody must have carried inside the store from outside the mall. She did not say anything and kept scratching her arm. After we reached her car, she took out the Caladryl lotion from her car and put some on her arm, and we went home.

After we arrived home, I went upstairs and rested. Rosie and Edward stayed in the kitchen and talked with Susong; once in a while, I could hear them arguing about something in the kitchen. Then Sabrina and Adam came home. Susong came upstairs to tell me she would take us to the steak house for dinner at five o'clock. I said OK, then I took a short nap. And then I heard Susong calling me from downstairs to get ready. After I got ready and went downstairs, I saw Susong pouring American ginseng juice that she had been cooking the whole morning in cups for all of us to drink; then she gave one cup to each one of us. After we finished drinking American ginseng juice, I went upstairs to get my small CD bag. I saw Adam come out from his room into the hallway, holding a jacket, so I asked Adam why he had brought the jacket with him. Adam said it would be cold inside the restaurant with the air-conditioner on. Then I told him I should get my outfit shirt too, in case I needed to use it when I felt cold, so I went back to my room to get my outfit shirt and went downstairs.

Susong took all of us to the steak house in King of Prussia. I cannot recall the name of the steak house in King of Prussia that we went for our dinner, but it was a small steak house; there were not too many people inside the restaurant at the time when we were in the restaurant. The waiter took us to a round table and seated us. Then we ordered food. I ordered a combination of beef, shrimp, and mashed potato. The food in that restaurant was OK for me. We could not stay too long inside the restaurant, because Sabrina and Adam had to pack to get ready to go back to New York the next morning. After we finished our dinner, Susong took out her credit card to pay. Rosie had said those two women, the mother and daughter, had jobs to feed their men in their household. I did not know what she meant. I did not say anything. I was just looking at her. Then the waiter came and gave them the receipt to sign. Sabrina signed the receipt and gave the receipt back to the waiter. Then we came out of the restaurant. On the way back from the restaurant, I told Sabrina about how to make cakes and breads. We went back to Susong's house. Rosie and Edward went home.

Before Edward went home, he reminded me to get ready tomorrow morning; he would come early to take us to New York. I went upstairs to my room to rest, because I needed to put up my swollen legs on the pillows. Then I received a telephone call from Sirena; she told me she was home with the dogs. She suggested that I talk to my dogs since they missed me a lot. My two dogs were happy to hear my voice on the telephone when I talked to them; they kept quiet and behaved well after they heard my voice on the phone. Sirena told me she had bought GenTeal eye gel from the CVS store for Lady Star to help her get relief from her dry eyes. She said she had to use a wet tissue to clean the hard layer in Lady Star's eyes before she applied the GenTeal gel in her eyes. She also told me she would be home every day after work to take care of them until I came home. I said I was relieved to hear she was taking good care of them. Then we ended our conversation.

On Tuesday morning, August 4, 2009, Edward came to pick me and Susong at 6:00 a.m. to go to New York. We stopped in Acme supermarket to get four bundles of flowers to take to the cemetery for our parents. After we bought flowers from Acme supermarket, Edward got on New Jersey Turnpike to go to New York. He took more than two hours to arrive at Manhattan Cemetery in New York. When we went to our parents' graves, it was a very quiet morning; no one was in the cemetery

241

except us. We put the flowers in front of our parents' graves and prayed. I saw one family had kept the dead lady's picture on the headstone. I was very scared to see the lady's picture on the headstone in the cemetery. I did not think it was a good idea to keep pictures of dead people on their headstones, making people so scared. They should keep the pictures of dead people privately, either inside their coffins or on doors created on the headstones so that they can open the door when they come and visit them. We stayed in the cemetery for half an hour. Then Susong suggested that Edward should take us to Sabrina's apartment in Upper Brooklyn to visit Sabrina. On the way to Sabrina's apartment, I suggested that we should find a better place to bury ourselves together; then we could move our parents out from that cemetery to be buried with us. Susong said that was a good idea, but who was going to arrange to buy the land? I told her we'd discuss that when we had time in the future.

Then we arrived in Upper Brooklyn near Sabrina's apartment at 10:30 a.m. Edward parked his car on the roadside, looking for the car parking meter to pay for the car parking fee. I told Susong about our great-great-grandmother and our great-grandfather's story; then Susong went to a bakery store, and she came out with a bag of food from the bakery store and she gave it to me. I did not know what was inside that bag, so I refused to take it. Then I walked to the front door of that bakery store to see what kind of baked items they were selling; when the men from the store saw me looking inside their store, they blocked me from inside the store. So I walked back to Susong, who was near the sidewalk waiting for Edward. When Susong saw Edward, she gave the food bag to him. Edward took it and started eating from the bag.

We walked to Sabrina's apartment. I told them, on the way to Sabrina's apartment, about the strange incident that had happened to me when I was in front of elderly Catherine's house in Pleasanton. I told them I had seen a big black van that I had never seen in my life blocking my car from behind, to protect me when I came out from elderly Catherine's house in Pleasanton. They were probably very scared to listen to my story; they prevented me from continuing to tell them about my scary story by walking fast to Sabrina's apartment. Once we reached Sabrina's apartment, we stayed there for an hour; then Edward took us to the nearby Thai restaurant to have luncheon. After we ordered lunch for all of us, Adam came in and joined us in the restaurant to have lunch with us; he told us he had just come back from an interview with a professor to discuss about the analysis of the bridges. After luncheon, we dropped Sabrina and Adam at their apartment; then we went to New York Chinatown to buy some groceries and went back to King of Prussia. Susong cooked shrimps and bitter melons for our dinner. After she cooked, she called Rosie and Edward to have dinner with us. After I ate my dinner, I went upstairs and left Rosie, Edward, and Susong in the kitchen, as they continued eating their dinner.

On August 5, 2009, Wednesday morning, Susong warmed up the leftover Burmese fish noodle soup. Rosie and Edward came and ate Burmese fish noodle soups with us. We did not have anything to do at home, so we went to the CVS store on Henderson road to shop after we ate our breakfast. Edward, Susong, and I went inside the CVS store, but Rosie said she did not want to shop, and she stayed inside the car. I walked around inside the CVS store for a while; then I came back out from the CVS store alone and I went inside Giants supermarket next to the CVS store to use the restroom. After I came out from the restroom, I saw fresh corn in Giants supermarket, and I bought five pieces of corn and carried them out in my right hand from the supermarket. Suddenly, I felt the weight of those corns pulling the right side of my body down, causing a lot of pain on the right side of my stomach. When I saw Susong and Edward loading the cosmetics inside the car trunk, I walked to them and called Susong to take over my corn bag. I told them I had a lot of pain in my right stomach and we had to go home. Susong took over the corn bag from me and put it inside the car back trunk, and we went home. I asked them how they cooked corn, on the way home. Susong said she boiled corns with water inside a pot as usual. I said I would show them how to cook corns in a microwave oven to get them ready to eat within five minutes. Susong said it would create more work for us if we used the microwave oven to cook corns; I said no.

After we arrived home, Susong unloaded the corns and all the stuff that she had bought at the CVS store from the car and put them on the table in her kitchen. I took one piece of corn out from the corn bag and put it in the microwave oven to cook for five minutes. Susong took the rest of the corns from the table, peeled the corn shells one by one, then broke each corn into two pieces and put them inside a pot. Then she poured water inside the pot and cooked on her stove. At that time, I heard the *pee pee* sound of the microwave oven, and I took out the corn from the microwave oven and put it on the table. Then I peeled the corn shell and left it on the plate, waiting for the corn to cool down a little bit more. I saw Susong was still cooking her corns on the stove. After my corn was cooled down a little bit, I was just about to break my corn into half when Edward came in from outside and called us to go to Bed Bath & Beyond store in DeKalb Pike to buy an electronic toothbrush for him. Rosie was rushing me and Susong to go. I left my corn on the kitchen table and rushed out to the front door, getting inside the car. Edward took us to Bed Bath & Beyond store in DeKalb Pike.

After we arrived at Bed Bath & Beyond store, Edward went inside the store with Susong to the home care section to look for an electronic toothbrush. Rosie and I walked around in the front section near the cashier counter, looking at the merchandise that was displaced in the front section. I saw Riddex electronic device packages were displayed in the front section near the cashier counters. These devices had been advertised on television for a decade that they used sound waves to kill cockroaches, termites, ants, mice, and spiders. Since I did not know whether this device would really work to kill all the insects that they described on the packages, I just bought one for myself and one for Susong to try out the devices at home. Then I told Rosie and Edward that Susong needed one in her house, because she had a lot of ants inside her house and in her yard. I asked Rosie to get one each for her and Edward to try in their houses to get rid of insects and mice. She said she did not have too many insects in her house, but she would check if she needed to get the device and she would get it later from the store. After Edward bought the electronic toothbrush at Bed Bath & Beyond store, we went home.

On our way back home, Rosie suggested going to Costco store to see her friends and taste the food that Costco store was offering the customers. She said she usually went to Costco store to taste all kind of food that they offered to their customers. Edward said he needed to buy vitamins and agreed to go to Costco store. So we went to Costco store, and Edward and Susong went to the health care section to get vitamins. Rosie took me to see her friends, who worked in Costco store; when her friend saw us she offered a whole ice bar to us. Then we met another friend of Rosie in Costco store. Rosie introduced her to me, she was really happy to know I had come back to King of Prussia again. The people from King of Prussia town were very friendly, just like the time when my family lived there. Susong came and rushed us to go to the cashier counter, to line up to pay for the vitamins that Edward had bought. I went with Susong to the cashier and paid for all the vitamin products that they bought from Costco store. Then we went home.

After we came back home, Susong turned on her stove to continue cooking the corns. I took my microwave oven cooked corn that I had left on the table and broke it into half. Then I saw Rosie looking at me, so I offered half of my corn to her so that she could taste my microwave-oven-cooked corn that was very sweet. She took the corn and ate it. She said my idea was excellent; the microwave-oven-cooked corn was sweeter than the corn that was cooked with water in the pot. Rosie and I finished eating our corns. Susong was still cooking her corns; she got mad on seeing that we had already finished with our corns. So I asked her which way was better. They all laughed. We ate the leftover Burmese fish noodle soup in the refrigerator for our dinner. Then Rosie and Edward went home.

On Thursday morning, I went to Acme supermarket in DeKalb Pike with Susong to buy groceries. After we came back home from Acme supermarket, Rosie came and suggested going to Norristown mall to shop. So we went to Norristown mall to walk around inside the mall. I saw there were a lot of empty stores; there were not too many people shopping inside the Norristown mall. We bought lunch inside the mall, shopped there for a while, and went home. After we arrived home, I went upstairs and rested for a while; then I came back down. I saw Rosie and Susong sitting in the living room and talking. I went to them and told them I had a lot of pain in my stomach muscle after carrying the corns. Then I told them about the accidents that had been happening to me in California for the past eight years after I went back there in 2001. I went back to my room to take my cellular phone and came back down to show them the pictures on it about the accidents that I had got in front of Pleasanton KPMC facility and the bad allergies that I got from my neighbor's birch tree. I told them I had bought a lot of different kinds of accident insurances from the bank to protect myself. I told them that since we could not predict our own lives about what would happen to us and who could set up on us to make us disabled or die, we should have insurance to protect ourselves. I explained to them about AIG insurance company, which was offering through the banks all kinds of accidental disability insurance benefits, including physician visiting fees, emergency and hospitalization fees. They said they would look into it. Then they mentioned about the Medicare system that we had in the United States; the system made it harder for all the elderly people to take out extra money to buy extra coverage for Part B that Medicare did not provide for cover. It was not easy for elderly people to have to pay over one hundred dollars to buy extra coverage each month. I suggested that I would find a way to help all the elderlies in the healthcare system if I could step up as the president of the United States. They asked me how I wanted them to help me at that moment. I told them I did not want anything from them, but I was experiencing a lot of pain at that moment, since I was surrounded with bad allergies and sickness in my environment at home; I just needed to get antibiotic medicines to keep at home for protecting my life. My doctors from Kaiser Permanente medical group did not provide me any antibiotic medicines to protect me. I needed to take antibiotic medicines when I got sick.

After I talked to them for a while, I went back upstairs to my room, put away my cellular phone, and rested for a while. I came back down downstairs because I heard some arguments in the kitchen. I saw Rosie and Edward sitting in the kitchen. Susong was cooking dinner. Edward and Susong were arguing something about politics and were saying that they could not accept the things that the politicians were doing. I yelled at them from the living room to stop arguing; then I walked in the kitchen. After they saw me, they stopped their argument. I saw the Riddex electronic device package was lying on the kitchen floor, so I picked it up and opened the package with a knife. I put the device in the family room's wall outlet to test it. I told Rosie that I had never used this device before and that I did not know whether this device would really work to kill insects or not by using the waves of electronic sound, but it would not hurt us to test the electronic device. I told Rosie to find out later from Susong whether that electronic device really worked. Then I told Susong to leave the device in the wall outlet for testing. Then Ivy came to Susong's house after work to have dinner with us. After we ate, I went back upstairs; Rosie and Edward went home. Ivy stayed in Susong's house for the night. Susong came upstairs to tell me they would take me to New York on Friday to see Harvey to check up my stomach pain. I said OK to her. Then she went back to her room.

On Friday morning, Ivy went back to work. Rosie, Edward, and Susong took me to Harvey's clinic in New York. When we arrived in Harvey's clinic, there were only a few patients in the clinic. After he was done with the patients, his assistant asked me to go into his office. I went into his office; his face showed that he was very uncomfortable to see me, since the last time he had issued a wrong allergy letter for me. I told him he should not feel uncomfortable, because he was not the only doctor who did not know that the white birch trees could cause itching and make people get bad allergies and sickness. A lot of people were misled and did not even know that birch trees had allergic fruit-like cluster flowers. Then Harvey asked me to lie down on the patient bed and pressed the right side of my stomach under the ribs up and down many times and asked me where the pain was; once he pressed on the section that caused me a lot of pain. I told him I felt pain; he said that was muscle pain. He prescribed me Tylenol pain-reliever pills and asked me to take two tablets, three times a day for my pain. He also gave me a lot of Chlor-Trimeton allergy tablets and Tetracycline antibiotic tablets to take home to safeguard me and my family. He gave B12 vitamin injections to my sisters and brother. I did not take vitamin B12 injection, because I was taking a lot of American ginseng root at home every day. We sat in Harvey's clinic for a while. Margaret took us to a Chinese pastry restaurant to eat Chinese pastries for breakfast. After we finished eating our breakfast, she took us to her new apartment. Her apartment house was only a few blocks away from their clinic and it was very convenient to commute. There were a lot of restaurants and stores nearby. They just had to walk down to the stores and buy any clothing they liked from the stores or buy any food they liked to eat from the restaurant. She cooked Burmese fish noodle soup for our lunch in her apartment house. After we ate, I fell asleep on the sofa for a couple hours. When I woke up, it was already 3:00 p.m. Rosie suggested going back to King of Prussia. Margaret said she would take us to the parking lot, and we left her house and went to the parking building where we had parked our car. She bought some steamed pork buns for us to take home to King of Prussia; then she went back to Harvey's clinic. After we were in the parking building, Edward said he was going to stay in New York, and he asked Susong to drive us back to King of Prussia in his car. Susong said OK and she took us back to King of Prussia.

When we arrived home, Susong unloaded all the food from the car and took them inside the house. Then Ivy came to have dinner with us. After dinner, Rosie suggested that I go with them to drop her home; on the way to her house, she wanted me to look at the house where I had lived before in King of Prussia. I went with them to drop her home. Ivy drove her car and waited in front of Edward's house. After we dropped Rosie at her house, we went to Edward's house to put his car in his garage. When we arrived at Edward's house, Susong drove Edward's car inside the garage and locked the garage door. I went out to look at the big white birch trees that were planted in front of Maryann's house since they had moved into that house in 1979, to make sure they were white birch trees in front of their house. The trees in front of Maryann's house were really white birch trees and the trunks of the trees were still white. They had all kinds of problems after they moved into this house; her son had died of eye cancer disease in this house. Susong asked me whether I would like to go in and visit Maryann. I told her I did not want to visit MaryAnn at this time. Then we went back to Susong's house.

On Saturday morning, August 8, 2009, I woke up late, because I was very tired after we came back from New York. Ivy came to my room and told me she had to go back to her New Jersey home; she had a lot of cleaning to do at home. She wished me the best of luck for going back to California and she left. I got up from my bed and went to the upstairs bathroom to clean up myself; when I flushed the toilet, the tissues in the toilet bowl would not flush away. I tried to flush the toilet a couple of times, but the water in the toilet water tank did not have enough pressure to push the tissues down and there was clogging inside the toilet bowl. Then I went downstairs to try the toilet in the family room; the toilet downstairs was clogged just like the one upstairs. I told Susong to use Clorox liquid to pour inside the toilets and keep it inside the toilets for an hour. Susong said she would take care of it and she asked me to eat my breakfast that she had prepared for me. Then she poured Clorox liquid inside the toilets. After an hour, I asked her whether she had poured Clorox liquid inside the toilets. She said she had already done. So I tried to flush both toilets downstairs and upstairs. It worked well and cleared out the clogged toilet pipes; the toilet water came out with strong force and cleaned the toilets perfectly. Richard came home with two plastic trash cans. As soon as Susong saw him, she asked him where he had gone the whole morning. He said he had gone to the store to buy two small trash cans to keep in the bathroom. Susong told him they did not need trash cans any more. The toilets worked well now. Richard said he would return the trash cans back to the store if the toilets were working well. I went to the family room to check the electronic device that I had kept it in the family room outlet yesterday. I found the device was gone; somebody had taken it out from the wall outlet. I asked Susong who had taken the electronic device out from the wall outlet; she said she did not know. I put the Riddex electronic device back in the family room wall outlet.

I went outside to her backyard to check on the ants. I sat down on the concrete porch under the old tree for a while. Then I looked up at the sky and the roof. I remembered I had seen tiny green plants' spot on the siding wall near the upstairs window last time. I wanted to know what kind of green plant was it on the siding wall. I walked to the porch corner near her kitchen window and looked up at the siding wall where the tiny green plants' spot was. Then I tried to trace where the green plants' spot came from by looking at the surroundings of her backyard. Then I saw a white seashell on the ground outside her backyard near her kitchen window. I stepped down on the ground from the concrete porch and picked up the seashell. It was a very beautiful, perfect seashell. I took the seashell inside the house and I asked Susong why she had thrown this beautiful seashell in her backyard. She said she did not know anything about it and that she had been very busy lately preparing for her daughter's wedding. I went inside the kitchen. I washed the seashell with my hands in the kitchen sink. But the black soil inside the seashell did not come out right away, so I asked Susong to give me a bucket to keep the seashell in water to sop the soil out from the seashell. She gave me a pot to keep the seashell in water. Then I washed my hands. I reminded Susong not to take the electronic device out from the wall outlet in her family room again. I asked her to check the device frequently whether that device could really work in getting rid of ants, spiders, and rats. She said OK. I went upstairs to my room to pack all my stuff in my luggage bag to get ready for tomorrow to go back to California. While I was putting my clothing inside my luggage, my left hand started to itch. I scratched a little bit and then I ignored the itch.

Rosie came to Susong's house at 11:00 a.m.; she said she wanted to take us to eat Chinese food in King of Prussia mall, so we went to the King of Prussia mall. After Susong parked the car in the King of Prussia mall's parking lot, we went to the restaurant section; on the way to the restaurant section inside the mall, I told them the ugly things that were happening in California. Rosie got upset and she went home by herself. Susong and I went inside the mall to the restaurant section to have lunch.

When we were in the restaurant section, I did not see too many people eating lunch. Maybe it was still early. We got a table for ourselves easily in the aisle in front of the Chinese restaurant. We went into the Chinese restaurant. Susong ordered chicken fried rice and I ordered beef fried rice. After a few minutes, the food was ready, and we took our food to the table that we had reserved in the aisle. The food was not that great, but it was OK. After we ate, we went back home.

Rosie came to Susong's house in the evening to have dinner with us. After dinner, Rosie gave me a red bag full of money to wish me a good trip to go back to California. After Susong washed all the dishes and cleaned up the kitchen table, she took out the game cards and suggested that we play cards; we all agreed and we set a twenty-dollar limit for each of us for the card game. If one of us lost all the money when we played the card games, we would end the game. We took out twenty dollars each to start playing the cards. We played all kinds of card games. Susong and I were winning all of Rosie's money. Rosie was upset about her luck. At that time, Richard came home to tell Rosie that he would take her home and asked her to get ready. So we ended the card game, as Rosie had lost all her money. Richard took her home. I went back upstairs. My left hand was getting itchy again. I kept scratching my hands. When Susong came upstairs to my room to check on me and ask me if everything was OK, I asked her to give me some lotion to stop the itching on my hands. She went to her room and got a small tube of Caladryl lotion; she helped me to put it on my hands and asked me to keep the lotion tube for later use. I felt much better after I put Caladryl lotion on my hands. Then I put the rest of my clothing inside my luggage bag. I laid down on bed for a while and went into the bathroom to brush my teeth. Once I washed my hands with water and soap, the itch came back in my hands. I went back to my room and put more Caladryl lotion on my hands, and I went to sleep.

On Sunday morning, August 9, 2009, at 5:30 a.m., Susong woke me up and asked me to get ready to go to Philadelphia airport, because my flight would take off at 6:51 a.m. I said OK to her and got up right away, went in the bathroom, brushed my teeth, changed my clothing, and put all my accessories inside my luggage bag. Susong warmed up the breakfast for me; then she came upstairs to my room to tell me to go down to eat my breakfast. She saw my luggage bag was already zipped and ready, and she took it down to the kitchen for me. I followed her to the kitchen. Then she gave me a bundle of game cards. I opened my luggage bag and put the bundle of game cards in my luggage to take back to California. I zipped and locked my luggage bag with a small key. Susong asked me to eat the pork buns that she had already warmed up for me. I took one pork bun from the kitchen table and told her I would eat it on my way to the airport. Richard was loading my luggage bag in his car trunk. After he was done, he asked us to get in the car. After Susong and I got inside Richard's car, he drove us to the Philadelphia airport. Susong and Richard took me inside the airport to the United Airlines ticket counter to get an air ticket with seat number. After he got an air ticket from the United Airlines clerk, he told me to use my credit card to pay for my luggage bag carrier fee. I gave him my credit card, and he helped me to use my credit card to pay for my luggage bag carrier fee in the machine. Then he took the receipt from the machine, and he gave the receipt and the airline ticket to me; he asked the airline clerk to take care of my luggage bag. Then they took me to the entrance of the United Airlines security departure gate to check in. After I checked in the security gate, I went to the departure gate of United Airlines and waited for the flight to depart. After half an hour, I heard the United Airlines flight attendant announcing that the passengers had to get ready to go inside the flight. I went to line up with the other passengers. I moved slowly to the flight attendant. Then I handed out my ticket to the flight attendant. I took back the small portion of the ticket that had the seat number from the flight attendant. I went inside the plane and settled myself on my seat. The United Airlines flight took off at 6:55 a.m. and arrived in San Francisco airport at 9:00 a.m.

The flight attendant opened the flight door after the plane connected with the arrival gate, and they let all the passengers leave the flight. I left the plane, and I went out from the arrival gate to the pickup luggage bag section. After I was in the pickup luggage bag section, I started looking for Shaun, but I did not see him. I called Shaun on my cellular phone; he responded to me and told me he was waiting for me in the flight passenger arrival section. I told him I was already in the pickup luggage bag section and asked him to come down and meet me there. He said OK and hung up the phone. After a few minutes, I saw Shaun come down from the escalator. As soon as I saw him, I called him, and he came to me and told me he was waiting for me at the arrival gate. I asked him where Sirena was. He said he did not know where Sirena was. He had come directly from Davis to San Francisco airport to pick me up. It took us ten to twenty minutes to wait for my luggage bag to come out from the luggage carrier machine. When Shaun saw my luggage bag rolling out from the luggage carrier machine, he picked it up from the carrier machine. We went to the airport car parking lot, and he loaded my luggage bag inside his car's trunk and we went home. He took me to Chinatown, Oakland, to have lunch on the way back home. After we ate lunch, we went home. We arrived home at 12:30 p.m. I met my two dogs that I had missed the most in my life, which were in my kitchen; they looked great under the care of Sirena. As soon as they saw me, they started wagging their tails and welcomed me home. They were very happy to see me home and kept wagging their tails and following me around in the kitchen while making a lot of noises. I played a little bit with them. Then Sirena came home from work. She showed me the eye lotion that she had used on Lady Star's eyes. I was very pleased to see the way Sirena had taken care of them very well. After they settled me at home, Sirena and Shaun went back home after 6:00 p.m. Since I was very tired, I went to bed early and let my two dogs stay in the kitchen.

Next day on August 10, 2009, Monday morning, the weather was very hot in California. I went out to my backyard and began watering all my plants. While I was watering the plants, my hands came in contact with water and a bad itch developed. I stopped watering the plants and went inside my house. I washed my hands with soap and water; then I applied Calamine lotion on my hands to stop the itch, but the itch did not stop, especially my right fingers which were getting so itchy and made me keep scratching them. Then I saw small pimple rashes had formed on my right fingers. I applied more Calamine lotion on my fingers to make them stop getting itchy. The itch stopped for a while, but it came back again. I kept scratching and scratching my fingers, and all those pimple rashes on my fingers turned into big blisters. After a couple of days, the blisters on my fingers broke and the blisters started spreading all over my palms and my hands. I took Chlor-Trimeton 4 mg pill every four hours besides the Fexofenadine allergy pill that my doctor had prescribed for me to use daily. After I got this bad allergy, I realized I should use soap and water to clean my hands to get rid of the blisters. I used soap and warm water to clean my hands from time to time. I applied Calamine lotion on my hands to get rid of the itch. After a week, the blisters on both my swollen palms and hands started to dry out a little bit, but when the blisters broke, the fluid kept spreading on my palms and hands, forming new blisters on my palms and hands. I decided to checkup with my doctor if my itch did not go away after a week. On Saturday, I called Susong and asked her why she had thrown that seashell in her backyard. She said she did not know anything about that seashell. She asked me where I had found the seashell. I told her that I had found that seashell outside her backyard near her big kitchen window. I told her I had never seen this seashell in her house before. But I had seen a lot of this kind of seashells when I was in Bahamas. I knew the people in Bahamas used this kind of seashells as horns. I kept asking her about the seashell. She kept telling me she did not know anything about the seashell in her house.

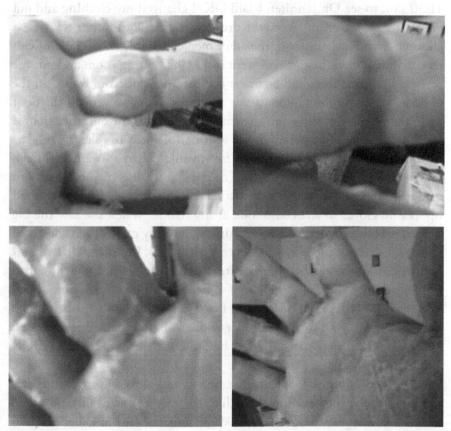

Top: Big blisters formed on my hands.
Bottom: Big blisters on my hands dried out; the hard skins started peeling.

On August 19, 2009, Wednesday, since the blisters on both my hands were getting worse and spreading all over my hands, I decided to call Dr. Jennifer. I called Pleasanton KPMC adult medicine clinic at 9:00 a.m. in the morning to leave a message for Dr. Jennifer, informing her that I had got very bad poisonous blisters on both my hands and I needed to get a cortisone shot right away. I requested her to let me checkup with her today as soon as possible and that I would like her to look at the kind of poisonous blisters that I had got on my hands. I also indicated to her that the blisters on both my hands were drying a little bit in some areas, but some areas were still getting worse and spreading badly. The nurse in Dr. Jennifer's clinic called me back after an hour to ask me to go in at 11:30 a.m. to see Dr. Jennifer. I said OK. I changed my clothing and put on plastic gloves on my hands. I drove myself to Pleasanton KPMC to checkup with Dr. Jennifer in the adult medicine clinic. I checked in with the front desk clerk first; then I went inside the waiting room and put the receipt slip inside the small box near the entrance door and waited in the patients' waiting room. When I saw the medical assistant open the door and take the receipt slip from the small box next to the entrance door, I went to her and let her know I was waiting for them to take me in. The medical assistant asked me to wait for a while. I had to wait for fifteen to twenty minutes in the waiting room; finally the medical assistant came out and took me inside the patient room. She asked me to take off my plastic gloves so she could look at my hands. When she saw the big blisters on both my hands, she exclaimed, "Oh my god!" Then she asked me how I had got those bad blisters on my hands. I told her that when I had picked up the seashell in my sister's house backyard, I got those bad blisters on my hands, and they were so itchy that I kept scratching them. She asked me what kind of seashell; I told her it was just a seashell. Then she asked me to wait for Dr. Jennifer and left. Before she left, I requested her to give me a new pair of gloves before I left the clinic. She said OK and left.

After ten minutes, Dr. Jennifer came in and looked at my hands and the big blisters; she exclaimed just like the medical assistant and asked me the same questions that the medical assistant had asked me. I told her about the seashell again, and she asked me what kind of seashell it was. I did not know how to tell her what kind of seashell it was, because I did not know what had happened to that seashell. I said it was just a seashell. Then she asked me to wash my hands with soap to get rid of the Calamine lotion from my hands. I went to the sink and washed both my hands with soap and water twice until the Calamine lotion was gone from my hands. Then I showed my hands to her and told her the fluid from the blisters kept spreading on both my hands after I kept scratching them. She looked at my hands and told me not to scratch my hands. Then she prescribed me Prednisone 20 mg for five days and asked me to take one tablet a day for five days. Then she left the room. The medical assistant came in and gave me a pair of new blue plastic gloves. I put on the gloves on my hands and left the clinic. I went to South Two pharmacy store to pick up my Prednisone pills and I went home.

After I came home, I took one Prednisone tablet right away. I made myself a big cup of warm tea, thinking how I was going to prevent those bad blisters on my hands from not spreading to the nearby areas to form new blisters on my hands. I decided to wash my hands every two hours and wear the gloves when I cooked. I kept washing my hands with soap and water every two hours to prevent it from spreading for almost a couple of weeks until the hard skin layer on my palms started to peel and new meat had formed after the hard skin layer had peeled. Some of the corners of the hard skin layers were very sharp and were poking the new meat, and my hands got infected again. It took a couple of months for the blisters on both my hands to completely dry out; the hard skin started peeling and new meat formed.

On August 24, 2009, I called Walnut Creek KPMC Gastroenterology department to reschedule my appointment from September 17, 2009, to November 2009, because I felt that I should not go anywhere after I had got those bad poisonous blisters on my hands. But the scheduling clerk told me that Nurse Joan's appointment schedules were fully booked till the end of November this year. If I wanted to reschedule my new appointment with her, it had to be January 2010. Since I did not want to wait that long, I told the scheduling clerk just to keep my appointment on September 17, 2009, and that I would try to make it on that day, and I hung up the telephone. After one week, I received the fecal-hemoglobin stool test package from the mail that Dr. Jennifer had sent out to me. I opened the package and read the instruction first; then I opened the small tube cap in the package. I went to the restroom and put a small amount of bowel material inside the tube as instructed. I sealed the package and mailed it to Kaiser Permanente laboratory. I received the stool test result from KPMC laboratory after a couple of weeks. KPMC laboratory indicated that my stool test was negative. I called Pleasanton KPMC adult medicine clinic on September 7, 2009, to leave a message for Dr. Jennifer, informing her that my stool test result was negative, and I asked her whether I still needed to go take my colorectal cancer screening test on September 17, 2009. Dr. Jennifer's assistant called me back to tell me to keep my colorectal cancer screening test appointment in Walnut Creek KPMC gastroenterology department on September 17, 2009. She insisted that I should go to take the screening test. I said OK to her. After my car accident in 1998, I was scared to drive, so I called Sirena to take me to Walnut Creek KPMC on September 17, 2009, at 3:00 p.m. Sirena called me back to tell me she would take me to Walnut Creek KPMC on my appointment date for my colorectal cancer screening test.

On Thursday, September 17, 2009, Sirena came home from work to take me to Walnut Creek KPMC at 2:00 p.m. We left home and arrived at Walnut Creek KPMC at 2:30 p.m. Sirena dropped me in front of the entrance of the KPMC building. I went up to the gastroenterology department on the second floor by myself; then I went to the front desk clerk to check in for my appointment at 3:00 p.m. with Nurse Joan for my colorectal cancer test. The front desk clerk asked me whether I had prepared for my colorectal cancer screening test as instructed on the preparation sheet. I did not understand what she was asking me. I told her that Dr. Jennifer did not give me any instruction sheet to prepare anything for my colorectal cancer screening test. I had repeatedly asked her what kind of preparation I needed to do before I came here. She had repeatedly told me that I needed to prepare sigmoidoscopy for my colorectal cancer screening test. I kept telling her that I was not told to prepare sigmoidoscopy before my colorectal cancer screening test. She handed out the flexible sigmoidoscopy preparation sheet to me, I looked at the sigmoidoscopy preparation sheet and I told her I had never received this kind of sheet from my doctor. Then the front desk clerk told me to pay $25 for co-payment. I paid her with my credit card. After she was done with the paperwork, she asked me to sit on the chair in front of her counter and wait for Nurse Joan's assistant to come out and take me in to see Nurse Joan. Sirena came into the waiting room to tell me she would be waiting outside in the hallway, and she asked me to meet her in the hallway after I was done. I said OK to her, and she went back out to the hallway. I sat patiently in the waiting room, waiting for Nurse Joan's assistant to take me in. Nurse Joan's assistant came out and took me to Nurse Joan's screening test room at 3:00 p.m. I went in with her. I met Nurse Joan, who was waiting for me inside the room. When she saw me, she asked me whether I had done the flexible sigmoidoscopy preparation for my colorectal cancer screening test. I told her I had just gotten better from the poisonous allergy on my hands. No one told me I needed to prepare anything for this screening test. I got my stool test result back from KPMC laboratory and it indicated that I had a negative for my stool test. I had checked with my doctor on September 7, 2009, to make sure I still needed to come there to take the colorectal cancer screening test or not, and my doctor had insisted I had to take this test. But she did not mention anything to me about the preparation for this screening test. Nurse Joan handed out the flexible sigmoidoscopy preparation sheet to me again, and she said that without preparation of this procedure of cleaning up the stool from my colon, she would not able to do the colorectal cancer screening test for me. She asked me to go back to the front desk clerk to reschedule another appointment to come back and do the test. She told me since she was not performing any screening test on me I should get my co-payment back. Then she went inside the back room of her clinic to inform her manager to take care of my case. The manager came out and took me to the front desk clerk and asked the front desk clerk to refund my co-payment back to me and reschedule another appointment date for me to come back for my colorectal cancer screening test. Then she left.

The front desk clerk refunded the money back to me; then she went inside the office to inform the lady manager to reschedule the colorectal cancer screening test for me. The lady manager came out with her and asked me to go in her office to reschedule the appointment date. I went inside her office with her, and she set up another appointment date for me with another sigmoidoscopy examiner. But I refused to accept the new sigmoidoscopy examiner. I told her I would like to set up another appointment with Nurse Joan. She said Nurse Joan's schedule was full until November; she said she would call me back as soon as she got Nurse Joan's new appointment schedule with open dates. She asked me all the information that she needed to know from me, and she told me they would call me back to set up another appointment as soon as they got the open appointment dates for Nurse Joan. I said OK. She asked me who had set up this appointment for me. I told her Dr. Jennifer's assistant had set up this appointment for me a couple months ago. She said if my doctor had made this appointment for me, my doctor was supposed to take responsibility of giving me the preparation instruction sheet before I came here to take the colorectal cancer screening test. I told her that maybe my doctor was a new doctor and she did not know it was her responsibility to give me the preparation instruction sheet for this screening test. Then she gave me the instruction sheet again to make sure I knew my responsibility to prepare for the procedure for this screening test before I came next time. I told her OK and I thanked her. I left the office and met Sirena outside the hallway. Sirena took me home and she went back to her office.

The scheduling clerk from the gastroenterology department in Walnut Creek KPMC called me back in the first week of October 2009 to reschedule my new appointment date on Wednesday, December 2, 2009, with Nurse Joan. I accepted this appointment date with Nurse Joan for my colorectal cancer screening test. Then I took out the flexible sigmoidoscopy preparation sheet from my file and read it carefully to prepare for my colorectal cancer screening test. I entered the date and time in my cellular phone to remind myself before I went to Walnut Creek KPMC Gastroenterology Department for my colorectal cancer screening test so that I would not forget to apply the medicine on myself before I went to take the screening test.

Since I had got bad blisters on my hands, I stayed inside my house, except when I went outside to my yard to water my plants in the morning. I tried to be very careful not to touch anything to prevent my hands from getting worse. My backyard was surrounded with many cypress trees. I found I had a lot of moths and other insects in my backyard. I decided to cut out the bottom parts of the cypress branches to get rid of all the insects from my yard. Then I called Pleasanton KPMC adult medicine clinic to set up an appointment to checkup with Dr. Jennifer in the second week of November 2009. The scheduling clerk set the appointment on November 4, 2009, Wednesday, for me. But I requested to schedule my appointment on November 11, 2009, Wednesday; the scheduling clerk said OK for setting up the appointment on the day I had requested. I went in Pleasanton KPMC laboratory department on Monday, October 26, 2009, at 1:30 p.m. to take my blood test to find out the changes in my diabetic data in my blood after I got those bad poisonous allergy blisters on both my hands. There were quite a number of patients in the laboratory waiting room. I went to the front desk clerk to check in for my blood sample test; then I asked the clerk where Grace was. She told me Grace was at lunch. So I did not say anything and waited for the laboratory technician to call me in. I saw Grace come out from the laboratory room and call the patient's name. The patient answered her, and she took the patient inside the laboratory room. When I saw Grace come out, I told the lady who sat next to me that Grace was a very good technician; no technician could draw blood sample from my right arm. I did not know the reason they could not draw blood sample from my right arm; the technician had to draw my blood sample from my left hand. The lady responded to me and said to me that everyone was a good technician and left. After a while I went to the laboratory entrance and looked inside the laboratory to check what were all the technicians doing. When Grace saw me, she asked me to go inside the laboratory room to have a seat. I went inside the room and sat down on a chair, waiting for Grace to finish with the patient that she was taking care of. The lady technician came to me after she took care of the patient, and she pulled up the table and said this was a better way to draw my blood sample. I heard Grace saying that she was good too. But I did not have any confidence in her, as I had never met her before. Most of the technicians would earlier search for the veins in both my arms to draw my blood sample. That made me lose confidence in them. I told her I was waiting for Grace to take care of me. After I refused to let her draw my blood sample, she laughed and went to another patient. After Grace was done with the patient, she came to me and asked me to put my right hand on the table so she could draw my blood sample. I did not say anything to her. I just let her draw the blood sample from my right arm. She could not draw any blood out of my right arm. I told her that she had forgotten she should not use my right arm to draw my blood sample. Then I put my left hand on the table, and I told her to draw the blood sample from my left hand. She drew the blood sample from my left hand, and she collected two bottles of blood from my left hand. Then I told her that the last time I was in the laboratory department, I had set up the rule for all the technicians that they were not allowed to inject the needle repeatedly to draw my blood sample from my hand twice. If they did, they would get hit on their heads. So I hit her head with my finger softly and told her she should get hit too just like any other technician; she laughed. I liked Grace a lot, after I became friends with her for so many years. I had been drawing my blood sample in this laboratory since 2006. We had good and bad times together in all those years in the laboratory. She remembered about my allergy and asked me whether my neighbors had already cut their white birch tree. I told her not yet. Then I left Pleasanton KPMC and went home.

On October 28, 2009, I received a phone call from the adult medicine clinic. Dr. Jennifer's assistant asked me to change my appointment date from November 11, 2009, to November 4, 2009. I said OK to her for changing my appointment date from November 11, 2009, to November 4, 2009, at 10:30 a.m., since Dr. Jennifer had already gotten my recent blood test results. Dr. Jennifer's assistant rescheduled my appointment date on November 4, 2009, at 10:30 a.m. for me to checkup with Dr. Jennifer. Then I hung up the telephone. On November 4, 2009, Wednesday at 9:30 a.m., I went to Pleasanton KPMC South Two pharmacy store to buy two Fleet enemas and one 10 oz bottle of magnesium citrate for my colorectal cancer screening test preparation; then I went to the adult medicine clinic to check in with the front desk clerk. After I paid my co-payment and the front desk clerk issued me the payment receipt, I went inside the clinic. I left my payment receipt inside the small box next to the entrance door of my doctor's clinic and I waited for Dr. Jennifer's assistant to take me inside the clinic. There were a lot of patients that day, waiting for their doctors to call them in. Some patients were reading magazines and newspapers; some were waiting patiently for their doctor's assistants to call them in. After a while, I saw a lady nurse walk in and out of both sides of the clinic. I did not know what she was doing in the hallway to go in and out from one side of the clinic to the other side of the clinic. I felt her action very strange. But I ignored her and just sat there, waiting patiently for my doctor's assistant to call me in. I saw some of the patients cover their mouths with a cloth and come in and sit far away from the other patients. I had been waiting more than an hour in the waiting room. Once in a while, I would get up and check inside the clinic through the small glass window to see what kind of activity was going on inside the clinic and why they did not come out and get me yet. Then I saw my doctor's assistant open the clinic door and take the payment receipt slips from the small box. I went over to her quickly to let her know that I had been waiting there for more than an hour. My doctor's assistant told me not to worry and asked me to wait patiently. She would get me after Dr. Jennifer was done with the patient. I said OK.

I went back to my seat and waited for my doctor's assistant to take me inside the clinic.

After fifteen minutes, my doctor's assistant came out from the clinic to call me to go inside with her. I responded to her, and I went inside the clinic with her. This time she took me to the patient room directly, and she asked me how I was doing. I told her I did not have any more blood in both my arms for the laboratory technician to draw my blood samples. She told me to tell that to Dr. Jennifer when she came in. Then she left. After a few minutes, Dr. Jennifer knocked on the door and came inside the room; it seemed like she was very busy taking care of the patients. After she came in, she told me she had got my blood test result and asked me how I was doing, I told her the laboratory technician could not draw my blood sample from my right arm; she said it was OK to draw my blood sample from my left hand. Then she looked at the computer and told me my diabetic HGBA1c data range was 6.2 percent, a little bit higher than normal, but overall my blood test result was still good. Then she measured my blood pressure herself; she looked at my swollen legs, and she suggested putting up my legs on the pillow at night. Then she said everything was OK with me. Then I told her that my right ribs were causing me plenty of pain when I carried the groceries at home. She asked me to lie down on the patient bed, and she checked the right side of my stomach near my ribs by pressing with her hand up and down. I cried out loudly, "Ah!" Then I told her I had a lot of pain when she pressed the muscle near my right lower side of the rib bone; she said it was muscle pain that I had got from lifting heavy stuff. I told her about the incident when I had carried five pieces of corn in my right hand in King of Prussia; it had caused me great pain. Since then the pain in my right rib muscles was on and off, which made me very uncomfortable. She told me to take Advil pills to get rid of my pain. Then I told her I had got the medicines in preparation of the colorectal cancer test. I checked with her whether I should use the whole bottle of magnesium citrate to prepare for my colorectal cancer screening test; she said yes. I mentioned to her again about yellow fluid flowing out badly from my left ear and forming a big cyst on my left throat near my left ear after my last poisonous incident. She checked my left ear and throat, and she advised me to call Dr. Sara to get my ear surgery done as soon as possible to prevent the infection from getting worse. Then she told me to come back to checkup with her after three months. I told her I would, and she released me. I went to central hallway, and took my doctor's checkup statement and my blood test result paper from the nurse and I went home.

After my bad poisonous incident, I stayed inside my house most of the times watching television, because both my hands were just getting better from the poisonous blisters and forming new meat and soft skins. I got a lot of information about the accidents that were happening recently in California from the television. The most heartbreaking cases were the accidents that had caused people to die in the new Bay Bridge after Caltrans engineers replaced a new section of the bridge there. Since the first weekend of September 2009 was the Labor Day weekend, the television reporters were reporting how Caltrans engineers had laid out the structure of the Bay Bridge to fix it by cutting out one old middle section of the it and replace it with the new middle section, attaching the half of the new bridge that was built from Oakland city to San Francisco city. After they had successfully joined the new bridge to the old bridge with the new middle section, the bridge became an "S" shaped curl in the joint section. The mayor of San Francisco opened the Bay Bridge to allow the people to commute from San Francisco to Oakland city in the upper deck of Bay Bridge. After they opened the new section of Bay Bridge, there were so many accidents happening in the new "S"-shaped curl section of the upper deck. After a few months, the television reporters had already reported forty big and small cases of accidents that had already happened in the Bay Bridge after the bridge was joined with the new middle section of the bridge. Different-sized vehicles were involved in accidents in the "S"-shaped curl section of the Bay Bridge. The last accident was when one of the trucks fell on the ground from the upper deck bridge in the "S"-shaped curl section of the Bay Bridge; both the truck driver and his wife were killed in that accident. After I heard about the last accident that had happened in the Bay Bridge, I was very upset at Caltrans engineers. I did not understand why Caltrans engineers did not have any consideration about the safety of the commuters before they opened the new section of Bay Bridge and why they did not take any action to prevent the accidents after so many accidents had already happened in the new joint section of the Bay Bridge. I was getting very annoyed with the accidents that had happened in the Bay Bridge. I needed to stop and prevent this kind of bad accidents that were continuously happening in Bay Bridge. I tried to find a way to stop the accidents at night. I knew all the commuters were driving their vehicles at high speed in the Bay Bridge; there was no warning sign to remind them to slow down their vehicles on the bridge, and the commuters did not know when and where they should decrease their vehicles' speeds to drive carefully in the Bay Bridge, thus preventing an accident. I remembered when we were in New York, when we drove our car to pass Manhattan Bridge, as soon as we passed the section that was laid out with metal boards on Manhattan Bridge road, we would hear the metal bumping sound that came out from the metal boards, forcing the drivers to decrease their vehicles' speeds as it reminded them to drive carefully. So I told Sirena to remind the Caltrans engineer to lay out the metal sheets on the section of the Bay Bridge before the "S"-shaped curl, thus reminding the commuters to decrease their vehicles' speed before they would drive through the "S"-shaped curl in the Bay Bridge, or to do something to make the vehicles slow down their car speed. After I asked Sirena to remind the Caltrans engineers to lay out a technique to slow down the vehicles to avoid an accident in the new Bay Bridge section, Caltrans engineers closed down the left-end lane, thus making all the vehicles slow down their vehicles' speed before they entered the "S"-shaped curl to avoid an accident. This technique worked so well for the commuters of Bay Bridge, as it made them to slow down their vehicles, thus preventing accidents in Bay Bridge. Finally, all kinds of accidents in Bay Bridge stopped.

On November 27, 2009, Friday, Shaun came home and cleaned all the gutters in my house; after he was done, he was ready to put away the metal ladder in the garage. When I saw him put away the metal ladder, I stopped him and told him to leave the metal ladder in my backyard. I could use it later when I had to cut down the cypress branches. He left the metal ladder in the backyard for me to use. Then I cooked some beef and vegetables for our dinner. I asked Shaun to take the garbage cans out after dinner. Shaun said OK, and he took the garbage cans out on the sidewalk and then went home.

On December 1, 2009, while I was eating my lunch at noontime, I tried to avoid eating food with seeds and red and purple colors as instructed in the sigmoidoscopy preparation sheet. I forgot I should not have eaten anything after noontime. When I saw one small piece of persimmon fruit left on the counter plate, I picked it up and ate it at 3:00 p.m. After I ate the piece of persimmon fruit, I realized that I should not have eaten anything after noontime, but as I had already eaten it, I could not do anything to change it. I decided to continue my colorectal cancer screening test. I took 10 oz of magnesium citrate at 4:00 p.m. After two hours, the medicine caused me diarrhea, so I had to go in and out the restroom for the whole evening to clean up my stomach. Next day, I woke up in the morning at 8:00 a.m. I let my two dogs out as usual. I took them back in the house and fed them their breakfast. At 9:15 a.m. and 9:35 a.m., I gave myself two Fleet enemas as instructed in the sigmoidoscopy preparation sheet. Then I changed my clothing and I left my house at 10:00 a.m. to go to Walnut Creek KPMC.

After I arrived in Walnut Creek KPMC Gastroenterology Department, I checked in with the front desk clerk; the front desk clerk asked me whether I had prepared for my colorectal cancer screening test. I told her I did, but I did not tell her I had forgotten about my colorectal cancer screening test and that I had taken one small piece of persimmon fruit at 3:00 p.m. before I took magnesium citrate. After I checked in, she asked me to sign the agreement paper to let Nurse Joan screen my colon. I signed the paper in front of her; she asked me to give this paper to Nurse Joan's assistant when he came out to get me. Then she told me to wait in the waiting room. Nurse Joan's assistant came out' at 11:15 a.m. to take me inside the colorectal cancer screening testing room. I gave him the agreement paper when I saw him. He took the paper from me and asked me to follow him to the room where the colorectal cancer screening test would be performed. He explained to me the procedure and asked me to change and lie down on the patient bed to get ready for Nurse Joan to perform the colorectal cancer screening test. I did the way Nurse Joan's assistant told me. I laid down on the patient bed and waited for Nurse Joan. Nurse Joan came out with her assistant; when she saw me, she said she still remembered me from last time when I was in the clinic without having done any preparation for the colorectal cancer screening test. I told her I remembered her too. She sat down on the chair next to my patient bed and asked me to turn my body to face the computer on the left. Then she explained to me how she was going to put a small pipe with a camera inside my colon and how she would pump air into my colon to screen it. She put the small pipe with the camera inside my colon, and she pumped in air to enlarge my colon; she was carefully screening the colon with the small camera pipe. I felt a lot of pain when she moved around the pipe inside my colon; the pain was just like stomach pain. I saw my own colon on the computer screen. I did not have any cut or infectious areas. Then she pushed the small pipe in and pumped in air again and again. I kept telling her, "Done! Done! Done!" But she did not stop pushing the pipe in and out. Then I heard her saying that the older you got, there was less possibility of getting colorectal cancer. She was pushing the small pipe in again and carefully screening. After she was sure that I did not have any cut in my colon, she finally pulled out the pipe from my colon and told me I did not need to screen my colon again for another five years. I was so relieved; I thanked her and wished her Merry Christmas! I also told her I would like to see her again, but this would be one and only time for her to screen my colon; she or any other technician would not be allowed to screen my colon for the colorectal cancer screening test again. She smiled and left the room. Her assistant told me I could get up to change into my regular clothing. I got up from the patient bed with tremendous pain in my colon and changed into my regular clothing. Then I checked with her assistant regarding the location of the restroom; he told me I had to go outside this room and the restroom was next to this room. I opened the door and went outside to the restroom. I cleaned myself up. After I felt I was clean enough to go home, I went out from the restroom to the hallway, my body bent because of the pain that I had during the colorectal cancer screening test. The receptionist in the hallway near the elevator saw me bent over with pain. She asked me whether I needed any help from her. I thanked her and told her I believed it would go away after a while. Then I asked her where the head and neck surgery clinic was. She told me it was on the third floor. I took the elevator to go up to the third floor. I went to the head and neck surgery clinic and asked the front desk clerk to set up a January appointment with Dr. Sara for my ear surgery. She checked the January appointment dates of Dr. Sara on the computer and told me it would not open until Friday. She suggested that I call back on Friday. So I took the elevator to go down to the first floor and walked to the parking lot in pain. I drove myself home. On the way home, I stopped at 99 Ranch supermarket and bought some vegetables, then went home. I put away all the vegetables in the refrigerator after I reached home. I made myself a cup of hot tea and went to bed early and rested.

I felt very uncomfortable and my swollen anus felt itchy after I came back from the colorectal cancer screening test. I kept cleaning my anus with water, but the itch would not go away, so I had to use soap and water to keep cleaning it. After two weeks, my swelling came down and was gone. On Friday, I went out to my front yard in the morning and brought all my garbage cans into my side yard and locked the side gate door. Then I decided to cut the branches of the cypress trees on the left side of my building, which were growing so big and so close to my house. I was afraid the cypress trees would damage my house, so I moved the metal ladder close to the cypress trees, and I climbed up the ladder and cut out all the small-sized cypress branches. Then I cut the main tall cypress branches into 1½ inches diameter. When I cut one of the 1½-inch-diameter branches to 1¼ inches, I saw the branch starting to fall. I tried to move and turn my body slowly to face the ladder, to prevent myself from getting hit by the falling branch that would fall on my head. If I tried to avoid the falling branch by stepping down the ladder quickly or moved my body to any side, I would fall from the ladder and hurt myself badly. So I just stayed on the ladder and let the bottom part of the cypress branch hit and stop on my left shoulder. I used my right hand to push the cypress branch from my left shoulder to the left-side ground. After the cypress branch fell on the ground, I carefully stepped down from the ladder and removed all the branches to the other side of my house. I cut out all the small branches piece by piece and dumped them in my green recycle can. I left all the big branches there for Shaun to come home and cut into small pieces, to use them later as firewood in my house. Then I went inside my house and sat down on my sofa and rested. I felt my left shoulder become numb when I touched it. I did not feel like going to the minor injury clinic to check with the doctor, so I took two Advil pain-reliever pills and went to bed. Next day, my left shoulder had swelled up, causing a lot of pain. I called Rosie and Susong to let them know I had got hit on my shoulder by the falling cypress branch while I was cutting the cypress branches. They asked me whether I had gone to the minor injury clinic to see the doctor. I told them I did not go, because I was very tired to drive myself to the minor injury clinic, and I had just taken Advil pain-reliever pills at home. I told Sirena when she was home on Sunday about my incident. She told me to be careful and asked me not to do it again. Then she cleaned up the kitchen floor, and she took both the garbage cans out on the sidewalk for me. After she was done, she went home. Every week, I tried to cut down the bottom part of the cypress branches to fill up my green recycle can. Sometimes when I was cutting the branches, a few branches fell in my neighbor's yards. I saw my left-side neighbors cleaning the cypress branches from their yards. I went over to them to say thanks for their generous act in helping me to clean the cypress branches that dropped in their yards. After I cut down all the bottom part of the branches from the cypress trees, my backyard looked wide open, and I could see all my neighbors' houses, and it made me felt good. I could not get rid of my allergies and sickness without my neighbors cutting down their white birch trees. My lips, ears, and body still itched badly after I came back inside the house from outside my yard.

On Monday morning, December 7, 2009, I called Pleasanton KPMC head and neck surgery clinic to set up an appointment with Dr. Sara. The scheduling clerk set up an appointment on January 8, 2009, at 4:00 p.m. for me. I asked her whether I could get the morning hour for my appointment. She said she would check and asked me to wait. After a while, she said the appointment would be on January 21, 2010, if I wanted the morning hour. I told her I did not want to wait that long, because my left ear was infected badly. So she set up an appointment on January 8, 2010, at 4:00 p.m. for me. After the accident, I stayed inside my house until my shoulder pain was gone. Since I did not have anyone to help me at home, I had to do all my lawn jobs by myself. I got bad allergies and got sick again and again. On Sunday, December 13, 2009, both Sirena and Shaun came back home, and they took me to Costco store to buy two bags of rice and food. After we came home, they helped me put away all the groceries and they both went home.

On December 23, 2009, I went to Safeway supermarket, and I bought vegetables and two boxes of tangerines and then went home. After I was home, I saw the gardener Martin and his guys were working in my front yard. I opened my garage door and drove my car inside my garage. I took out all my groceries and put them away. Then I heard somebody knocking on my front door, and I went to my front door; when I opened my door, I saw Martin standing on my front door, and he asked me whether he could use my garbage can to dump out all of the lawn waste. I told him I had got hurt last week and I had not done anything this week, so my garbage can was empty, and he could use my garbage can to fill in his lawn waste. Then I told him the city of Pleasanton had restricted us, not allowing us to use big garbage cans for the green waste anymore. I did not think this medium-sized garbage can was big enough for us to dump the green waste every week. Then I took him to my backyard to show him all my cypress trees and I asked him if he cut trees. He said he did cut trees and accepted the contract from other people to cut trees. I asked him to give me an estimate to cut the top portion of my cypress trees. He calculated and told me the estimate right away. I told him I needed to discuss it with Shaun. If Shaun agreed, he would call him. He said OK. I let him take out the empty green garbage can and let him continue his work. I requested him to leave my garbage can on the sidewalk after he had filled in all the lawn waste in the waste garbage can. Then I went inside my house.

On December 24, 2009, I went to Chase bank in Pleasanton downtown to deposit the check that I had got from my brother Edward; after I deposited my check in the bank, I went to Safeway supermarket and bought over fifteen pounds of pork meat and two boxes of tangerines and I went home. When I carried the pork meat into my kitchen from my garage, I found I had great pain in my left wrist. When I checked my left wrist, I found the middle metacarpal bone on my hand was pulling away from my wrist carpal bone and it had left a very deep area in between the carpal and metacarpal bones. I could see the edge of my wrist bone very clearly.

Shaun came home at 8:30 p.m. on Thursday night and told me he had bought a new cellular phone for me. He asked me to give him my old cellular phone. I gave him my old cellular phone. He took out the phone card from my old cellular phone; then he replaced the old phone card in the new cellular phone and tested whether the pictures on the old phone card showed up on the new cellular phone. But the pictures on the old phone card did not show up in the new cellular phone, because the brand of the new cellular phone was different from the old cellular phone; he said he could not use the phone card from the old phone in this new phone, so he would return this cellular phone and get me another cellular phone of the same brand as my current cellular phone. Then he switched the old phone card back from the new cellular phone, and he gave my old cellular phone back to me. I took my old cellular phone and told him I needed his help in transferring all the pictures from my old cellular phone that I had taken in the past couple years to my home computer. I did not know whether it could transfer the pictures from the cellular phone to the home computer. He said he would help me transfer the pictures from my cellular phone to my home computer when he came back home next time, because he said he needed a device and program to transfer the pictures to the home computer. Since he had just came back home, I asked him if he had already eaten; if he had not eaten yet, I had pork meat ready in the oven that I had baked for him in the evening. He said he had already eaten a little bit, and he went to his room and slept. I put away all the food in the refrigerator and cleaned up my kitchen. Sirena had told me she would go to her friend's house for the Christmas party and she would be home after the party. So I did not wait for her to come home. I went to bed.

On next day, December 25, 2009, when I woke up in the morning, I prepared fried noodles for my children to eat when they got up. After I was done frying the noodles, I went outside to my backyard and watered my plants. They both got up after 10:00 a.m. and ate the fried noodles that I had prepared for their breakfast and lunch. After they had eaten, I asked Shaun whether he had found out the technique to transfer files from the old small computer to my new home computer. He said he had, and he went to the living room to work with the computers to help me transfer all my files from the small old computer to the diskette; then he transferred all my files from the diskette to my home computer. After he was done transferring all the files, he found the device in his room to transfer the pictures from my cellular phone to the home computer on the table; he hooked up the device on my cellular phone and home computer, and he tried to transfer the pictures from my cellular phone to my home computer for me, but he did not successfully transfer the pictures from my cellular phone to my home computer. He called me and explained to me that he needed another software program to transfer the pictures from my cellular phone to my home computer. He said he had the program in his laptop to transfer the pictures, but he had left his laptop in his apartment and he would bring it next time he came home. I said OK. Then he left and went home. Before Sirena went home, I reminded her to come home next Sunday a bit earlier. I wanted to take her to Macy's store to get some clothing for her New Year presents. She said OK and went home.

On December 27, 2009, Sunday, Sirena came home and gave me a new sportswear set as my New Year present. It was a very beautiful sportswear set that she had bought for me. Then we went to Macy's store in Pleasanton Stonebridge mall to look for clothing for her. On the way to Macy's store, I showed Sirena the big caps on my wrists between my hand bones and my wrist bones, which had pulled apart and dislocated, causing me a lot of pain when I carried the pork meat to the kitchen. She told me to checkup with the doctor. I told her I wanted to wait for another month to see whether my wrists would be getting better. Then we walked around inside Macy's store, looking for her clothing. After we walked around for a while, she said she did not want to buy any clothing anymore. I insisted her to get some new clothing. She went to the women's clothing department to choose two blue jean pants and one winter coat for herself. I paid with my credit card and we came home. Then we had dinner together. I asked her to feed the dogs for me after dinner. She took out the chicken, and she cut the chicken into small pieces, mixed it with rice; then she warmed up the chicken and rice in the microwave oven and fed the dogs. Then she cleaned the kitchen for me. After she was done with cleaning the kitchen, she went home. Next day I went to Walmart store to get clothing for Shaun as New Year present. I did not know the size of clothing that he usually wore. I was unable to get anything for him. I went home, and I called Shaun to ask him about the size of his clothing. He said he would go to Walmart store with me next time when he came home. I said OK and hung up the phone.

On the last day of the year of 2009, December 31, I was home alone. I prepared pound cakes, fried chicken noodles, and some baked chicken for myself and my dogs to celebrate the last day of the year of 2009. After I finished making the food, I fed my two dogs baked chicken first. Then I ate my hot, delicious fried chicken noodles and baked chicken. I turned on the television after dinner to watch news. I did not know how I fell asleep on my sofa. I woke up at 9:00 p.m. I let the dogs out into my backyard and waited for a while to let them come back inside the house. After they came inside the house, I went to bed. Next day I woke up at 8:00 a.m. as usual, but the year was different. It was the newest year of "2010" and the date was January 1, 2010, Friday. When I looked at my cellular phone, I found there were two text messages from Sirena at 12:06 a.m. and 1:00 a.m. She had sent out the text messages to me last night to wish me Happy New Year! She had said she was going to be in her friend's New Year's Eve party; she must have been still in her friend's house when she sent out those text messages to me. I had been very tired and gone to bed early last night. I did not even know when she had sent out text messages to me. This was the first time I had missed New Year's Eve program. I had never missed any New Year's Eve program before in the past twenty years. I must have been sleeping soundly. I did not even hear the cellular phone ring when Sirena sent out text massages to me. After I read her text messages in the morning, I sent out text messages to both my children to wish them Happy New Year! Then I received Shaun's text message wishing me Happy New Year. Sirena came home and suggested taking me out to eat for our lunch on New Year's Day. Since I had not been to Chinatown, Oakland, for so long, I suggested going down to Chinatown in Oakland to have some hot noodle soup and to buy American ginseng roots if it was not raining. Actually, I wanted to wait for Shaun to come home to go down to Chinatown in Oakland together, but the weather television channels were announcing that it would be raining on New Year's Day. I told Sirena I had already sent out a text message to Shaun that we were not going to Oakland because it was going to rain. He had already sent back a text message to me to let me know that he would not be home on New Year's Day but that he would be home on Monday, January 4, 2010, on his day off. I told Sirena to take a chance to go down to Chinatown, Oakland; hopefully it would not be raining until we came back home. She said she would like to take me and drive down to Oakland. So we went to Chinatown in Oakland. We parked our car in the underground parking building in Chinatown, Oakland. We went to the Chinese restaurant that we usually went. The restaurant was very busy as usual, filled with customers. When we arrived in front of the restaurant, there were some customers there, already waiting outside to get tables to go inside the restaurant. We went to the entrance of that restaurant to give out our names for getting a table for ourselves. When I saw one of the waiters come out and take the names and numbers of the customers that were waiting outside the restaurant, I told him we were two people, and he told us to wait for a while. Then an old lady waitress from the restaurant came out to ask Sirena how many people we had. Sirena told her, "Two people." Then the old lady waitress told Sirena they had two unoccupied chairs at the corner table and we could go in and be seated if we did not mind sharing the table with other customers. Sirena told her it was OK for us to share the table with other customers. So the old lady waitress took us to the corner table near the kitchen; a customer was already seated and having his noodle soup. We pulled the chairs out and sat. When the lady on the next table saw us, she tried to help us rearrange the stuff on the table to let us have more space to eat our lunch. I thanked her; then I asked her where she was from. She said she was from Laos and introduced her mother-in-law, her husband, and her daughter to us. I told her she was a very nice lady to take her mother-in-law out for lunch. Then we ordered our food. I ordered a bowl of hot noodle soup. Sirena ordered fried noodles with beef and a plate of fish cake. We did not have to wait long to get the food that we had ordered. After we got our food, we ate and enjoyed our food until we finished all of it. After we finished our food, we paid and left the restaurant. We walked around Chinatown for a while and bought some vegetables from the nearby stores; then we went to "New Day" Chinese grocery store on the Ninth Street. On the way to this store, I saw some of the old stores were closed and replaced by a lot of new banks and new stores. When we arrived at the "New Day" store, we went inside. The front part of this store was really big and was selling a lot of different kinds of Chinese groceries. Now I saw that this store had rented half of their store to other businessmen. All the stores were not busy, and there were no customers inside the stores; the economy must be very bad lately in Chinatown, Oakland. I met the lady cashier who had taken care of me when I had been in that store before. As soon as the lady cashier saw me, she asked me where I had been all these years; she said she had not seen me come down to Oakland for a long time. I told her I had got a bad allergy and was sick all these years, so I did not get a chance to come down here. I said that today my daughter had come home and brought me down to Oakland to have lunch and buy American ginseng roots. She showed me different grades of American ginseng roots, and I told her I wanted to buy four pounds of media grade of American ginseng roots for myself to use at home. She took a paper bag and tried to put four pounds of American ginseng roots from the tank into the paper bag. She weighed the American ginseng roots in a paper bag and indicated to me that it was more than four and a half pounds. She tried to take out some pieces of American ginseng roots from the bag. Then she put them back all in and asked me to take all of it. I said no problem and gave her my credit card. She took my credit card and gave it to another lady cashier; the lady cashier charged the cost of American ginseng roots to my credit card. Then she packed the American ginseng roots in the paper bag and gave it to me. I took the bag and we left the store. We walked around a little bit on the street; there were not much people on the street. I saw some empty building spaces had put up the sign "To rent." After a while, I felt tired and told Sirena I wanted to go home. We walked to the pay parking booth in the small shopping center. Sirena went over to the pay parking booth to line up with other people. I sat on the side concrete bench, waiting for her. After she paid the parking fee, we took the elevator and went down to the floor where we had parked our car. After we got our car, we took 580 Highway to go back home. There were not too many vehicles on the highway. All the people must have been watching the Rose Parade show on television at home on New Year's Day.

After we arrived home, Sirena took out all the groceries from my car and put them in the kitchen. Then she told me she was tired and she would like to take a nap, and she went into her room to take a nap. I put away all the groceries that we had bought from Oakland on the shelf. After I was done, I went inside my room and took a short nap. I felt much fresher after I woke up. It was good for me to get out from my house once in a while and take a short trip to other places. When I looked outside, it was getting dark, and the clock showed five o'clock. I went in Sirena's room to wake her up and remind her she had to go home before dark. She told me to give her half an hour to get up. So I went out to the family room and watched television. After half an hour, I still did not see Sirena come out yet. So I went in her room and saw she was still sleeping, I woke her up again, and she told me to give her another half an hour to get up and go home. This went on and off until it was 6:30 p.m., and finally she came out and told me she was going home; she kissed me and took her purse and the food that I had prepared for her to take home. She opened the front door and was just about to go out when I remembered she had not taken the garbage cans out for me yet, so I got up to stop and remind her to take the garbage cans out to the sidewalk. She said OK; then she asked me to help her open the garage door, and she put away all her stuff inside her car. I opened the garage door for her. She went out from my side garage door, opened the side gate, and took all the garbage cans to the sidewalk for me. Then she closed the garage side door and went out to her car from the garage and left. I closed the garage door and went to my family room. I turned on the television and watched it until 9:00 p.m. Then I left the dogs out into my backyard and made myself a cup of hot coffee. After a while I saw both my dogs waiting outside in front of my sliding back door. So I left them, came inside the house, and went to bed. Next day I sent a text message to Shaun to make sure he would be coming home on Monday. He sent back a text message to me that he would be definitely coming home on Monday. On Sunday morning after I woke up, I took out coconut chicken noodle soup from my refrigerator to cook for Shaun to take home. After I finished cooking, I put them inside a jar for Shaun to take home on Monday.

On January 4, 2010, Monday, when Shaun came home in the morning, I asked him whether he had got the software program to transfer all the pictures from my cellular telephone to my home computer; he said yes. Then he said he needed to load the Samsung software program from his laptop to my home computer first. Then he went out to his car to get his laptop. After he took out his laptop from his car, he came back inside the house and started working on the computer in the dining table. I warmed up a bowl of coconut noodle soup for him to eat first. After he ate, he went in the dining room to load the software program from his laptop to my home computer. After he was done loading the software program on to my computer, he asked me to give him my cellular phone. I gave him my cellular phone and I told him I would take a shower. I went inside my room. After I finished taking the shower, I saw he was sleeping in his room. I woke him up and asked him whether he had finished transferring the pictures from my cellular phone to my home computer, and he said he had already done. Then he told me to let him sleep for a while. I said OK and told him to let me know when he had finished loading all my pictures in my home computer. He said he would and he went back to sleep. Since I did not want to cook, I took my dogs to McDonald's restaurant to buy sandwiches for all of us. I bought French fries, two Big Mac sandwiches for me and Shaun, and two double cheeseburgers for my dogs from McDonald's restaurant. When I reached home, I fed the double cheeseburgers to my dogs; they loved to eat them. Then I made myself a cup of hot coffee and ate my Big Mac sandwich. I woke up Shaun at 4:30 p.m. to tell him he had to go home before dark. After a while Shaun came out to the family room; he asked me to look at the pictures on my cellular phone that he had transferred to my home computer in the dining room. I asked him to eat the Big Mac sandwich and French fries that I had got ready for him to eat; then I gave him a cup of hot American ginseng soup to drink. He finished his Big Mac sandwich and American ginseng soup. Then he showed me all my pictures on my home computer. I saw all my pictures were looking clear on the home computer than on my cellular phone. Then I told him he needed to help me transfer the videos from my cellular phone to my home computer; he said he would try and he worked on transferring the videos from my cellular phone to the home computer. After he was done, he called me to show me the videos on my home computer. I was so happy to see that all the pictures and the videos from my cellular phone were on my home computer. Earlier I was worried I would lose all the pictures and videos on my cellular telephone if it broke. Now I did not have to worry about them anymore. Then I went in the kitchen to pack all the food that I had cooked for him in plastic bags to take home. He played with the computer for a while in the dining room; then he went to his room and worked on his laptop. After I packed all the food for him in plastic bags, I went to his room to remind him he had to go home before dark. Shaun got up from his bed. When I saw Shaun get up from his bed, I showed him I had tried to clean up his room and helped put away all his books inside the boxes. I tried to organize his room for him. While I was organizing his room, I saw there were two pictures that he had hung on the walls with pins. One of the pictures was of his 1992 baseball team group and another picture was of Mr. Roger Staubach from Dallas Cowboys football team with his signature on the picture that he had given Shaun when Shaun was in Amador High School baseball team. Every time he came home, I did not get a chance to tell him to get frames for these two pictures. I told him those pictures were very valuable pictures and that he would never get them back again in his life if he ruined them. I told him I would get picture frames for both pictures from the frame store. I asked him to take down the picture of his baseball team from the wall for me. I wanted to take this picture to the picture frame store to get the right size of the frame for the picture. He said he did not want me to spend money for his picture; he asked me to leave his pictures on the wall. I told him I would like to get a picture frame for his baseball team picture to make it last forever, as a remembrance of his coach and all his baseball teammates from Amador High School. I reminded him again he should get picture frames for all his pictures that he had taken all these years, and he should value all the pictures from his young age and keep them in picture books. He looked at me and said, "OK, Mom."

Baseball game was very popular in Tri Valley. Almost all the boys in the Tri Valley joined the baseball teams; they were very good at baseball games. Every Saturday all the parks in Tri Valley would be filled with those young baseball players playing baseball; their parents would watch them playing the games. Shaun had joined the baseball team when he was in elementary school until he graduated from Amador high school in Pleasanton. I still remember that I would take him to the baseball field to practice his baseball games every Saturday. Every time when his team played and competed with other teams from Tri Valley, most of the times his team lost, which made them very unhappy. When their team won, their coach took them out to McDonald's restaurant for their lunch to celebrate. I asked him whether he still remembered his baseball team when he saw those pictures. He said, "Yes, Mom." He got up from his bed right away to take down the picture for me. Then I stopped him from taking down the picture, because it was getting dark. I did not want to ruin the picture after he took down the picture from the wall and put it on the desk. I told him he had to get ready to go back to Davis and that I would find a way to take down the picture from the wall myself and take them to the frame shop to measure the right size of the frame for that picture. I asked him to shut down his laptop and home computer in the dining room and to organize all his stuff to get ready to take home. I went out to the kitchen to get all the food ready for him to take home. He shut down his laptop and organized all his stuff in the dining room; he put his laptop and his stuff in his big bag and took them to his car. After he put away his bag in his car, he went to pick up the mails from my mailbox, which was two houses away. He came back with all the mails and gave them to me. Then he went to the dining room to shut down my home computer for me. I found there was a letter from Kaiser Permanente insurance company, informing me to increase my health care rate, and I gave it to him. He took the letter and put it in his pocket. I told him each year all these insurance companies kept increasing the medical insurance rate, leading to people not being able to afford to buy them. We had to do something about it to stop them from increasing the health care rate. He shook his head and said he knew it. Then he went home. Next day on Tuesday, January 5, 2010, at 12:39 p.m., Shaun called me to let me know that PG&E had approved my application to get a discount on the PG&E electric bill.

I had lived in California for so many decades; no matter how hard I worked for our family to build the company, a group of bad hearted people kept after me, creating and setting up bad accidents for me, to get me killed. When I set up the deal with the city of Pleasanton and the people from America and all over the world to search out the proof that the birch trees were the allergic trees that were causing the people to get bad allergies and sickness in the residential areas, and after I spoke out that the birch trees were the allergic trees causing the people to get the bad allergies and sickness, a group of bad-hearted people used dried birch powder to poison me. Both my children were working hard and they were financially supporting me so that I could live in this house comfortably all these years. We never gave up hope for ourselves for standing up to struggle for our lives to survive in this country. Luckily God is up in the heaven, watching us, taking care of us, and saving our lives.

On Friday, January 8, 2010, I had an appointment to go to Walnut Creek KPMC to checkup with Dr. Sara for my ear surgery in the head and neck surgery clinic. I kept an eye on the weather and watched the weather channel to find out the weather in these few days in preparation for my appointment in Walnut Creek. I was very happy I would not have to drive my car to Walnut Creek in the rain after I heard the weather channel reporting it would not be raining on Friday. But on Thursday, the weather channel reported the weather was changing again and that it would be raining on Thursday and would have morning showers on Friday. I got up early in the morning on Friday. I looked at the sky; it was dark and the weather was very cloudy, but I did not see any rain yet. I was a little bit worried about driving my car in the rain to Walnut Creek. Then I remembered I had to prepare for Dr. Sara the list of medicines that I had recently started taking daily, so I took out all my medicine bottles and wrote down all the prescription names on a piece of paper on the kitchen counter. After I was done listing all my prescription names on the paper, I checked the outside weather again. I saw there were a few raindrops falling outside. I sat down in my family room and watched television; after a while I checked the outside weather again, and the rain had stopped. I took a shower at 12:30 p.m. and got ready to go to Walnut Creek. Since my appointment with Dr. Sara was at 4:00 p.m., it was still a bit early to go to Walnut Creek KPMC, but I did not want to checkup late with Dr. Sara. I would rather wait in KPMC if I arrived there early. So I left my house at 2:30 p.m. and took 580 East Freeway exit from Santa Rita Road, then 680 North Freeway to go to Walnut Creek city; the sky was very unpleasant, but when I passed San Ramon city, I saw the sun coming out, and it was sunny all the way to Walnut Creek. I took South Main Street exit from 680 North Freeway and went straight; after I passed two traffic lights, I turned left to go into KPMC parking garage. Since it was evening, the parking garage was full. I could not find any parking space inside the garage, so I had to drive my car all the way to the fourth floor, and then I saw a car pull out from the parking space and leave. I parked my car in that parking space. I took the elevator to go down to the ground floor and I went into the medical center next to the parking garage; then I went to the restroom on the first floor of the medical center building; someone was inside the restroom when I arrived there, but I just had to wait for a while. The lady came out from the restroom and told me to go in. I went inside the restroom. I did not know why the floor was so sticky. I felt my shoes were sticking on the floor. I washed my hands after I used the restroom, and then I came out. Since I was an hour early, I had nothing to do inside the medical center building. I went back and walked around outside the medical center building, I read all the signs that were posted outside. There was a small shopping center across the street next to the Walnut Creek KPMC. There were not too many people on the streets or in the small shopping center. I felt I should go back inside the main medical building, so I walked back to the medical center building. I took the elevator to go up to the third floor to the head and neck surgery clinic. But the front desk clerk was busy talking on the phone, so I had to wait on the floor mat, which indicated the patients to wait. After a while, the front desk clerk asked me to check in with her. I told the clerk that I had an appointment with Dr. Sara at 4:00 p.m. She asked me to give her my home address; I gave it. Then she asked me to pay for my co-payment. I gave her my credit card; after she entered my payment in the computer, she gave me my receipt. I took my receipt. I sat on the chair, waiting for Dr. Sara's assistant to take me in the patient room. I was still half an hour early; no patient was waiting in the waiting room except me. The television was not on, and it was very quiet, so I went to the front desk clerk to ask her to turn on the television for me. The front desk clerk turned on the television for me. I sat on the waiting room chair, watching television. Suddenly I remembered I did not know how it worked if I needed to stay in the hospital for one night, so I went to the front desk clerk to find out how the hospital arranged for the patient to stay one day at the hospital; she told me it was just like staying in the hotel; one day meant allowing the patient to stay one night in the hospital. Then I asked her if the surgery was done at night, the patient had to stay two nights; she said she did not know. She suggested that I check with my doctor. I said OK to her. Then I told her the reason I had asked her this question was to prepare for my hospital stay on the night after my ear surgery. Then I told her I should have gotten that surgery done a few years ago. But every time the surgery scheduler called me for my ear surgery, I had to keep refusing the surgery scheduler to go in for my ear surgery, because I did not know how to come to Walnut

Creek or Antioch KPMC. The surgery scheduler had suggested that I take the bus to go to Walnut Creek KPMC, but I did not know where the bus station was, so I refused to take the bus to go to Walnut Creek KPMC. I had told the surgery scheduler that he should call me three or four days ahead to give me time to find out how to go to Walnut Creek KPMC. When I received the phone calls from the surgery scheduler, I called my children and left a message for them to call me back, but I never received any return call from my children. When I asked my children when they came home why they did not return my calls, they told me they were very busy. At that time, I was also getting treatment from my physical therapist to fix my shoulder after the accident, which I got from diabetic medicines that made my joints dry out and made my shoulders stiff. Then I told her about the bad poisonous blisters that I got on both my hands in August 2009 after I came back from Pennsylvania. Last time when Dr. Jennifer insisted that I must go to Walnut Creek KPMC to get my colorectal cancer screening test done, I had no choice but to ask my daughter Sirena to take me to Walnut Creek KPMC to take sigmoidoscopy screening test in the gastroenterology department. After Sirena took me twice there, I put my feet down on the ground to learn how to come here. She said she understood it was hard to go to a new place without knowing the direction which way to go there. While we were talking, the phone rang, and we stopped our conversation. I went to sit down on the chair in the waiting room for Dr. Sara's assistant to take me inside Dr. Sara's clinic.

Dr. Sara's assistant came out at 3:59 p.m. and took me to the patient room, asking me to sit inside the room and wait for Dr. Sara. Before I sat down, I gave her the prescription list that KPMC had left me in a message to prepare for Dr. Sara. She advised me to give the prescription list to Dr. Sara myself when she came in. Then she left the room. After a while, Dr. Sara knocked on the door and came inside the room. As soon as I saw her I gave her the prescription list; she took the prescription list from me and she sat down on a chair next to me and looked at it. Then she asked me about my ear infection. I told her I had a lot of yellow fluid flowing out from my left ear after I got the bad poisonous allergy accident recently when I picked up the seashell in August. I told her I did take the pictures of my swollen hands, but I had already transferred it to my home computer and I was unable to show her the swollen blisters on my hands on my cellular phone. Then she asked me whether I was ready to do surgery. I told her yes, I wanted to get my ear surgery done as soon as possible. Then she suggested that I not smoke one month before the surgery and one month after the surgery. I said to her that I had two ears; if my left ear infection was caused by smoking, then why did my right ear not get infected? I did not think it was fair for her to ask me not to smoke. Then she suggested that she would look at my right ear first, and she moved her chair closer to my right side of the chair to look at my right ear. After she was done, she told me my right ear condition was good. Then she moved her chair to my left side to look at my left ear. After she checked my left ear, she said my left ear infection was not that bad. I told her fluid was flowing out badly from my left ear last night and I had just cleaned it this morning before I came to see her. I showed her the cyst on my left throat; then I told her that my cyst was getting bigger each day, but after the fluid flowed out from my left ear, I could feel that the cyst on my throat was getting smaller. She checked the cyst on my throat. Then she told me that I had to wait till March to perform surgery on my left ear, because there were so many patients waiting to get surgeries done. I told her Dr. Jennifer had suggested that I get my left ear surgery done as soon as possible while my glucose fasting result in my two recent blood test results was within in the normal data range, 88 mg/dl in July and 97 mg/dl in October. I insisted that this would be the best time to perform my left ear surgery while my glucose fasting data was in the required normal data range. Then she asked me whether I had got my hearing test done recently. I told her not yet. I asked her whether I needed to take another CAT scan X-ray of my ear; she said no, because the radiation would hurt me more if I kept taking CAT scan X-ray. She brought up the result of my hearing test from last year on the computer, which Cara T. had performed in Pleasanton KMPC head and neck surgery clinic for me; then she checked all the data in the graph table. I requested her to arrange my ear surgery as soon as possible. She wrote down "Herbal," the name of the surgery scheduler, and their telephone number on her business card for me to call the surgery scheduler if I did not hear from them after two weeks. I took her card and told her I would call the surgery scheduler if I did not hear from them after two weeks. Then we left the room. I gave her the prescription list again in the clinic hallway on my way out to go home. She said she had already written down all the information on her sheet and gave it back to me. I insisted on her keeping the prescription list, because I had a note written on the prescription list about Dr. Jennifer insisting that I must get my ear surgery done as soon as possible. I was pushing her really hard this time to get my ear surgery done as soon as possible. Then I pouted my lips in front of her, telling her loudly that I had been with her for over two years and I was the senior most patient of her and that she should take care of me first. I told her she should ask her other new patients to wait, because the ears of her new patients were not infected badly; she laughed and said OK. I was very happy to hear that she had promised to take care of me first. I came out from the clinic and went over to the front desk clerk to say good-bye and went home. I drove my car carefully, and I was happy to be home smoothly.

On Saturday, January 9, 2010, I wanted to prepare ahead for all the things I needed for my ear surgery, so I sent out a text message to Sirena whether she would be home on Sunday, because I needed to buy detergent and extra dog snacks for my dogs from Costco store. She sent back a text message at 11:33 a.m. on Sunday to let me know she would be home at 1:00 p.m. to take me to Costco store. After I got her text message, I changed my clothing to wait for her to come home. When Sirena came home, we went to Costco store. I told her to order pizza from Costco restaurant on our way to Costco store. She said OK, and she called Costco restaurant and ordered combo pizza. We bought eggs, yogurt, and detergents from Costco store. Costco store did not have dog snacks; then we picked up the combo pizza from Costco restaurant, and we went to the Costco gas station to fill up gasoline in my car. Then we stopped in Safeway supermarket to buy groceries and then went home.

After Sirena put away all the groceries at home, she took one piece of pizza from the pizza box and sat down on the sofa, and she turned on the television and watched it, at the same time eating her pizza. I remembered I still needed to pick up my tuna fish cans that I had ordered from the CVS store; before I went to the CVS store, I called the CVS store to make sure they had forty-eight tuna fish cans for me. The CVS store manager told me they had enough tuna fish cans for me and asked me to come and get them. So I told them I would come in tomorrow to get the tuna fish cans. After I hung up the phone and watched television with Sirena, I realized I should buy the tuna fish cans today when Sirena was home; she could help me put away all the tuna fish cans in the cabinet shelf for me, so I asked her whether she could take me to the CVS store to get tuna fish cans. She said I had already told the CVS store to get tuna fish cans tomorrow and I would get them tomorrow. Then I asked her to feed the dogs for me before she went home. She got up and went to the refrigerator, took out steamed chicken, chopped it, and mixed it with rice and fed the dogs. She said it was not enough meat for the dogs, so she took another big piece of pork meat from the refrigerator, chopped the pork meat, and fed the dogs again. She washed all the dishes in the kitchen sink for me. Then she said she was going home; she gave me a kiss and then picked up her purse from the living room floor and left. After Sirena left the house, I continued watching different programs on television. When I felt tired, I went in my room and laid down on my bed. But I could not sleep, so I came back out to the family room at 11:30 p.m. I turned on the television and switched from one channel to another channel to find a good program to watch. When I switched the channel to Discovery Channel, I saw the program was about space and I heard a scientist reporting about the incident in Siberia long time ago. I realized this was the same program that I had been watching before about a big stone falling from the space to the ground, leaving a big round shape, the size of a football field, with no materials left on the ground in Siberia. I was very pleased to watch the whole program again and found out the name of the country was Siberia. After the program was over, I went inside my bedroom and slept the whole night. Next day I woke up feeling quite fresh at 8:00 a.m. and watched television as usual. Then I went to the CVS store to get the tuna fish cans that I had ordered yesterday at 12:30 p.m. After I bought the tuna fish cans, the cashier took out a big plastic bag to put all my forty-eight cans of tuna fish. I requested her to put the tuna fish in small separate bags for me so that I could carry them out from my car when I was home. She helped me put the tuna fish cans in separate small bags to make it easy for me to carry. I took the tuna fish can bags to my car and loaded them inside my car. Then I went to Safeway supermarket to buy meats, carrots, and mayonnaise; then I went home to make myself a delicious tuna fish sandwich for lunch.

On Monday, January 25, 2010, I tried to call the surgery scheduler Herbal from KPMC head and neck surgery clinic, but no one answered the telephone. I just had to leave a message for Herbal to call me back. I called Pleasanton KPMC adult medicine clinic to leave a message for Dr. Jennifer to call me back about the pain on my left wrist and to let her know the situation about my ear surgery. Dr. Jennifer's assistant called me back in the evening. I told her about the deep gaping area in between my middle metacarpal bones on my hand and the wrist carpal bones that were pulling apart. I told her my sister had told me I needed to take an X-ray of my wrist after I talked to her. Dr. Jennifer's assistant told me I was supposed to report to Dr. Jennifer instead of my sister. I told her I knew. But I was used to talking to my sister and brother and listening to their suggestions all these years. I just had a habit of telling them what was happening to me. She said Dr. Jennifer needed to examine my wrist first before she could advise me to take an X-ray. Then the nurse asked me how long ago this incident had happened to me. I told her it was a month ago on Christmas Eve when I had been lifting over fifteen pounds of pork meat with my left hand that I had found my left wrist was in great pain. I tried to fix my wrist myself by massaging my wrist; after a week, I felt much better, but when I carried the groceries again, the pain came back. So she said I needed to set up an appointment to see Dr. Jennifer. I told the nurse I would but that I wanted to wait till April for my six months' checkup. I wanted to get my ear surgery done first. She said OK. Then I told her about the Fexofenadine allergy pill that I had ordered from Pleasanton KPMC South Two pharmacy store, but they had not sent it to me. She said I had to buy my allergy medicines from the counter; Kaiser Permanente medical insurance company would not provide any allergy medicine for their patients anymore. I told the nurse I did not understand the reason my medical insurance company could not provide allergy medicines to me anymore; then I told her I would talk to the pharmacist from KPMC pharmacy department and I hung up the phone.

I pulled out the letter that Dr. Jennifer had sent to me from my files, in which she had indicated to me to switch my allergy medicine pills from Fexofenadine to OTC Cetirizine because it was cheaper to use than the Cetirizine pill. After I received Dr. Jennifer's letter to change my allergy medicine from Fexofenadine to OTC Cetirizine or Zyrtec allergy pills, I tried to use and finish all the sample allergy pills that I had at home. Holly used to send me all kinds of sample allergy medicines that she got from the pharmaceutical company. I used up all the medicines that the doctor had prescribed to me. I just kept all the sample medicines that my sister and brother had given me in my medicine box. When I ran out of the medicines that my doctor had prescribed to me, I used the medicines from my medicine box. After I used and finished all the sample medicines from my medicine box, I used Chlor-Trimeton allergy pill that Harvey had given to me recently when I was in his clinic in New

York. After I took Chlor-Trimeton, I felt very drowsy and sleepy. I called KPMC pharmacy store to talk to the pharmacist as instructed by Dr. Jennifer to ask her about the OTC Cetirizine allergy pill. The pharmacist explained to me the difference among the allergy pills such as Cetirizine, Chlor-Trimeton, and Fexofenadine. She said Fexofenadine pill was the only allergy pill that did not cause drowsiness; Chlor-Trimeton pill and Cetirizine pill caused drowsiness, but Chlor-Trimeton pill had stronger strength than Cetirizine pill that caused drowsiness. The pharmacist suggested that I try out Cetirizine pill for thirty days and to let my doctor knew the effect of Cetirizine pill after I tried it, and if I did not feel comfortable with Cetirizine allergy pill, she would suggest that Dr. Jennifer changed my allergy pill back to Fexofenadine allergy pill. I said OK to the pharmacist and hung up the phone. I tried to stop taking the allergy medicines, but I felt very itchy all over my body and big allergic pale spots formed on my legs after I stopped my allergy medicines. I could not do anything about my neighbor John Clark's white birch tree. John Clark kept refusing to cut down his birch tree every time I sent out Charlene to talk to him. He kept complaining to Charlene that they got the bad allergy from their right-side neighbor's birch trees too. I called Renee and Marlene to complain about my allergy again, but they both were not in their offices, so I left messages for them. But I did not get any return calls from them.

On January 26, 2010, I received a phone call from the surgery scheduler Herbal from KPMC head and neck surgery clinic to let me know that they were arranging my ear surgery in early April. I told her I needed this surgery as soon as possible. She said she would schedule my ear surgery on an earlier date, and if she could arrange earlier for my ear surgery, she would let me know. I kept pushing her to schedule my ear surgery earlier, because I did not want my ear infection to get worse. She said OK. Then I called Pleasanton KPMC adult medicine clinic to leave a message for Dr. Jennifer about changing my allergy medicines. Dr. Jennifer's assistant called me back after they got my message. I told her I had talked to the pharmacist from KPMC pharmacy store about my allergy medicines and they had referred me to talk to Dr. Jennifer to prescribe me Fexofenadine allergy pill again for my allergy. I indicated to her that Cetirizine allergy medicine made me very drowsy. She said she would talk to Dr. Jennifer and call me back. In the evening, I received a voice mail from Dr. Jennifer's assistant to tell me that Dr. Jennifer had already sent out a message to Pleasanton KPMC South Two pharmacy store to prescribe me sixty tablets of Fexofenadine allergy pill for thirty days. I called Pleasanton KPMC South Two pharmacy store to mail order the Fexofenadine allergy pill.

On Sunday, February 7, 2010, I woke up as usual, cooked, and waited for Sirena to come home. Sirena came home at 11:45 a.m. with a big bag of Chinese pastries that she handed out to me and asked me to eat. She said she had bought all those pastries at the restaurant near her work for me; she wanted me to try the pastries from that restaurant and told me they were really good. I asked her whether she already had lunch; she said she had. I took out one piece of pastry from the bag and ate it. Then we went to Safeway supermarket to buy groceries. After we came back, I showed her my DMV letter and asked her how to set up an appointment to go to the DMV to renew my driving license. She said she would find out whether I could just call in to set up an appointment to renew my driving license. She asked me to wait until she had found out the information and called me back. I said OK. Before she left, she went to the mailbox to get the mail for me. I received the letter from AIG, in which they indicated that they needed the proof of the description of my treatment from my physician visit on January 8, 2010. I called Pleasanton KPMC head and neck surgery clinic to get the phone number for contacting Dr. Sara. I told the operator that I needed to get Dr. Sara's phone number to call and get my doctor's visiting treatment description from her for my insurance company. The telephone operator gave me Dr. Sara's Walnut Creek KPMC telephone number for me to call, and I hung up the phone after I got Dr. Sara's telephone number.

On Monday, February 8, 2010, I woke up after six in the morning. I tried to call AIG insurance company to find out what kind of description information they needed from Dr. Sara, but I could not get through the customer service of AIG insurance company. Then I called Walnut Creek KPMC head and neck surgery clinic to request them to talk to Dr. Sara to get a statement for my last physician visiting information; the clerk told me that Dr. Sara was on vacation and she would not be back until February 17, 2010. She asked me to leave a message for her and she would call me back after she came back from her vacation. I left a message for Dr. Sara to inform her that I needed the description statement from my last visit with her on January 8, as my insurance company required me to send it to them for my doctor-visiting claim and I hung up the phone.

After I left a message for Dr. Sara, I sat in my family room. I did not feel like watching television or doing any other thing; then I remembered I still needed to renew my driving license at the DMV, so I decided to go to the DMV to renew my driving license instead of waiting for Sirena to call me back to tell me how to set up the appointment through the phone to go to the DMV to renew my driving license. I got up at 10:30 a.m. I went to the DMV to renew my driving license. I saw a lot of people were lining up in front of the DMV building to get in there. After I parked my car in the DMV parking lot, I came out of my car. I went to the lady who was the last person on the line and asked her why all those people were lining up in front of the DMV building; she said all those people were lining up to get in the DMV building to apply or to get their driving licenses or car licenses. So I stayed behind her. I told her I had come there to renew my driving license. The people were moving slowly to go inside the DMV building. I was a bit of afraid I would not pass my eye test, because sometimes I could not see well after I twisted my back when I was carrying heavy objects or when my diabetic data was high. I tried to read the big and small words on the papers that were stuck on the DMV building door. I could not read some of the small letters. I did not understand what they said, so I asked the lady in front of me whether she could read those small letters; she explained to me those words were Spanish words. When it was my turn to go inside the DMV building and I saw the size of the DMV letters on the ceiling computer that was required by the drivers to read for testing their eyes, I was very happy to see those letters were big enough for me to read all of them so clearly from a distance. I knew that I would not have any problem in passing my eye test. The people were moving in slowly to the receptionist to get the number slip inside the building. When it was my turn, I went to the front desk receptionist and showed her the letter that I had received from the DMV; she took the letter and read it; after she read it, she issued me a number G089 slip and clipped it on the letter for me. She gave me back the letter and asked me to sit in the waiting section to wait for the DMV clerk to call my number. I took my letter and went to the empty chair on the back row and sat on it.

After I sat down in the waiting section, I did not know when it would be my turn to go to the counter to renew my driving license, so I asked the lady who sat next to me how to find out when it would be my turn to go to the counter to renew my driving license; she looked at my letter, and she guided me to look at the computer on the ceiling to make sure my number showed up on the computer screen. I told her I had just come to renew my driving license. I had not come to this DMV building for almost fifteen years. I was very pleased to see the new system of DMV, which made it very convenient for people to renew their driving licenses or their car licenses. Then I showed her my DMV letter, which indicated I had been renewing my driving license twice through the mails. She looked at my letter and gave it back to me. Then I looked at the computer screen every time I heard the DMV clerk announce the issued numbers and the counter numbers. After a while the lady who sat next to me left when she heard the DMV clerk calling her number. I had been waiting there for half an hour when finally the DMV clerk called my number to go to Counter 11, and I looked at the computer to make sure my number showed on the computer. After I saw my slip number and counter number were on the computer, I went to Counter 11 and handed out my DMV letter to check in with the clerk; she took the letter from me and processed it. Then she asked me to read the letters on the ceiling board. I read them clearly as she instructed me to read. Then she asked me to give her my old driving license. I took out my old driving license from my wallet and gave it to her. She looked at my driving license and asked me my home address. I told her my home address; then she asked whether I was still living in the same address; I said yes to her. She asked me whether my weight was still 125 pounds. I said my weight was more than 125 pounds; it was 140 pounds now. She said 140 pounds was OK. I said OK; so she typed in the information in the computer and asked me to go to the picture-taking section. I went there and waited for her. After she was done entering all my information in the computer, she came and asked me to put my right thumb in the small computer box to take my thumbprints, and she took two prints of my thumb, telling me some of my thumb lines were faded. I laughed and told her I would be sixty-two next month and how much did she expect for me to get clear thumbprint lines. Then she laughed; when she saw my teeth as I laughed, she said I had very pretty teeth. I said no more to her, and I opened my mouth to show her the empty spaces on both sides of my mouth. I told her I had lost my teeth when my baby dog's eye was ruptured and I cried a lot. Then she told me to stand in front of the screen to take my picture. I stood there to let her take my picture. After she was done taking my picture, she asked me whether I liked to donate any of my organs to any hospital; I told her no thanks, I didn't want to donate any of my organs to any hospital. I told her all through this year I had even saved all my falling teeth at home to bury with me at the time I died. She laughed and asked me to sign the paper. I signed the paper for her in front of her. Then she gave me the receipt and told me I would receive my driving license in the mail. I thanked her and went home. I was happy that I had passed my driving license test. After I was home, I called Rosie to tell her about the organ donation that the DMV was asking people to do to the hospital. Rosie told me that she would never donate her organs to any hospital. I said to her how I could donate my organs to the hospital. I tried to be careful in taking good care of myself, because I wanted to die with a perfect body with my hands and legs attached to my body. I even saved all my falling teeth to be buried with me when I died. I had taken good care of myself and my children all these years. I had two big car accidents in my life before, but they were because of other people's faults. I also told her how I had guided my children not to get upset, not to hurt themselves and others. They had to do things carefully and drive their cars carefully. Then I ended the conversation with her and hung up the phone.

On Thursday afternoon, February 11, 2010, I went out to get my mail from my mailbox and came back home. I found the medicine package from KPMC pharmacy store in my mail. I opened the package. I was glad that I had finally received Fexofenadine allergy pills again from my doctor. Next day, I called KPMC pharmacy store at 9:00 a.m. to inform the pharmacist that I had received the Fexofenadine allergy medicine package that they had sent out to me. I told the pharmacist the reason I had called was the previous pharmacist that I had talked to had suggested that I call back after I received the Fexofenadine allergy medicine package from them. The pharmacist told me she would talk to Dr. Jennifer to have her change my prescription for Fexofenadine allergy pill from sixty tablets to two hundred tablets each time I ordered. I told them I needed this medicine as long as my neighbor was still keeping their white birch tree. She said OK and hung up the phone.

I got a phone call from Dr. Sara on February 17, 2010, after she came back from her vacation; she told me that she got the description statement ready for my physician visit, and she asked me whether I had a fax machine for her to fax it to me. I told her my fax machine was broken and I would like her to mail it out to me. She said she would mail it out to me. I said OK to her. I thanked her and I hung up the phone.

When I received the description statement from Dr. Sara on February 25, 2010, I faxed out the description statement of my physician visit to AIG insurance company on the same day that I received the description statement from my doctor.

On March 5, 2010, I called Pleasanton KPMC adult medicine clinic to set up an appointment with Dr. Jennifer on April 5, 2010, for my six months' checkup. On March 17, 2010, the surgery scheduler Herbal from KPMC called me to inform me that my ear surgery date was arranged on April 20, 2010, in Antioch KPMC. I told her I did not want to go to Antioch Kaiser Permanente Hospital to have my ear surgery done, and I preferred Walnut Creek Kaiser Permanente Hospital to have my ear surgery done. Then she rescheduled the date for my surgery on May 7, 2010, Friday, at Walnut Creek Kaiser Permanente Hospital. She advised me to take my blood sample test and EKG test before my ear surgery. I said OK to her; then I asked her when and how I should go in the hospital on my surgery day. She said she would inform me before my ear surgery date when and how to go in the hospital. On March 28, 2010, I was waiting for Sirena to come home to go to the supermarket. She did not show up in the morning, so I went to Safeway supermarket myself to buy groceries for my ear surgery. After I came back from Safeway supermarket, Sirena was already home; she told me she had to work today and she had come home late. I baked beef and vegetables for our dinner. After dinner, she went home. Then I didn't eat after 8:00 p.m. to prepare for my blood sample test tomorrow.

I went to Pleasanton KPMC laboratory department for my blood sample test on March 29, 2010. When I was inside the laboratory, I saw Grace was taking care of a patient. I went to the numbering machine to take the number slip and then waited for the front desk clerk to call my number. When the front desk clerk called my number, I went to the front desk clerk to check in for my blood sample test. Then one of the technicians from the laboratory called me to go inside the laboratory room to draw my blood sample. As soon as I sat on the chair, Grace was done with the patient; she came to me and I put my left hand on the table to let her draw my blood sample from it. She asked me how I was doing lately. I told her my ears, lips, and body were still itching very badly and I felt very uncomfortable and sick most of the time and sometimes I could not breathe well. She advised me to use the inhalation pump to help in my breathing. I told her I did use the inhalation pump to help in my breathing. Then she injected the needle into my left hand to draw the blood sample; when she saw the speed of my blood flow was very slow, she said my blood was very thick; she had to wait for a while to get three small test tubes of my blood sample. After she was done, she released me and I went home.

On March 31, 2010, both my children called me to wish me happy birthday, and they said they would take me out to eat to celebrate my birthday when they come home on Sunday, but I told them I would like to visit Colma city on Sunday, because I had never been to Colma city before. They said they would take me to Colma city when they came home. On April 4, 2010, Sirena and Shaun both came home after 12:30 p.m. and told me to get ready to go to Colma city as they had promised to take me. But it was raining very heavily. I told them it was not a good idea to drive down to Colma city when it was raining so heavily. I suggested canceling this plan and stay at home. They said they would like to take me to watch the movie *Clash of Titans* in Dublin Movie Theater for my birthday. I said OK to them; then I told them to have their lunch at home before we went to watch the movie in the movie theater. They ate their lunch at home and we left home at 1:50 p.m. We reached the movie theater in Dublin at 2:25 p.m. After we arrived in the theater in Dublin, they both went to the ticket booth to line up with other people to buy the movie tickets. I went to wait for them near the theater entrance door. When I stood in front of the movie theater, I felt the ground under my feet vibrating very strongly. I went to my children to ask them whether they felt any underground vibration, and they said they did not notice any vibration from the ground. Then I went back to the place where I was standing before. I did not feel any more underground vibration at the place that where I was standing before. After my children bought the movie tickets for the three of us, we went inside the movie theater and sat in the front seats in the back section. It was a scary movie and more than one and a half hours long. I enjoyed watching this new movie in the theater. After the movie was over, we found it was raining heavily outside, so they both suggested that I eat out in a restaurant for my birthday. But I did not feel like going out to a restaurant to have dinner on my birthday in this kind of weather. So I suggested taking out sandwiches from the Burger King restaurant for our dinner. Shaun drove us to the Burger King restaurant, and Sirena ordered whopper sandwiches and French fries for all of us and double cheeseburgers for our dogs. We waited there for a while; after we got the sandwiches and French fries, we went home. After we ate the sandwiches and French fries for our dinner, Sirena vacuumed the carpets and Shaun cleaned the kitchen floor for me. After they were done with their cleaning jobs, they went home.

On April 5, 2010, I got up early in the morning as usual. When I turned on the television, I heard the town between the border of the United States of America and Mexico had been struck by an earthquake yesterday again. I presumed the ground vibration that I had felt in front of the theater must be related to the earthquake in the border town between the United States and Mexico. I turned off the television and prepared for my doctor's visit. I decided to run my errands first before I went to checkup with my doctor. I left my house and went to Walmart store to shop for a while; then I went to 99 Ranch supermarket in Dublin. But the supermarket was not open yet, so I went to the CVS store next to 99 Ranch supermarket and shopped. Then I went to the Chase bank to deposit my check. The banker Annie Lee at the Chase bank helped me to deposit my check for me. Then she recommended me to get a better credit card from the Chase bank. I said OK, and she helped me to fill up the application form to apply for a new Chase credit card. After she was done, she told me I would receive my new Chase credit card within two weeks. I thanked her and I left the Chase bank at 9:30 a.m. I went to Pleasanton KPMC adult medicine clinic to checkup with Dr. Jennifer for my 10:00 a.m. appointment. I checked in with the front desk clerk; then I went to the waiting room to wait for Dr. Jennifer's assistant to call me in. Her assistant, Brenda, took me inside the clinic at 10:00 a.m. and measured my blood pressure and weight; then she took me inside the patients' room and went over all my information on the computer with me, and then she asked me to wait for Dr. Jennifer. I waited in the patients' room for a while. Dr. Jennifer knocked on the door and came in. She was very happy to see me and she told me she had a look at my blood sample test result in the computer and said they were all good. All my diabetic HGBA1c, glucose fasting, total cholesterol, LDL cholesterol, and triglyceride data were within the required normal data range except the HDL cholesterol data range was still below the required normal data range. I told her I was happy to see all my blood test results were good. I told her I was still having bad allergies and pale spots had formed on my knees and legs. I had to drink a lot of water every day after I came back in from my backyard, but I was still getting bad allergies and got sick. Then I showed her the scattered pale spots on my knees and legs. I told her that I drank a lot of water to get rid of the poison from my body. Since I drank a lot of water every day, I could not even smoke a cigarette at home; the nicotine in my body came out of my system and made my mouth very bitter. I did not know why the right side of my neck, chest, and stomach ribs was having a lot of pain. Dr. Jennifer checked my blood pressure again; then she checked my neck, chest bone, and back spinal cord. Then she asked me to lie down on the patient bed to check my stomach. When she pressed on my right ribs above my stomach, I did not feel any pain, but when she pressed on my right ribs far more right, I yelled, "Ah-ah-ah," and I told her I had a lot of pain at the position she pressed. Then she asked me to get up. After I got up from the patient bed, I showed her the scattered pale spots on my left knee and leg. She pressed the bones to check my left leg all the way to my foot. I told her that earlier I had got an itch just like needles poking all the way to my toe. After Dr. Ma prescribed me Fexofenadine 60 mg allergy tablet to be taken twice a day, my toe itch was gone. I did not have any problem with my left toe anymore. Then I told her about my left wrist; she said I did not need to take any X-ray on my left wrist after she checked my wrist. She said she would give me the instruction sheet to take home to exercise, and she issued me the instruction sheet before I left. Then she told me I needed to make an appointment to check my eyes again in the coming year of February. She asked me to take from the nurse the fecal-hemoglobin stool test package home on my way out after she filled up the information in the blue form. After she was done with me, I asked her whether she had any patient that had changed their eye color; she said she had not seen any patient in her practice before that had changed eye colors. Then she released me. I went out to the hallway. Norma gave me my blood sample test result, my release statement, home exercise kit for my hands and wrists, and my stool test package. Then I took the kit and package from Norma and I went home. When I reached home, I read the instruction sheet on how to exercise my wrist, hands, and fingers. I exercised my wrist, hands, and fingers. Then I felt I did not want to stay inside my house, so I took my dogs with me inside my car and I drove myself to downtown Pleasanton and then I came home.

On April 6, 2010, at 11:00 a.m., I put some stool material inside the bottle as instructed after my bowel movement. I sealed the stool test envelope and put it in the mailbox to mail out to the KPMC laboratory.

When I walked back to my house, I saw a lot of dried birch flowers on my driveway. I felt so bad to see the allergic birch flowers on my driveway again, so I took pictures of the allergic birch flowers on my concrete driveway. Then I worked a little bit in my front yard to pull out some of the small kind of weeds near my tangerine tree, and I came back inside my house. I got so itchy again and I had to take two AllerClear Loratadine 10 mg allergy medicine pills every day. This was the way I had been living for the past decade in this house while dealing with the allergies and sickness from my neighbor's white birch tree. I kept complaining and taking the allergy medicines every day.

On April 25, 2010, Sirena came home with a big bag of pastries for me to eat, which she had bought at the restaurant near her house. I told her I would like her to eat with me, so we ate all the pastries together. Then we went to Costco store to buy some dog food and we came home. Sirena stayed and watched a little bit of television and she went home at 6:00 p.m. On April 26, 2010, I went to Pleasanton KPMC radiology department to take the EKG test at 8:30 a.m. After I arrived at the radiology department, I found there were so many people lining up to check in to take X-rays, mammogram X-rays, or EKG tests. After I checked in with the front desk of the radiology department, I put my receipt slip in the front box next to the EKG testing room and sat on the chair, waiting for the technician to take me in. While I was waiting there, a lady came to me and told me I should put my Kaiser Permanente membership card inside the box instead of my receipt slip. I told her I did not know I had to put my Kaiser Permanente membership card in the front box. I thought it was just like any other doctor visit and I only needed to put my receipt slip inside the box. She said no to me. Then I went to the box next to the EKG testing room to take back my receipt, and I put my Kaiser Permanente membership card inside the box near the EKG testing room door. I went back to sit on my chair. Then a gentleman came and put his Kaiser Permanente membership card inside the box and sat next to me, waiting for the technician to take him inside the room to do the EKG test. I just had to wait there for a while since a patient came out of the EKG room. The technician called my name. I went in with her in the EKG testing room. She gave me patient's clothing and asked me to change and lie down on the patient bed. After I was done changing my clothing, the technician asked me to lie down on the patient bed and performed the EKG test. After she was done, I got up from the patient bed and changed back to my clothing. Then she gave me a copy of the EKG test result sheet to me and asked me to give it to my doctor on the surgery day. I took the EKG test result and left Pleasanton KPMC South One building. I went to Chase Bank on Stonebridge road to deposit my checks and then I went home. When I was home, I put all the paperwork in my luggage bag to get ready for my ear surgery. Then I went to 99 Ranch supermarket in Pleasanton, bought groceries there, and went home. I put away all the groceries in my kitchen. I ate my lunch that I had bought at the supermarket. I did not feel like working on my computer. I went inside my room and slept for the whole evening. I had all the data for my recent blood test result and the EKG test result. I was ready for my left ear surgery and was waiting for the surgery scheduler Herbal to call me. I got a call from the surgery scheduler Herbal in early April 2010 to inform me that the ear surgery was arranged on May 7, 2010, Friday, with Dr. Sara, at Walnut Creek medical facility. I said OK; then she told me I had to be in Walnut Creek Kaiser Permanente Hospital before 8:00 a.m. She mentioned about the request that I had made with Dr. Sara earlier about staying overnight in the hospital after surgery. She said Dr. Sara had approved my request to stay one night in the hospital. I was allowed to stay overnight in the hospital. I had to go home before 11:00 a.m. on the next day, May 8, 2010. She advised me to be in the hospital on time and she hung up the phone. I called Sirena and Shaun to inform them that my ear surgery was arranged on Friday, May 7, 2010, and I was allowed to stay in the hospital overnight and I could go home on May 8, 2010, Saturday. Sirena called me back on Friday that she would take me to Kaiser Permanente hospital for my ear surgery on May 7, 2010, and would take me home after surgery on May 8, 2010. Then Shaun called me to inform me that he would be home on Saturday and Sunday to take care of me and that he would go back to Davis on Sunday night. I said OK, and he hung up the phone.

On Friday morning at 7:00 a.m., May 7, 2010, Sirena came home, and she took me to Walnut Creek Kaiser Permanente Hospital. After we arrived at the hospital, we parked our car in Walnut Creek KPMC car parking lot. Then we went to the Kaiser Permanente Hospital building, second floor, to register for my ear surgery with the front desk clerk. After I had done my registering with the front desk clerk for my ear surgery, the nurse took me inside the room to get ready for my surgery. Then two nurses pushed my bed to the surgery room at 9:00 a.m. I did not know how long it took for Dr. Sara to operate on my ear. The nurse in the surgery room tried to wake me up; after I woke up, I found myself in a hallway room. I heard Sirena calling me, "Mom, Mom." I also heard the nurse calling me and telling me that my ear surgery had been smooth and I could go home tonight. But I told the nurse that Dr. Sara had given me permission to stay one night in the hospital. After I told them I had got permission to stay in the hospital, they moved me to the hospital to stay overnight as an emergency patient in the hospital. There were a lot of patients in the hospital to stay overnight. I heard patients passing my room as they went to the bathroom in and out of the hallway the whole night, and that did not allow me to sleep the whole night. I did not know how I fell asleep. I woke up in the morning when the nurse came in and woke me up; she told me to clean up before Dr. Sara came to check up on me, and she said Dr. Sara would release me from the hospital. I told the nurse I wanted to go to the restroom, and she said OK. Then she took out the injected needle from my hand and pushed away the glucose bottle stand from my bed; then she helped me to get up from my bed. I walked to the restroom to clean myself up and then went back to my room. The nurse got breakfast for me and she left. I ate some pieces of bread with strawberry jam for my breakfast and drank milk and apple juice. After I finished my breakfast, Sirena came in and gave me my clothing to change. I took my clothing from Sirena and changed to get ready to go home. Dr. Sara came in, and she took out the big thick piece of cotton in my left ear and asked me about my ear. I told her I had pain. She told me the pain would go away after my ear healed, and she told me to come back on May 27, 2010, to checkup with her; then she released me from the hospital. I went home with Sirena. Shaun was waiting for me at home. I told my children that I was happy to be home and that I could not sleep in the hospital the whole night, because the patients were passing by my room and going to the restroom the whole night. Sirena and Shaun laughed; then Shaun brought me rice soup for my lunch. After I ate my rice soup, I went into my room to rest. Sirena went back to her office after she settled me in my room. Shaun stayed with me at home to take care of me.

On May 27, 2010, I went to Walnut Creek KPMC head and neck surgery clinic to checkup with Dr. Sara. When I was in the patient's room with Dr. Sara, she took out all of the cotton from my left ear; then she checked my left ear and said the ear surgery had gone well. She suggested that I set up an appointment for my hearing test and she released me. I went to the front desk clerk to set up an appointment on July 23, 2010, to have my hearing test done. I went in on July 23, 2010, to take a hearing test with Cara T. in Walnut Creek KPMC head and neck surgery clinic. Cara T. performed the hearing test for me. The hearing test included audiometry, comprehensive threshold evaluation, and speech recognition. After the hearing test, Cara T. set up an appointment for me to see Dr. Sara on September 1, 2010, for my final checkup. I checked up with Dr. Sara on September 1, 2010. Dr. Sara said my ear surgery had gone well and she discharged me.

I checked in to see Dr. Jennifer for the three months' follow-up on October 8, 2010. On January 6, 2011, I went to the ophthalmology department to check in to let Dr. Daniel S. G. to checkup my eyes for diabetic retinopathy disease. After Dr. Daniel carefully checked my eyes, he indicated to me that my eyes did not have any diabetic retinopathy disease; he reminded me to control my diabetes and he released me. Then I went to the adult medicine clinic to checkup with Dr. Jennifer for my three months' checkup. This way I had been in and out to check up with Dr. Jennifer every three months. Now I have Dr. Lakshmi M. as my primary adult medicine doctor. I take blood sample test and checkup with her every three or four months. I was getting tired of complaining about the allergies and sickness from my neighbor's white birch trees to my doctors. Even when I gave out the doctors' letters to prove that my allergies and sickness were from the birch trees, my neighbors would not cut down their birch trees.

Every time I received my blood sample test result from my doctor, I entered all the data from my blood test result in my computer to save them in "My diabetic and lipid data chart" as shown in Chart 4.1. I reviewed and compared the data of diabetic HGBA1c, glucose fasting, total cholesterol, HDL cholesterol, LDL cholesterol, and triglyceride from the recent blood sample test result with the previous blood sample test result; then I adjusted the food that I ate every day to keep all of my diabetic and lipid data in the required normal data range, but sometimes my mouth dried out so badly that I could not even open my mouth. I had to adjust myself to drink a lot of water every day to get rid of my dry mouth. Sometimes I had to use a little bit of sweet to get rid of my dry mouth. I took all the medicines in time to bring down my diabetic HGBA1c and glucose fasting data close to or within the required normal data range, but if I worked outside in my yard, my ears, lips, and whole body got itchy and my diabetic data went up. Before I had any diabetes, I could eat and drink sweet food; after I squeezed the birch flowers and tasted their fluid, I had diabetes and became very sick. I had to have medicines to control my diabetes and glucose fasting after this incident.

Blood sample test date	HGBA1c	Glucose Fasting	Total Choles-terol	HDL Choles-terol	LDL Cholesterol	Triglyceride
Required normal data range	4.6–6.0%	60–99 mg/dl	<239 mg/dl	>45 mg/dl	<129 mg/dl	<199 mg/dl
10/29/99	-	91	255*	51	172*	163
08/05/01**	-	95	255*	42*	162*	259*
08/09/02	-	-	260*	36*	177*	234*
05/03/06**	-	175*	-	-	-	-
09/12/06	6.9*	147*	-	-	-	-
11/30/06	-	-	193	39*	115	197
04/27/07	6.5*	-	248*	35*	172*	203*
07/31/07	6.1*	136*	168	41*	84	216*
11/30/07	6.0	-	-	-	-	-
02/18/08	6.1*	139*	-	-	-	-
06/17/08**	6.7*	-	201	40*	102	295*
09/23/08	6.6*	135*	201	42*	61	289*
01/05/09	6.3*	101*	150	38*	63	244*
04/06/09	6.1*	115*	139	38*	58	216*
07/07/09	6.3*	88	135	41*	55	194
10/26/09**	6.2*	97	140	34*	67	195
03/29/10	6.0	98	130	37*	63	148

Chart 4.1: Diabetic and lipid data chart

My blood sample test results of my diabetic and lipid data from 10/29/99 to 03/29/10 and the data of my diabetic HGBA1c, glucose fasting, total cholesterol, HDL cholesterol, LDL cholesterol, and triglyceride data from my blood tests results are listed in my diabetic and lipid data Chart 4.1

according to the dates of the blood sample tests. I have used the symbol (**) in my diabetic and lipid data chart to indicate the dates that I went in the laboratory to draw my blood samples after I got my bad allergy accidents. I have used the symbol (*) in my diabetic and lipid data chart to indicate the data of my diabetic, glucose fasting, LDL cholesterol, and triglyceride were above the required normal data range, the symbol (*) in my diabetic and lipid data chart on HDL cholesterol indicates that my HDL cholesterol data was under the required normal data.

My blood sample tests on 10/29/99 and 08/05/01 were taken by Dr. Harvey Chu in New York. My blood sample test on 08/09/02 was taken by Dr. Calvin in Pleasanton VCMC, California. Blood sample test results from 05/03/06 to 09/23/08 were taken by Dr. Ma, Pleasanton KPMC adult medicine clinic, and blood sample test results from 01/05/09 to 03/29/10 were taken by Dr. Jennifer in Pleasanton KPMC adult medicine clinic in California. My glucose fasting data was 91 mg/dl, which was within the required normal data range on 10/29/99, and my glucose fasting data was 95 mg/dl on 08/05/01, which was still in the normal data range. My HDL cholesterol data was 51 mg/dl on 10/29/99, but my HDL data gradually dropped to 42 mg/dl after I squeezed the birch flowers and tasted the birch fluid on my hands; then it dropped to under the required normal data range of 36 mg/dl on 08/09/02, but my other lipid data did not change much; they were above the required normal data range and my triglyceride data went up from 163 mg/dl on 10/29/99 to 259 mg/dl on 08/05/01. My LDL cholesterol data was 172 mg/dl on 10/29/99, 162 mg/dl on 08/05/01, and 177 mg/dl on 08/09/02; they had not changed much. I started to complain about my allergy and my lips were itching badly after I accidentally squeezed the fresh male white birch flowers with my fingers and tasted the birch fluid with my tongue. My glucose fasting data had gradually gone up to 175 mg/dl on 05/03/06. My glucose fasting data went up to almost the double amount of the required normal data range. After Dr. Ma prescribed me to take Metformin Hydrochloride 500 mg twice a day, Fexofenadine 60 mg twice a day, and Lovastatin 40 mg once a day, my glucose fasting data dropped back down to 147 mg/dl and my diabetic HGBA1c data was 6.9 percent on 09/12/06. My total cholesterol data dropped to 193 mg/dl, my LDL cholesterol data dropped to 115 mg/dl, my triglyceride data dropped to 197 mg/dl, and my HDL cholesterol data went back up to 39 mg/dl point on 11/30/06, and all of my lipid data were improving.

After I worked in my backyard more than four hours a day, I had a very hard time breathing. When I took my blood sample test on 04/27/07, my diabetic HGBA1c data was 6.5 percent, not much different from my previous diabetic HGBA1c data of 6.9 percent on 09/12/06; my total cholesterol data had increased to 55 mg/dl point, LDL cholesterol data had increased to 57 mg/dl point, and my triglyceride had increased to 6 mg/dl point when we compared the lipid data from 04/27/07 with the previous data of 11/30/06, which indicated all my lipid data were not improving and stayed above the required normal data range. My good HDL cholesterol data dropped from 39 mg/dl on 11/30/06 to 35 mg/dl on 04/27/07. But when I stopped working outside in my backyard, my diabetic data was reduced to 6.1 mg/dl on 07/31/07 from 6.5 percent on 04/27/07; then my diabetic data gradually dropped to 6.0 mg/dl on 11/30/07. But my glucose fasting data dropped to only 11 mg/dl compared with the data of 147 mg/dl on 09/12/06 to 136 mg/dl on 07/31/07. The diabetic data had not changed much from 07/31/07 to 02/18/08; they were 6.1 mg/dl, 6.0 mg/dl, and 6.1 mg/dl, but I had glucose fasting data of 136 mg/dl on 07/31/07 and 139 mg/dl on 02/18/08.

I went in Pleasanton KPMC laboratory department to take my blood sample test after two weeks of getting my bad allergy accident on 06/17/08. I found my diabetic HGBA1c data went up to 6.7 percent from 6.1 percent on 02/18/08. All my lipid data were increasingly changing from 07/31/07 to the data of 06/17/08. Dr. Ma increased my Metformin Hydrochloride prescription pill from 500 mg to 750 mg and instructed me to take it twice a day. After three months of this accident, my diabetic HGBA1c data was 6.6 percent, my glucose fasting data was 135 mg/dl on 09/23/08, my total cholesterol data, HDL cholesterol data, and my triglyceride data had not changed much, except my LDL cholesterol data dropped from 102 mg/dl on 06/17/08 to 61 mg/dl on 09/23/08. Because of my diabetes, my HGBA1c, glucose fasting and lipid data had not changed much; when we compared their data from 09/23/08 with the data from 06/27/08, it did not show any improvement, and their data were above the normal data range in three months, Dr. Ma increased my Metformin Hydrochloride prescription pill from 750 mg to 1,000 mg and instructed me to take it twice a day. After I continuously took the medicines and closed all my windows and stayed inside my house, my diabetic HGBA1c data went down to 6.3 percent on 01/05/09 and 6.1 percent on 04/06/09; my glucose fasting was 135 mg/dl on 9/23/08,

101 mg/dl on 01/05/09, and 115 mg/dl on 04/06/09. My LDL cholesterol dropped to 58 mg/dl, dated 04/06/09, from 102 mg/dl, dated 06/17/08. My HDL cholesterol data was 38 mg/dl on 04/06/09 and dropped to 4 mg/dl from 09/23/08. My diabetic data on 06/17/08 showed a tremendous increase in my diabetic HGBA1c data, which could prove my allergies and sickness were caused by my neighbor's bad white birch trees.

I got another bad allergy incident again on both my hands after I picked up a poisonous seashell from my sister's backyard in King of Prussia, Pennsylvania, on 08/08/09. Big bad blisters were forming on both my hands and palms and kept spreading. These types of blisters had formed on my hands all the time I was working at home in my backyard in Pleasanton, California. I checked up with Dr. Jennifer on 08/19/09 for this incident. Dr. Jennifer prescribed me Prednisone 20 mg medicine to be taken daily for five days, and all the bad blisters on both my hands dried out. I went to Pleasanton KPMC laboratory department to draw the blood sample on 10/26/09, and when we reviewed the test result, my diabetic HGBA1c data was 6.2 percent and had not changed much when compared with the previous 07/07/09 diabetic HGBA1c data, but my glucose fasting data had increased from 88 mg/dl on 07/07/09 to 97 mg/dl on 10/26/09; my good HDL cholesterol data dropped from 41 mg/dl on 07/07/09 to 34 mg/dl on 10/26/09, which went down 7 mg/dl far more under the required data range. My other lipid data had not changed much from 07/07/09 to 03/29/10. All my diabetic and lipid data were good when I reviewed my blood sample test results on 03/29/10; they were in the required normal data range except my HDL cholesterol data range was still 8 mg/dl lower than the normal data range. Even though I have good control with the help of the medicines that the doctor has prescribed for me, I still breathe in bad chemical substances from my neighbor's birch trees and get bad allergies; my ears, lips, body, and legs itch badly and pale spots form on my knees and legs. I have been using antibiotic medicines to protect my allergies and sickness all year round when I do not feel good after I stay outside and work in my yard.

I had stationed myself in one place in my house in California all these years, except when I went to East Coast to visit my sisters and my brothers in King of Prussia and New York. When I was home in Pleasanton, I went to the stores and supermarkets in Tri Valley to get all my daily needs food, groceries, and clothing. We had all good plants and good trees except the birch family plants, which were bad plants containing betulinic acid. By reviewing all the blood sample test results from my diabetic and lipid data in Chart 4.1, we can prove that the only bad poisonous chemical substances from the birch trees were in our environment, which made us get bad allergies and sickness. The acid from the birch trees burned and damaged our internal systems and led to us getting diabetes, ear infections, eye diseases, and it caused us to get bad allergies and sickness. It was a mistake for me to blame the 3 percent hydrogen peroxide that I used to clean my teeth when I gave out the excuse to Dr. Ma before indicating that my diabetic and lipid data with fasting were high because of it. Actually my glucose data with fasting was 175 mg/dl on 05/03/06, which was the glucose data that I had before I used 3 percent hydrogen peroxide liquid to clean my teeth and to treat my infectious ears. I have stopped using hydrogen peroxide liquid all these years to clean my teeth. If you keep using any chemical liquid inside your mouth, it does affect the glucose and diabetic data with fasting more or less in blood sample test result. If the chemical liquid that you are using in your mouth has the ability to burn and form pimple rashes inside your mouth, it will have the same ability to damage your internal system; it will affect the diabetic, glucose, and lipid data with fasting in your blood system. The strength of hydrogen peroxide is just like the strength of alcohol; they both have the ability to kill diseases in the infectious areas. I do not think hydrogen peroxide liquid will affect much the diabetic and glucose data in our blood sample test. If you keep breathing in any bad chemical substances from the air in your environment, they burn and form blisters rashes inside your internal system, just like when you come in contact with the same kind of bad chemical substances on your outer skin, which burns and form blisters rashes and damages your internal system. I hope you all will understand the concept how the chemical acid from the birch trees or any poisonous plants burns and damages your internal systems if you keep breathing them in your internal systems, causing your diabetic and lipid data to go up high in your blood sample test results.

Chapter Five

Experiments

I have been living in the same house in Pleasanton, California, since 1984. I have had good times and bad times in this house and in this city. I got to know a lot of good people in Tri Valley, especially the people and the counselors of Pleasanton Senior Supporting Group, who came to my house to help me prove the allergies and sickness were from my neighbor's allergic birch trees. I was invited to Pleasanton Senior Supporting Group luncheons in Pleasanton Senior Center every quarter when Charlene would visit me. I enjoyed meeting all the young and old people of Tri Valley and nearby cities, who came to the luncheon parties in Pleasanton Senior Center. I enjoyed and missed Marlene's cooking very much; she always liked to prepare the food herself for all the people. They entertained their guests with live music, using different kind of instruments to play music. They had different programs, activities, and performances in Pleasanton Senior Center. I went to group dance classes in Pleasanton Senior Center every Friday to learn Western dance. I got a lot of exercise from Western dance with the natural movements straightening my neck nerves and body. Sometimes I had to be very careful in some dance movements when I danced; otherwise I would twist my chest bone and my backbone and develop a lot of pain. The worst thing for me when I was in the dance class was that I could not hear the music well; I could only pick up the dance steps from the dancing instructor by looking at the instructor's dance steps. After my left ear was infected twice when I lived in this house, I went through the ear surgery many times in my infectious left ear, caused by my neighbor's birch trees, and finally I could hear well with my left ear. But every time

302

I went outside to my yard, I had to use cotton to block both my ears to prevent it from getting infected again. Unfortunately, I stopped my dance lessons after I got in an accident in front of Pleasanton KPMC main building parking lot on November 25, 2006.

I enjoyed going to the farmer's market in downtown Pleasanton on Saturdays to buy vegetables and fruits. I met some children there who came with their parents to the farmers' market to help their parents sell their goods there. I talked to these children and I explained to them to stay out of the sun at noontime; when the sun heated up, the toxic chemical fluid in the dumped trash vaporized and stayed in the air; either they directly contacted or breathed into their body toxic chemical moisture, gases, or dried toxic chemical powder from the air, and they would burn their system and get bad allergies and sickness. In particular in hot weather, they would get sickness like leukemia cancer and the doctors could not help to save their lives. I cared about all those children, so I reminded the farmers to protect their children by letting them stay inside their houses when the weather was very hot.

Because of the expansion of the city of Pleasanton and Dublin, a lot of wild species like wildcats, mice, rats, squirrels, raccoons, hawks, and all other kind of small and big birds started migrating into our community after the builders cleaned the areas to build houses. We had a lot of hawks in Tri Valley. All the animals and small birds were afraid of the big hawks. When they saw big hawks flying above the sky, either they ran or flew away to places where they could hide their bodies. My two Pekinese dogs, Sir Space and Lady Star, were afraid to go out in my backyard after they got attacked and grasped by big hawks several times. One afternoon, when I took my two dogs out to my backyard, I saw them run into the bushes and hide themselves inside the bushes. I did not know what was happening to them, so I went over to the bushes to pull them out from their hiding place. I saw that they both were shaking. When I took them inside my house, the shaking in their bodies would not go away, and they kept hiding themselves in places where they could cover their bodies inside the house. I saw Sir Space hiding under the table next to my sofa, where I usually sat. Lady Star kept following me and sitting next to me, weeping in a low voice. I did not know what was happening to them. I just ignored them and sat on my sofa as usual, watching television. At nights, I took both of them in my room, letting them sleep on the floor near my bed. Next day when I woke up, I heard Lady Star was moaning and weeping in a low voice again; it seemed like she was having a lot of pain on her body. I sat down on the floor with her and checked her body. I saw she was trying to squeeze her body and moaning. I put her down flat on the floor to check her body. I heard her breathing sounds were loud and fast, so I laid my head down to her body and tried to listen to her heartbeats, and I found she had very fast, irregular heartbeats. I did not know what had made her have that kind of fast heartbeats suddenly. I fed them with good nutritious food every day, and they were both really strong and healthy. When I usually pushed them away with my hands, I could feel that they were really heavy and strong. I was surprised to hear her moaning and her irregular heartbeats. I decided to take her to checkup with her doctor to find out what was happening to her. I thought maybe she was pregnant.

Next day, I called HAH to set up an appointment with Dr. Eliz; the doctor's assistant told me to bring Lady Star to HAH right away. I took her to HAH. Dr. Larry was in the hospital. I told Dr. Larry that Lady Star had a lot of pain in her body and she had irregular heartbeats and I believed she was pregnant. Dr. Larry asked me about Lady Star's last period. I told Dr. Larry that I had seen Lady Star's period last month. Dr. Larry checked on her by listening to her heartbeats; then he said he did not think she was pregnant, because there was only one kind of heartbeats in her body. But he would take an X-ray to find out what was causing her to get such kind of pain in her body, if I agreed to let him take an X-ray of Lady Star. I said yes to Dr. Larry. Dr. Larry asked me to wait in the clinic room, and he took Lady Star inside the back room to take an X-ray of her spinal cord. After he reviewed the X-ray film, he came back out with Lady Star and told me he had found a swollen spot between Lady Star's two bones in the middle of the spinal cord area. I asked him what was causing Lady Star to have this kind of swollen spot between two of her spinal cord bones and also the pain in her back. He said it was caused by Mother Nature. I disagreed with Dr. Larry about that. I remembered I had used the stick to strike on the bushes to find them when I was looking for them in my backyard, so I told Dr. Larry that maybe she got hit by my stick when I was striking the bushes to look for them, but Dr. Larry said it was not the stick that had caused the wound. He prescribed pain relievers and antibiotic medicines for Lady Star and discharged us. I took Lady Star home. After I was home, I fed Lady Star the medicines that the doctor prescribed for her, then I tried to figure out how Lady Star got the swelling in her spinal cord, which caused her great pain.

After a couple of weeks, when I took Sir Space and Lady Star inside my house from my backyard, I did not see Sir Space in the family room. I looked in every corner inside the family room for him, and finally I found he was hiding behind the sofa corner next to the stereophonic table. I pulled him out behind the sofa, and I yelled at him not to hide himself behind the sofa in the family room. He was squeezing his body; it seemed like he had a lot of pain in his body. So I checked his body and I gave him ¼ pill of aspirin and antibiotics to get rid of his pain. Next day, he was hiding under the table next to my sofa again, and it seemed like he was afraid somebody might attack him from behind him, so he was hiding himself in a place that could cover his whole body. I did not know what had happened to my dogs lately; they both were in pain and were squeezing their bodies. I did not see any sign that they were fighting with each other or they were fighting with any other animals outside in the backyard. I tried to figure out what was causing them to have this kind of pain, by squeezing their bodies and hiding themselves in places that could cover their bodies. I decided to search Sir Space's body to find out the truth. When I held him up and touched his back, he moved his body away; it seemed like he had a lot of pain in his back when I touched it. I took my time in looking at Sir Space's body to find out what was causing him to have pain in his back. I searched and searched all over his body, but I did not find anything on his body except a tiny round-shaped scar with a black spot on top of it near the middle portion of his spinal cord. I tried to find the material or small branches to match the tiny round-shaped scar on his swollen back, inside and outside my house, but I could not find any. So I tried to think of something to match his tiny round-shaped scar, but I could not think of anything that could have hurt his back. I kept an eye on both of them every day when I took them outside to my yard. I kept an eye on all outside activities to figure out what kind of animal could attack them.

One day when I was sitting on my sofa and looking outside to my backyard, I saw a big hawk land on one of the branches of my cherry tree. I stood up from my sofa and went near the window to look at the hawk clearly; when the hawk saw me near the window inside my house, he suddenly flew to the window, attacking me and trying to grasp me with his claws. But luckily as the clear glass of the window was blocking him from getting into my house, he could not attack and grasp me. I only heard the loud sounds on the window when the hawk flew to the window and his claws hit it. I saw very clearly that one of his legs had hit the window glass and he flew away. He was a big hawk; his claws were big and strong. I found that the tiny round-shaped scar on Sir Space's spinal cord matched the size of one of the hawk's claw nails. The hawk must have used his claws to grasp Sir Space's middle portion of the spinal cord meat when the dogs were outside in my backyard. The weight of each of my two dogs was over fourteen pounds, so it was impossible for the hawk to grasp and take them away. Once I knew the hawk had tried to grasp my dogs, I kept an eye on them every time I left them out in my backyard. I got a lot of information from either the advertising papers or newspapers that there were a lot of people looking for their missing small pets in the lost-and-found sections, and sometimes they went out themselves door to door, looking for their pets. I did not think the people in our neighborhood were aware of how their small pets were missing. I did not think they knew we had big hawks that grasped the small animals in our neighborhood for their food. All these hawks are very dangerous species. I do not think the biologists in the Tri Valley give any consideration to the people's safety, as well as the safety of young children and small pets in the neighborhood, to prevent them from getting attacked by those big hawks when they let all those hawks out in the fields. When those big hawks do not get enough food in the wild open fields, they migrate to the residential areas to attack and grasp all the small pets for their food, and sometimes they attack people. All these wild animals and wild birds are creating a lot of environmental disasters, forcing us to live in a very uncomfortable situation. We cannot enjoy our lives in our own homes with all these dangerous species and allergic trees surrounding us in our community.

After I found my two dogs had been attacked so many times by the big hawks in my backyard, I studied my dogs' bodies and their movements closely. I found their pain and sickness was not caused by Mother Nature; they were caused by outer objects. When I studied the color of their eyes, I found their eyes contained a mixed color fluid, depending on the location, lights, and positions that they stayed. When I looked in Lady Star's eyes, I found her eyes had a dark brown color, and Sir Space's eyes had a strong light brown color. The color of the eyes depended on the color of the eye fluid that was mixed inside the eyes. We have so many different eye colors. Some people have blue eyes, some have green eyes, some have brown eyes, some have dark eyes, and so on, just like when the painters use different colored liquids to mix and produce the colors that they like to use in their paintings. No matter what color are human eyes, they all are healthy eyes. I never knew animals' eyes could change to another color until I was in AECH in Fremont. During Lady Star's doctor visiting, I saw some of the dogs' eyes were changing from their original eye color to blue color; when I asked the technicians about the dogs with blue eyes, they told me that those dogs' eyes had diseases, and their eyes changed from the original color to blue color. When I asked Dr. Deborah about these blue-eyed dogs and their sickness, she told me she did not know what was in the air that made the dogs' eyes turn to blue color. After they treated the dogs' eyes with medicines, if the color did not change back to their original eye color, the doctor would have to perform surgery to remove their diseased blue eyes.

After we performed corneal surgery on Lady Star to repair her ulceration that had ruptured in her left eye, her left eye also changed to a light blue color just like the sick dog's eyes in AECH. After I found out her damaged left eye's color had changed to light blue color, I got concerned and I started feeding her with American ginseng roots, with which I cooked soup for myself every week, and the light blue color of her left eye slowly changed back to her regular dark brown color just like her right eye after a certain period of time. I did not know how long she had been eating American ginseng roots to make her left eye change back from light blue color to her regular dark brown color. Unfortunately, Lady Star's both eyes became very dry, and the discharge in her eyes started forming a hard layer, covering her eyes so that she could not see well. I had to use a tissue to clean out the hard layer discharge in her eyes and I used GenTeal gel to apply in her eyes to get rid of the dryness every day. Sometimes the hard layer discharge in both her eyes transformed to a milky cloud gel fluid after I applied GenTeal gel in her eyes. I had to apply Moxifloxacin hydrochloride ophthalmic solution on her eyes to get rid of the milky gel fluid. Sometimes I gave her ¼ tablet of Tetracycline antibiotic pill, and then she got better. Usually when she got itchy, she put her face on the carpet and kept scratching her face and she would use her back leg to keep scratching her body. Sir Space also got itchy and kept scratching his face and body on the carpet just like Lady Star. I just could not find any solution on how to help them get rid of the itches from their eyes and bodies. Lately, there had been so many big wildcats that had migrated to my backyard; when they saw the big wildcats in my backyard, they would be afraid to go outside my backyard without me. I had to take them outside my yard every day so that they could urinate. I got a bad itch and got sick after I came back from outside. I just didn't know how to get rid of the allergies and sickness without letting my neighbors cut down their allergic white birch tree.

I had been doing a lot of interesting projects at home in this city all these years. I never gave up studying, researching, and comparing the environment in different communities to search about the allergies and the sickness for the people. I spent a lot of money and time on my projects. I had studied and raised birds and livestock before. I had researched about allergies and sickness at home after my car accident. I set up a deal with the city of Pleasanton to prove that white birch trees were the allergic trees. I grew different plants and trees to find about their ingredients and their chemicals. It took years and years to learn and study how the trees grew in different environments. I bought most of the soil from Home Depot store. The employees at Home Depot store helped me load the soil in my car. Since they knew I was not strong and healthy enough to lift heavy things, sometimes they got mad at me and would be upset to see me doing these heavy projects, but they still did their best to help me. Sometimes I unloaded the soil from my car myself after I bought them from Home Depot store, but most of the times I left them in my car till my children came home to unload them for me and take them to my backyard. I had never seen the leaves and flowers of the fruits that I was eating before. I did not know what the leaves and flowers of the fruits looked like. I went to the supermarket and bought a lot of different kind of fruits. I used the seeds of the fruits to grow fruit plants; at the same time, I searched the environment in our neighborhood to find where all those allergic substances were coming from. After I planted the seeds inside the pots, I did not see any fruit plants come out from the seeds in my backyard. I did not know how all those seeds had disappeared, but I did get a lot of small white birch plants from the seeds that flew in from my right-side neighbor's birch tree and small maple plants from the seeds that flew in from my left-side neighbor's maple tree. I hated so much to see those two kinds of plants growing in my backyard. It took me a lot of time to plough them out from my backyard and throw them away; it was not an easy job. I had to keep plowing them out and throwing them away in the trash. I never complained to my left-side neighbor who had so many maple trees, because maple trees were not allergic trees. But I kept complaining to my right-side neighbor because of their allergic white birch trees, which were causing me bad allergies and sickness almost every day.

Even though I did not get any plant from the fruit seeds that I grew, I never gave up any hope to learn and try again. I bought different fruits again from the supermarket and put the fruit seeds in pots to grow fruit plants again. Another year passed by, but I did not get any fruit plants from the seeds again. I tried to observe the environment in my backyard carefully to find out why I did not get any plant from the seeds. When I observed the environment my backyard, I did not see anything wrong with it except I saw a lot of birds and squirrels running around in my backyard, digging out all the seeds and soil from the pots and spreading all over my backyard. The birds and the squirrels dug out all the fruit seeds from the pots and ate them all. Since I did not get any fruit tree from the seeds, I decided to grow avocado plants that had big seeds in my backyard. I bought fifty avocado fruits from the supermarket. I put the big avocado seeds inside the pots to grow avocado plants. After a few months, I saw most of the avocado plants had started growing and only a few avocado seeds were lying on the ground. I presumed the squirrels must be the animals that dug out the avocado seeds from the pots; they tried to eat them, but the avocado seeds were so hard for them to bite, so they left them on the ground. After a year I bought apples, peaches, and nectarines from the supermarket and used their seeds to grow plants inside the pots again; then I used plastic sheets to cover the pots to prevent the birds and other animals from digging the seeds out from the pots and eating them. A few months later, I saw all the seeds were growing inside the pots with beautiful healthy green leaves. Then I grew kiwi plants with their tiny seeds. Kiwi plants are fruits that Are not easy to grow from seeds, because their seeds are so tiny. I had to follow many steps to help the kiwi plants grow big. After so many years of researching on how to grow different fruit plants, finally I got a lot of tangerines; oranges; apples; apple pears; green, brown, and red pears; peaches; nectarines; and kiwi plants in my backyard. I also had mango plants, but it was not the right plant to grow in this neighborhood. I also had a lot of pink cherry flower trees and the palm type of trees with white flowers in my backyard.

Since I lived alone in the city of Pleasanton, I had to do everything myself. I used small cups to pour soil in the pots; then I transplanted the plants from small pots to big pots. After I was done transferring the plants from the small pots to the big pots, I had to move all the big or small pots by pushing or pulling them to the destination that I wanted to keep them. I watered them every day. When I moved around all those pots, sometimes I had a lot of muscle and back pain in my body. When I carried or pushed or pulled to move the pots, sometimes I twisted my back or my spinal cord disk slipped, hurting my back, and my right brain and right eye had a lot of pain. I took pain-reliever pills to get rid of my pain when I had it. Most of the times if the pots were too heavy for me to move I kept them aside, waiting for my children to come home and move them for me. I was lucky enough to have my children to come home and help me. My two children never refused to help me; they were always helping me whenever I needed them. But I knew they felt bad when they saw that I had to do those kinds of heavy jobs and get hurt. After they helped me, they also had a lot of pain in their bodies. They never told me they had pain in their bodies after they helped me; they did their best to help me so that I could search for the truth where all those allergies and sickness came from. I took care of all the plants and watered them with a pipe in my backyard every day. It was not an easy job to deal with plantation. Because I had made a commitment to the community to search for the truth about the allergies and sickness, even though I got into accidents and had so much pain while doing this project, I never gave up. I learned and studied the plants and trees until my projects were done. I never gave up hope on the things that I promised and set a deal with the people to prove where the actual allergies and sickness came from.

I studied different plants, their leaves, flowers, and pollens. All the plants have roots, veins, skins, woods, flowers, pollens, colors, odors, fluids, and chemicals. All the plants have their own structures of leaves, flowers, pollens, colors, odors, and chemical fluid. They are just like human beings; they need water to survive and they need vitamins to get stronger and grow. The plants spray moisture in the hot weather; the fluid from the plants transforms into moisture in hot weather and is transmitted into the air. Sometimes you find out the leaves and the flowers have dried out if the weather is very hot, because the fluid of the plants vaporize and dry out, and sometimes the plants die if they do not get enough water to absorb into their systems. When the plants absorb the water, they also absorb the chemicals dissolved in the water if the water has any chemical mixed with them. After the plants absorb the water mixed with chemicals, these chemicals are already in the plants. If the chemicals are vitamins, they make the plants grow stronger, but if the chemicals are toxic acid, they kill the plants. If the people eat the plants with bad chemicals inside their system, the bad chemicals from the plants cause the bad allergies and sickness to the people; sometimes it causes people to die.

I used the insect killer, ether chemical compound, for my experiment. I put a large portion of the insect-killer liquid inside a bottle and mixed it with water and watered one of the peach trees that I grew in my backyard. After a couple of weeks, I found out the top portion of the peach tree had slowly turned black and dried out. Then I dumped out all the water that contained the insect-killer chemical from the pot and the pot tray. I used fresh water to water them daily again; it took a while for the peach tree to slowly grow back, but the top portion of the branches of the peach tree had already turned black and dried out. This experiment proved that any plant or tree and their leaves and fruits could absorb the insect killer or any other kind of chemicals that was mixed with water; the plant and their leaves and fruits could be killed by insect killer chemicals or any other bad chemical that they absorbed from the water. If we eat the fruits of the trees that contained the insect killer chemicals, we could get their poison in our system and we could die if we got a large amount of the poison in our system. I heard the reporter on the television news station report that the lettuce farmers in California washed the lettuce in clean water three times before they put the lettuce in the markets, but people were getting E. coli disease from the lettuce, causing them to be very sick, making them throw up and having bad diarrhea; this E. coli disease in the lettuce caused a few people to die after they ate the lettuce that was grown in California. The farmers were using water mixed with insect killer chemicals to spray the lettuce and kill the insects. The lettuce plants absorbed the insect killer chemicals mixed with water into their system. No matter how many times the farmers washed the lettuce with clean water, they could not wash away the insect killer chemicals from their system, because the insect-killer chemicals were already inside the lettuce's system, and this was the reason the lettuce was causing people to get sick after they ate them.

If you eat the fruits, flowers, or leaves of the plants that contain the poisonous chemicals daily, these poisonous chemicals could get into your blood system, making your blood get thicker and thicker and making you get sick with black legs. The reason people have black legs when they stand up is because of the gravity of the earth; the thick poisonous substances in the blood system reside in the bottom part of the legs. A lot of people with poisonous black legs have died all over the world without knowing the cause of the death. No one was aware that people and animals could get poisoned from the vegetables and fruits that they eat every day. The doctors presumed this poisonous sickness was due to Mother Nature. Most of the sources of poisonous sickness are exposed either through the air or through the fruits and plants that people eat every day or through the acids that are produced inside the human body. Human body produces uranic acids in its stomach to digest food; if it does not have enough food in its stomach for the acids to digest, the acids will burn the surrounding stomach tissues, causing infection, leading to any type of sickness depending on the state of the sickness and causing stomach cancers. The livestock and animals are exposed to the sickness either through the air or the fruits and plants that they eat just like human beings. The researchers of different institutes have given different names for the diseases and sickness to make it a standard for future researchers and scientists to review. West Nile and mad cow diseases were found either from the direct bite of the mosquitoes or from the food that they ate or from what they breathed in from the air that contained bad chemicals. Monkey boxes and different viruses of Africa were exposed from animals to humans and humans to humans through the air.

I did the experiment repeatedly on my hands with the leaves and flowers of different fruit plants that I grew at home by squeezing the fresh fluid from the leaves and the flowers on my hands and rubbing them many times. I did not get any allergy reaction from the leaves and the flowers of the fruit trees. But when I squeezed the white birch flowers and applied their fluid by rubbing them on my hand, the area that I rubbed with white birch fluid would get very itchy, making me to keep on scratching, forming pimples and blister rashes on the area that I rubbed, and sometimes the small pimple rashes transformed into big blisters after I kept scratching my hands. The sizes of the pimples that were formed depended on the sizes and ages of the flowers from the birch trees. I repeated the same procedure to test on my hands with different sized birch flowers many times. I got the same kind of results, forming the same kind of pimples and blister rashes depending on the sizes of the birch flowers. If you get poisonous pimple blisters on your hands, the water could make your hands get a bad itch if you used water to wash your hands, and the blisters on your hands would spread all over your hands. My ears, lips, face, and whole body got a bad itch every time I came in from my outside yard; sometimes I got a lot of red rashes on my face. My lips and ears would have a bad itch; pale spots would appear on my knees and legs very distinctly, and most of the times I found that both my legs turned black when I stood up for a long time. When my lips would itch, I tried to use water to clean my face to get rid of the itch from my lips, but it did not go away. I had to take allergy medicine to get rid of the itch every day. I did not know the reason how I got the itch on my lips and body every time I passed the white birch trees, how my legs turned black, and how pale spots formed on my knees and legs. I tried to get the answers with the three most important words "what," "why," and "how." The environment made my lips and ears so itchy and led to the formation of pale spots on my knees and legs after I passed the white birch trees. I knew that the white birch trees contained a bad toxic betulinic acid, which was causing me to get burns on my skins and get a bad itch. But I did not know how they got into my system to make my lips and ears get a bad itch and led to the formation of pale spots on my knees and legs, even when I did not touch the birch trees and their leaves and flowers. I kept thinking and I used all kinds of techniques to dig out the answer to explain how and why they made my lips and ears get itchy right away after I passed the birch trees or I stayed inside my house. Finally I got the answers from the experiments that I tried, by using a perfume bottle and the concept of spraying perfume inside my house.

I used different perfume bottles to do the experiments at home, when I was very sick. I used a perfume bottle to spray perfume inside my family room to help myself get better when I was sick. After I sprayed perfume in the air in my family room, I smelled them and then I felt much better. I did the experiment by spraying one type of perfume on my left hand and I tried to smell it. When I put my left hand closer to my nose, I could smell the good scent of the perfume, and when I put my left hand away from my nose, I could still smell the scent of the perfume, but the scent was not that strong. I tried to use different types of perfume bottles to spray the perfume in the air in my family room. I could smell the scent of the different perfumes in my family room. So I figured out there must be some reason I could smell the scent of the perfume in different experiments. Then I figured out how the perfume scent from my body was transmitting to the air when I sprayed the perfume on my body; then the scent of the perfume in the air was transmitted to my nose, and this was the reason I could smell the scent of the perfume on my body. I also thought of how I could smell the scent of the perfume on my body if this perfume did not have any scent or was odorless. I figured out if my body did not have any odor, I could not smell any odor on my body; only if my body had an odor, then I could smell it. Then I figured out when I passed the people in supermarket, I could smell some of the people having a bad odor that made me dizzy and feel like throwing up. Then I figured out even though I did not have any odor on my body, I still could smell and feel the moisture; that meant my body was still spraying odorless moisture to the air and the moisture in the air was transmitting it to my nose; my senses told me my body did not contain any odor. This concept is similar to the concept that you can feel the heat of my body; if my body has heat, you can feel my body producing heat, and if my body is odorless, you will not smell any odor from my body. The same concept can apply to good, bad, or no odor of the plants, just like good, bad, or no odor of the human body. All these odors are from the chemical moistures that are sprayed out from my body. If my body moisture contains rose scent, the rose scent moisture from my body is transmitted to the air. Then from the air they are transmitted to my nose, and then my sense tells me I smell of rose scent. If there is another person standing next to me, the rose scent in the air is transmitted to that person's nose just like it is transmitted to my nose and the person standing next to me will smell the rose scent just like me. Even though all human bodies contain the same type of chemical fluid in their bodies, depending on the body heat and the reactions of the chemical fluids, they produce different kinds of odors depending on the level of the heat from their bodies. When the human body is heated up due to hot weather, the chemical fluid from the human body transforms into the moisture state; then the moisture from the human body is transmitted into the air. When you pass by a person with any odor, your nose comes in contact with the chemical moisture in the air of the person that you pass by. Your nose will breathe in the same type of chemical moisture from that person into your body system; then your senses will tell you that you smell the odor from this person. If this person does not have any odor, you will not smell anything, but you will still breathe in the same type of chemical moisture from this person through the air into your system. In particular, when you are in a crowd with so many people, you will feel warm, because of human bodies' heat against each other, making the air warm. When you pass by a person who is sick, your senses will tell you that person is having strong heat in his or her body, and you will feel the same kind of heat from that person and it will make you feel sick just like the sick person that you pass by. The chemical fluid from human bodies contains different PH data level of chemicals, producing different levels of heat inside your body.

We can use the same concept of human body's odor and heat that are produced inside the human body to apply on plants and trees. We can smell the scents from the plants and trees just like we can smell the scents from the human body. The different kinds of plants and trees have different kinds of chemical fluid with different kinds of odor. If the trees contain a good chemical fluid with good odor, no matter whether you smell their flowers, leaves, or the wood of their branches or trunks, your sense will tell you they contain a good smell with the same kind of odor. Some trees have a bad odor, and your sense will tell you these trees contain a type of chemical with bad odor. We can use the same concept to apply for the odorless trees, just like the trees with odors. Different types of trees contain different kinds of chemicals and different kinds of scents. No matter whether the trees contain good or bad chemicals with good or bad odor or are odorless, the chemical fluid from the trees is transmitted into the air by the hot weather. If the weather is hot, you will see the trees heating up, the chemical fluid and oil from the trees leaking out from their skins, and you can smell the odor from the trees if they have a scent. If the weather is cold, you can still smell their scent from the trees if they have a scent in the surrounding areas of these trees. Just like the scent from the trees, the chemical fluid from the tree's trunks, branches, leaves, and flowers transforms into moistures or the gas state, transmitting into the air all year round whether the weather is hot, warm, or cold. If the trees contain harmless chemical fluid with good odor, we can smell the good odor from the trees in the surrounding areas and they make us feel better. If the chemical fluid of the trees is a bad toxic chemical fluid, they will make us feel itchy, dizzy, and sick all year round. In particular, in the hot weather, you can feel the strong moisture and their odor if these trees contain a strong odor. Otherwise you cannot smell anything if these trees are odorless. If the weather is cold, the chemical fluid of the trees will be still in the surrounding environment, and you can still smell their mild odor or no odor in the surrounding areas of the trees. Even if the trees have no odor, you cannot presume that the surrounding environments are free of the chemical acids from the trees. If the trees that contain the toxic chemical acids grow in your areas, your areas will be surrounded with all these kinds of toxic chemical acids from the trees; they can be in solid, liquid, moisture, and gaseous state. The toxic chemical acids from the trees can burn your skin in any state and form pimples and redness rashes with or without blisters on your skin, depending on the strength of the chemical acids from the trees. If the type of chemical acids from the trees contain the ability of burning your external skin just by contact, then they have the same ability to burn your internal system when you breathe in these chemical acids from the air in the state of solid powder, liquid, moisture, or gas form. If you breathe in this type of toxic chemical acids in the state of moisture and gas from the air into your body, they will dissolve in your blood system and spread all over your body, burning your internal organs inside your body, which will make you have a bad itch on your lips and your body, and you will find pale spots forming on any portion of your body, knees, and legs and sometimes your legs may turn black. We can use the rose plant to describe as a good plant and white birch tree as a bad plant to make people understand the concept of how our body gets so itchy and how pale spots are formed on our bodies, making us get bad allergy and sickness by the toxic chemical fluid from the birch trees. The rose plant does not contain the type of chemical acid that can cause you any allergy or sickness, but they have good acid with good odor to make people feel good on smelling their good scent; they can even help sick people to get better when they smell the rose scent. The white birch tree is an odorless plant and has a white trunk and white branches. As they look pretty and seem like a good tree, the people never suspect that the white birch tree with a white trunk and white branches contains the type of toxic acid that can cause people to get a bad allergy and sickness.

After I got the bad blister rashes on both my hands, caused by the poisonous acid from the birch tree, it made me understand that the fluid from the bad blisters was just like the poisonous acid from the birch tree, which burned and spread all over my hands after the blisters broke, and the fluid from the blisters burned the nearby skin of my hands and also dissolved in my blood system, spreading inside my body system and damaging it. Because I breathed in the bad poisonous acids of birch trees from the air, the bad poisonous acid of birch trees burned and formed blisters and infection spread all over my body, showing pale spots and hives type of symptoms on the skin of my knees and legs. After I understood this concept, I started getting concerned and afraid of getting infections and cancers in my internal system, and I stopped working outside in my yard to protect myself. But I had so many plants growing outside my backyard that every day I had to force myself to go outside to water the plants in the morning. When I went outside to water the plants in the morning, I still felt that I breathed in more and more bad toxic chemical moisture and gases from my neighbor's big white birch tree, because a lot of pale spots and hives were still forming on my knees and legs, and sometimes both my feet would turn black when I stood up for long. Even though I tried to cut down all my cypress branches to open my backyard so as to clean up the bad air, I still could not stay long in my backyard. If I stayed long, pale spots and hives formed on my knees and legs, my lips, ears, and body got a bad itch, and sometimes I felt dizzy and very sick with my whole body itching.

There are other types of skin diseases that cause pale spots to be formed on human faces and bodies. We can distinguish its causes: On some people's faces, only one pale spot is formed. Some people have big or small pale spots formed on the back of their bodies. Some people have big pigment loss on their faces and bodies. The doctors believe the pigment loss on their faces and bodies is caused by the sun. I do not believe that, because most of the people who get pigment loss on their faces do not even stay under the sun before the pigment loss occurs on their faces. I believe the pigment loss from the people's faces or bodies is, most of the times, caused by the salty chemicals from their own sweat. Some people have big or small pale spots on the backs and these are mostly washed away by the salty fluid of the sweat; if the patients keep changing their clothing after they get sweaty and wet, they can make the pale spots on their back go away. Sometimes they can hot boiled eggs to rub on the pale spots until they disappear; the heat from the hot boiled eggs can kill the diseases from the pale spotty skin. I just shared the information with the readers about the techniques that I had learned from the elderly on how to get rid of the pale spotty skin diseases. I do not guarantee it will work for all the people in getting rid of all kinds of pale spotty skin diseases, but it will work for some pale spotty skin diseases in some people. Since the researchers have already found the type of chemicals in the human skin could change the human skin's color, I believe dermatologists can help these people to get rid of their pigment loss or pale spotty skin diseases on their faces and bodies. In my case, the pale spots on my knees and legs that showed very distinctly were caused by the burning of the toxic chemical acid from my neighbor's birch tree, which I breathed in from the air while I was working outside my yard. I got very sick every time I came back in from outside my yard. I took antibiotic pills to protect myself all the year round to prevent my allergies and sickness from getting worse.

The doctors and the researchers kept telling people that the allergies and sickness were caused by the pollens from the flowers of the weed plants, but they did not indicate in detail the type of pollens and which flowers, which weed plants, which portion of the flowers, leaves, and branches of the plants were causing the allergies and sickness. If they were unable to indicate the type of plants that produced bad pollens in the flowers or any portion of the plants, they should not keep telling people that the pollens from the flowers of the plants were the main source that caused people to get allergies and sickness. Instead of telling people about an uncertain source, the doctors and the researchers should search out more to find out about the plants' ingredients and their chemicals in the analytical laboratory; then they should test on animals' bodies to verify the true cause of allergies and sickness. The pollens, the flowers, and any portion of the plants and trees that contain bad toxic chemicals can cause the same kind of bad allergies and sickness all year round whether the people come in contact with them or breathe them in. The pollens, the flowers, and any portion of the good plants and trees that contain good chemicals can help people get healthier if they breathe them in all year round.

All the plants and trees have male and female flowers. Some have both male and female petals in the same flowers. On each male flower, they have a lot of active pollens; maybe a few inactive pollens will form in the male flowers. When the active pollens from the male flowers come in contact with the female flowers' petals, they form fruits with seeds on the female flowers. When I observed the fresh pollens on the male flowers in different plants and trees, the pollens were so tiny; some had round shape, some had egg shape, and some had long shape. The fresh tiny pollen contain tiny amount of fluid of tiny weight; it cannot blow too far away by the wind, but if the pollens, flowers, leaves, and broken branches of the plants and trees dry out, all the dried powder or broken pieces of dried flowers and leaves of these bad plants and trees, blown far away by the wind, could cause a lot of people to get bad allergies and sickness and could lead your skin to have big or small different sizes of red rashes with or without blisters on your face and your body, even if the people do not live closer to the areas that have a lot of bad allergic trees. Most of the allergies and sickness of the people develop depending on the seasons, and they get the allergies and sickness. If the community has a lot of bad allergic trees of the birch family, then the people in that community get the same kind of bad allergies and sickness all the year round. We can presume where all these allergies are from by studying the size of the external redness and spotty rashes on the people's faces and bodies.

While I was studying and researching the allergies and sickness in our community, I found most of the people, including my neighbor's teenage children's faces, were burned and approximately average size of ½ × ½ square inches of red spotty blister rashes formed on them. I met one of the elderlies in Pleasanton KPMC lobby; a spot on her face, near her ear, was covered with Band-Aid tape. I asked her what happened and she took out the Band-Aid and showed me the spot that had caused her to be very itchy, and she said when she checked up with the doctor, her doctor told her that that red itchy spot was skin cancer; if the itch did not go away on that spot, the doctor would have to burn that itchy spot. I asked her whether she knew how she had got the itch on that spot on her face, and she said she did not know how but the doctor had told her that it was caused by the sun when she asked the doctor. I told her I did not believe the itch on her face was caused by the sun. I told her that if human faces were burned by the sun, they would burn the big areas on the human faces that directly came in contact with the sun; it would not be just make one spotty area itch. Then I asked her whether she had a lot of birch trees in the community that she lived in. She said yes, she had a lot of white birch trees growing in the community that she lived in. I told her that I believed her itch was caused by the powder or the pieces of dried birch materials from the birch tree which burned her face to make her itch on that spot. I explained to her that if the itch on the spot was caused by the sun, then her whole face would lead to cancer because of the sunburn, because the same amount of sun heat would be distributed in her face. I told her about my left-side neighbor Linda's son, Kurt, who had also got scattered red spotty blister rashes on his face, of an average size of ½ × ½ square inches, after he cleaned the leaves and flowers on the right side of my bushes under my neighbor's white birch trees. My neighbor Linda's daughter got the same kind of scattered red spotty blister rashes just like her brother after she and her brother helped her father clean up their yard. She said this was terrible and that people should get rid of this type of bad trees in the community. I also talked to some of the elderlies that I had met in our community about the birch trees; when I asked them whether they had any white birch trees in their neighborhood, they said they did not have any. Then I asked them whether they had any skin cancer on their faces; they said no, they did not. Most of the elderlies who had birch trees in their neighborhood said they had skin cancer on their faces. I believed their itch spots on their faces were burned by the chemical fluid from the powder or the fiber pieces of the birch flowers and leaves. I suggested that the elderlies to beware of the birch trees; if they had any birch tree in their community, they should tell people to get rid of them as soon as possible. They shook their heads, smiles on their faces.

Most of the allergies and sickness are caused by toxic chemical fluid from the plants and trees that grow in the neighborhood. When people breathe in that toxic chemical fluid into their bodies, it makes them sick with different kinds of high fever virus sickness. When people get sick with high fever, depending on the strength of the chemical fluid in the air that they breathe into their body system, it burns and produces high fever inside their bodies, causing their bodies' temperatures to rise higher than the temperature of normal healthy people and making them very sick. The temperature of normal healthy people is in the range of 97–98.6°F. When people are sick, their body temperatures are varied; depending on the amount and strength of the toxic chemical moisture and gases in the air that they breathe into their body system, their internal organs get burned and their bodies burn with fever; the temperature range of the fever depends on the body heat produced and virus sickness occurring. The medical researchers have created and used different names to distinguish the different types of virus sicknesses. The chemical fluid in human bodies has different strengths and varied temperatures to transform into the moisture in their body and transmitting into the air, then transmitting to the person who breathes in this chemical moisture from the air. For example, a sick person named Jimmy had a high fever with a body temperature of 105 degrees and had a B kind of virus. The chemical compound X from the air, which made Jimmy very sick after he breathed it in and got burned, heated up his body system to 105 degrees or higher and cause virus B. If two persons named John and David went closer to Jimmy when Jimmy was sick and if John was not strong enough to resist the chemical compound X in the air, John would be sick and would get virus B just like Jimmy. But David did not get sick, because he was strong enough to resist virus B this time. Next time if David were to go near a sick person who was already sick with virus B just like Jimmy and if he did not have enough resistance, he would get sick just like Jimmy and John. Depending on David's body resistance, he will or will not get Virus B. Where did this chemical compound X come from and how did it reside in the air? The bad chemical compound X could be transmitted to the air either from the plants that have it or from the sick people who have already got Virus B. Even when you have recovered from the virus B sickness, no one can guarantee that you will not be sick again with virus B sickness if you do not have enough resistance to resist it. The doctors called the chemical compound X as virus B disease. This virus B sickness could get worse and transform into another state of sickness if these a bad chemical compound X, which would keep burning and creating bad infection inside your body; unfortunately, if the infection in your body got worse, kept spreading and damaging the tissues inside your body badly, and if the infection damaged the tissues of one of your internal organs inside your body, leading to cancer diseases, even the doctors and the medicines cannot help to get rid of the cancer disease from your body. Viruses are the primary state of sickness, and the cancer sickness is the secondary state of sickness. If the air contains a larger amount of the chemical compound X, it can cause secondary state of cancer sickness directly in people. This is the path how people get the different kinds of viruses and get sick by different bad chemicals either from plants or from sick people or from sick animals or livestock that transmit to the air. How can we get rid of the chemical compound X that causes virus B sickness? We cannot stay away from the environment that contains chemical compound X just by cleaning up our environment; we need to get rid of the chemical compound X by cutting down the trees and the plants that contain or producing it, and remove the factories that produce it. Then we can get rid of Virus B disease totally from our environment.

It took me years and years to study and figure out how the birch trees were making people get red pimple rashes with or without blisters, how the birch trees were making people get a bad itch on their lips, ears, and bodies, causing pale spots to be formed on people's faces, knees, and legs, and how the birch trees were making people get bad allergies and sickness all year round. The birch trees contain betulinic acid as mentioned in Chapter Three and they spray it from their trunks and branches all the year round. In summer, they spray the toxic chemical acid moisture and gases from their flowers, leaves, branches, and trunks when they were heated up in the hot weather. In fall, their flowers and leaves start to turn yellow and disintegrate from the tree and fall to the ground, and some of them dry out on the trees. In winter, most of the birch flowers dry out; some of them become rotten, either caused by the rain or the snow, and a big portion of the leftover dried birch flowers and leaves fall to the ground. In early spring, fresh new birch leaves grow; a few leftover rotten, dried birch flowers and leaves which are still on the trees disintegrate from the birch trees and fall to the ground. All these rotten dried birch flowers and dried leaves break into small pieces or get smashed into powder or small pieces of fiber by Mother Nature on the ground, and they blow all over the nearby neighborhood when the wind blows strongly. Another summer, fall, and winter pass by and in early spring, new small birch leaves grow and the leftover rotten dried flowers and leaves fall on the ground again; this way all the birch trees produce new branches, leaves, and flowers in their new lifecycle each new year. The white birch trees disintegrate their leaves and flowers in four seasons all year round. The old rotten dried flowers are crushed into powder or small pieces of fibers or chemical acid of the birch trees and their flowers and leaves heat up and vaporize in the hot weather and transform into a state of moisture or gases in the air. When the wind blows, all these toxic poisonous chemical moisture and gases spread all over the neighborhood and they get inside your house through the air ducts or screen windows if you open your window; these poisonous chemical moisture or gases inside your house can change into chemical crystal powder state when your house cools down at night and reaches the temperature that can transform them to poisonous chemical crystal state and then drop on uncovered food or any corners inside your house. A lot of tiny dried poisonous chemical powder can also blow inside your house when winds blow strongly through your windows if you keep the windows open;

some land on your uncovered food and some land in any corner of your house. If you eat that uncovered food, you will get bad burns and have a bad allergy inside your body and get very sick; if you come in contact with the poisonous chemical powder that blows inside your house, you would get burned and have a bad itch and rashes with or without blisters on any portion of your uncovered body, and if you breathe in all these bad poisonous chemical moistures or gases that have already got into your house, it could make you get a bad itch and become sick. All of this poisonous chemical crystal powder that already reside inside your house can transform back to poisonous chemical moisture or gaseous state if your house is heated up again, and if you breathe those in, you would get an itch, allergies, and become sick again. You cannot say you are safe even when you stay inside your house and that you will not get any allergy and sickness. If you have the bad poisonous allergic birch family trees in your areas or nearby areas, whether you are inside or outside your house, you will be repeatedly getting the allergies and sickness all year round, no matter how much you try to clean your house and your yard to avoid them all year round; your ears, lips, and body will be very itchy all year round, because all the poisonous chemicals from the birch tree can be changed into any form of solid, liquid, moisture, or gas state depending on the weather in your neighborhood. If you get rid of them from your environment by cutting down all these bad white birch trees, then your environment will be totally clean and you will be out of allergies and sickness, whether you are inside or outside your house.

You can use the following technique to perform an experiment on yourself to find out whether the plants or the trees can cause an allergy to you. First, you have to take fresh flowers or leaves from the plants or trees to rub and test on your skin directly; if you do not get any reaction right away, just let them stay on your skin for twenty-four hours and observe the reaction and the result. Maybe you will not get any reaction if you use young fresh flowers, because the strength of the chemicals in the fresh flowers depends on their sizes and their ages; the smaller the sizes of the young flowers, the lesser they will contain chemical strength. Second, you can use the powder or small pieces of the dried flowers of plants or trees to rub on your skin and observe the reactions and the results. In order to get the dried flowers of plants or trees, first you need to get fresh flowers or leaves from the plants or the trees; then clean them a couple of times in fresh water, store these flowers in a plastic bag or a container, and let them dry out themselves. After the flowers dry out in the plastic bag or the container, you can smash the dried flowers or leaves into powder and rub them on your skin a couple of times. After you apply the powder on your skin, if you get any reaction from the dried flower powder that makes you itch and cause pimples with or without blisters to be formed on your skin, it indicates that this type of plant or tree causes allergy to you. I used this technique to test white birch flowers on my skin, and I found out I got a bad itch and different sizes of blister rashes were formed on my hands. After I did the testing of the powder of birch flowers on my hands, I got very sick and my diabetic data range went up a lot higher than the required data range, because the betulinic acid from the birch trees was burning and damaging my internal system.

I watched a program on the Discovery Channel in which the researchers were talking about the river birch trees which were growing near a lake in California. The researchers said when they measured the PH data level of the water in the lake where river birch trees were growing nearby, it was 6.5; it was the same as the PH data level of the water of the city of Pleasanton that we were using, which was 6.5 as the chemist of the water department from the city of Pleasanton told me. The researchers mentioned that when they left live fishes in the lake where river birch trees were growing, they found all the fishes could not survive and died in this lake. I assumed in this case that even though they had the same PH data level of 6.5 in the water in two different places, they contained different kinds of chemicals in the water in these two different places. Because the river birch trees contained acid with a high carbon aromatic benzene ring, the chemicals of the discharging flowers and leaves from the river birch trees dissolved in the lake, causing the fishes to die in the lake.

When I watched the news on a Chinese television news station, I heard the reporter reporting that the people who lived in the northern part of China had raised over one thousand horses, but only over three hundred horses were left within a year. They said the people did not know the reason the horses were dying. While the reporter was reporting this news, I observed on the television the environment of the places where the people were raising the horses in the northern part of China, and I saw they had a lot of big white birch trees growing in the areas that they were raising the horses; all these horses must have died due to the bad allergic poisonous chemicals in the white birch trees in their neighborhood. I felt bad for all those people as they did not know the birch trees were the bad allergic trees that caused their horses to die.

I decided to talk to the people in my neighborhood to find out how much did they know about the allergies and sickness that were caused by the birch trees. I stopped at one of the houses, which had three big white birch trees on the side of their front yard next to my street. I went into this house and I knocked at the front door; the lady was holding a pair of gloves in her hands when she opened the front door. It seemed like the lady was working in her backyard, wearing the gloves. I asked her whether they had any problem with their white birch trees. She said no to me. Then I asked her how old were her white birch trees, and she said they were in her house since her family had bought and moved into that house fifteen years ago; her children had grown up in this house and they never had any problems with the birch trees. Then I asked her who took care of their lawn, and she said her husband took care of it; they had been just working in their backyard. I pointed my finger at her white birch trees' trunks and asked her whether she was aware that her white birch trunks were turning into black color, but she said she had not noticed it. Then I asked her whether she knew the birch trees could cause allergies and sickness, and she said no, she was not aware of it. Then I asked her whether she had got any itch. She said no to me, embarrassed. Then I asked her again if she had not got an itch, how come she had a big scratchy red area on her neck; she did not reply and just smiled at me in embarrassment. Then I suggested that she go inside her room after I left to check her neck in front of the mirror whether she had a scratchy area on her neck. Then she smiled at me in embarrassment again and asked me who I was. I told her I had been living on her neighboring street for more than so many decades. I was the first owner of my house. I would have liked her to come out to look at my neighbor's allergic white birch tree which was over twenty years old, the trunks of which were turning black. I told her those white birch trees were causing very bad allergies and sickness to us in our neighborhood and that my husband and my son had complained a lot about the allergies when they took care of the lawn in my yard. I had never complained of any allergy at the time when they were taking care of the lawn before, as I stayed inside my house most of the time. But after I took over the job to take care of my lawn, I started to complain about allergies and sickness just like my husband and my son. I wanted her to find out about the allergic birch trees and how the trees were causing the people to get bad allergies and sickness before it was too late. Then I asked for her permission to talk to her husband. She said no and refused to let me talk to her husband. Then she said she did not know that and she would find out herself. I advised her to go to Pleasanton Library to read my little book and check with the city of Pleasanton. Then I left and went home. After I came home that day, I realized that I should not be wasting my time going around the neighborhood to talk to the other housewives, because most of the housewives did not take care of their lawns and yards, so they could not tell you anything about the itch and the allergies from being outside in their lawns. The lady that I talked to did not even notice that she had a big red scratchy area on her neck; she responded to me as if she did not have any itch. Maybe she misunderstood the kind of itch that I had asked her about and made her smile at me in embarrassment.

When I talked to one of my friends about the allergies from the plants, she told me about her complaint regarding the odor from her neighbor's honeycomb plants. She said each time she went outside to her yard, she was very sick due to smelling the odor of the honeycomb plants in her neighbor's yard. Her neighbor refused to get rid of their honeycomb plants when she talked to her neighbor to request them to get rid of them. She said she had to take her neighbor to court to make her neighbor get rid of the honeycomb plants that made her very sick. I never heard that honeycomb plants could cause any allergy to mankind. Her body system must be changing for her not to be able to resist and accept the kind of odor from the honeycomb plants, making her very sick.

In late 1994, I found my body system was changing just like my friend that I mentioned above. I could not stand the odor of scallion when my sisters took me to a Chinese restaurant to eat noodle soup in Chinatown, New York. Usually I liked to eat scallion plants. I liked their smell very much. When I was in New York in late 1994, I could not tolerate the smell of scallions when the waiter put a plate of scallions in front of me. I pushed the scallion plate far away from me on the table. I did not know why I was getting so sensitive to the odor of scallion. I stopped eating scallions for a long time. I did not persuade anyone to get rid of scallion plants, because scallion was not an allergic plant. I understood that my body system was changing, which made me dislike the scallion odor. After a couple of years, when my body system was changing back to normal, I could smell and eat scallions again.

I talked to some of the dog owners during Lady Star's doctor visit in AECH about the birch trees that would make people get bad allergies and sickness; one of the dog owners shared his information about crabs that could cause bad allergy to people. He said when he was in a restaurant with his friend, his friend ordered a plate of hot crabs, and after the order arrived, his friend took one crab out from the plate and separated the crab's shell from the body; accidentally a drip of hot fluid from the crab dropped on his friend's hand. It formed a red spot, and he got a bad itch; he called it bad allergy. I explained to him that this was not an allergy symptom that I was talking about; this was only a minor burn by the hot fluid of the crab and the fluid from the fresh crab could not burn the external human skin. I told him crab's meat would cause bad allergy in some people only if the people ate crab meat and that the crab meat helped the infection to get worse inside the body. I explained to him again that the red spot his friend got was a burn by the hot fluid of the hot crab when he separated the shell from the crab's body. Then he shook his head and left the clinic.

Some people complained that the soaps caused them a bad allergy. The soaps that they were using were made of high carbon; these kinds of soaps had the ability to remove all the oil from the skin, making people have dry skin and get a bad itch. This kind of itch was an external minor itch. Once you apply lotion on your skin, the oil from the lotion restores the oil on your skin and this external itch goes away. The best soaps for people to use daily are the soaps that are made of low carbon hydroxide.

After I talked to a lot of the people in the neighborhood, I found out a lot of people misunderstood the meaning of "itch" and "allergy." They should not use these two words to describe in a state of nervousness or psychologically show their dislike to any person or any object. In this itch and allergy cases of the birch trees, I meant itch, scratches, burns form hives and pimples, redness, blisters, and rashes on human bodies because of bad toxic chemical substances from the birch trees; when those chemical substances come in contact with any part of the human faces and bodies, they make people get itchy, form hives and redness rashes with or without blisters either on the faces or on the bodies, and get very sick. Mostly the people who work in the lawns and yards are the victims of these kinds of bad allergies and sickness that are caused by the bad trees; they do not know where they get the diseases that make them very sick and die. No one suspects that the trees are one of the main sources of making people suffer with different kind of allergies and sickness and have bad infection with diseases in their bodies due to the bad chemical acid of the trees, making them very sick and die. The bad acid of the bad trees also causes people to get diabetes and eye diseases and go blind and infect the people's ears. Even though we all enjoy the beauty of the plants, the trees, and their flowers, unfortunately some of the plants and trees contain bad toxic chemical acid that makes people get bad allergies and sickness; they are the enemies of human beings, and we should not keep the bad toxic plants and trees in our environment. Once we get rid of all the bad toxic trees in our environment, the percentage of diabetic patients, patients with infectious ears, patients with eye diseases, and patients with bad allergies and sickness would reduce in our community.

When we first moved into this house, we believed when our neighbor told us that the white birch trees were good medicine trees. Siok believed him and he bought two paper birch trees and planted in our backyard. After a few years, Siok and Shaun were complaining a lot about the bad allergies in their bodies after they worked outside in the yard; they said they did not know what was in the air that made them itch badly and caused them a bad allergy. I found out the birch trees were the bad toxic allergic trees that were causing us bad allergies and sickness. I asked Shaun to cut down the two paper birch trees in our backyard after we found out the paper birch trees were the allergic trees. When I took over the job of cleaning our yard from my son Shaun, I found I got bad allergies from my neighbor's white birch trees. Charlene and I requested John Clark to get rid of his bad white birch tree, but he refused to get rid of it. I even gave him my doctor's letters to prove that the birch trees were causing allergy to me, but he refused to get rid of his birch tree; he said the people owed me money and they still had to pay me because of the deal that I had made with the city of Pleasanton to prove the birch trees were allergic trees. Then John Clark and his family moved out from my neighbor's house without cutting down his bad birch tree, and we had another new neighbor, Mr. Tom Fox, and his daughter, Jeanie, move in and living on my right-side neighbor's house. I went over to Mr. Fox to let them know he had to get rid of their bad white birch tree that was causing a bad allergy to me and to the people in our neighborhood. I told him our left-side neighbors on our street had complained a lot about the allergies that they were getting in their lawns and that they said they could not even lay their hands on their lawn, as their hands got a bad itch, which made them get bad allergies and sickness. When I told Cara that we should go to the court, she stopped me and she said she would talk to Mr. Fox. When she talked to Mr. Fox and his daughter Jeanie to cut down their bad birch tree, they ignored her. Because of my request, she kept calling Mr. Fox and his daughter Jeanie to ask them to act responsibly and cut down their bad white birch tree, but Mr. Fox kept avoiding responding to Cara. Finally Mr. Fox responded to Cara and told her that he did not want to deal with her and he would talk to my son, Shaun. He talked to my son Shaun, but Shaun did not tell me Mr. Fox had talked to him about his birch tree. When I talked to Mr. Fox to request him to cut down his birch tree, he told me Shaun had let him keep his birch tree. So I asked Shaun whether Mr. Fox had talked to him about his birch tree, Shaun said yes. I asked him why he had told Mr. Fox to keep his birch tree. Shaun said he had forgotten about our bad allergy from the birch tree and that he had mistakenly told Mr. Fox that he could keep his birch tree. Then Shaun said since we had Mr. Martin to clean and take care of our front yard, he thought that would help to prevent allergy from my neighbor's birch tree, just by cleaning up all the toxic discharge of flowers and leaves from the birch tree, but he was not aware that our allergies and sickness would not go away if my neighbor kept their white birch tree in our environment and he mistakenly told Mr. Fox to keep his white birch tree. I said no to Shaun. I showed him my doctor's letters from Dr. Ma and Dr. Young; both my doctors had indicated my bad allergies and sickness were from the birch tree. Then he realized he had forgotten about my allergies, and he said he would call Mr. Fox to inform him about my allergies and sickness from their white birch tree and would request him to cut down his bad birch tree on the my right side of my garage; then he suggested to me not to take Mr. Fox to the court. He and Cara kept calling Mr. Fox to cut down his bad white birch tree; they tried to explain to Mr. Fox that I had already got my doctors' letters, indicating that my allergies and sickness were from the white birch trees and that if we took them to court we just had to show my doctor's letters about my allergies from the birch trees and the court would order him to cut down his bad birch tree. They both requested him to solve this problem outside the court just by cutting down his white birch tree, instead of solving this problem in the court. But Mr. Fox has not responded to them till today. I told Shaun and Cara that Mr. Fox's right-side neighbor also had two big birch trees planted next to Mr.

Fox's house. My ex-neighbor John Clark and his family complained a lot about their right-side neighbor's birch trees; he said everyone in his family had been also getting bad allergies from their right-side neighbor's birch trees when they lived there. When I saw Mr. Fox's right-side neighbor remodeling their lawn and their house, I went over to the owners to talk to them, and I explained to them that the white birch trees were bad allergic birch trees. I suggested and requested to them to get rid of their two big bad allergic birch trees while they were remodeling their front yard lawn. They responded to my request, and they dug out and got rid of their two big white birch trees next to Mr. Fox's house. This helped prevent Mr. Fox and his family from getting bad allergies and sickness from their right-side neighbor's birch trees. I helped Mr. Fox ask their right-side neighbor to get rid of their bad allergic white birch trees, Mr. Fox should have responded to my request to cut down his bad allergic white birch tree to clean up the environment for all the people in the neighborhood. But unfortunately Mr. Fox ignored our requests. So I had to keep asking Shaun to keep calling Mr. Fox to inform him about removing his bad allergic birch tree. But we did not get any response from Mr. Fox yet.

On Thursday, May 15, 2014, my female dog Lady Star had a high fever and suddenly died at home. Sir Space and Lady Star were very healthy dogs; they did not have any disease and sickness, except that they had dry-eye problem in their eyes. On May 14, 2014, the weather was very nice outside. Lady Star and Sir Space liked to stay outside in my backyard, so I let them stay outside in my backyard more than three hours. As usual, I fed both of them chicken and rice for their dinner. I did not notice that Lady Star became very sick after she came back in from outside. On May 15, 2014, at six in the morning, I took Lady Star and Sir Space out to my backyard as usual, and at 9:00 a.m., I saw Lady Star opened her mouth and started breathing heavily; it seemed like she felt very hot, so I put a few drops of water inside her mouth. I fed her and Sir Space 1/3 of antibiotics as usual, and she felt better and she went to sleep on her bed. I woke both of them up at 12:00 p.m. to let them out into my yard. Then I fed both of them chicken and rice for their lunch and dinner at 12:00 p.m. and 4:00 p.m. as usual. After Lady Star ate her lunch at 12:00 p.m., I saw that she laid down on the floor and slept near the refrigerator. When I came out to take both of them out to my backyard at 4:00 p.m., I saw she was sleeping. I did not wake her up and I just let her sleep. I took Sir Space out to my backyard. Then when I came out from my study room at 9:00 p.m. to take both of them out to my backyard, Lady Star would not get up. I tried to wake her up, shaking her with my hand, but she did not move. I found she was dead, her mouth open. She must have breathed in a lot of the allergic birch acid that had caused her to get high fever and suddenly die, but Sir Space got better after I fed Sir Space antibiotics, but not Lady Star. I realized I had made a mistake in letting them stay outside in my backyard for more than three hours on May 14, 2014. I felt very upset at my neighbor that I could not do anything to make them cut down their white birch tree. I felt very upset to see Lady Star get sick with high fever and die; it was very hard for me to lose my baby dog Lady Star. When she was two years old, she got enough suffering when her left eye became blind because of the birch acid, and now she had got sick and died by breathing in the birch acid from the air only to get high fever. She was only eleven years and ten months old. This was very unfair to us; because of my neighbor's bad allergic birch tree, we had to suffer with allergies and sickness. I do not think this will be a good neighborhood if all the people do not get rid of their bad allergic birch trees. We all should be united in cleaning up our neighborhood to provide a healthy environment for all the people who live in our community. This is one of the biggest environmental disasters that the people do, by mistakenly planting the bad allergic birch family trees in a residential community.

Chapter Six

Environmental Disasters

I felt very upset to hear that we got all kinds of environmental disasters in the past decades created either by wild species, mankind, or by Mother Nature in our community, in our country, and all over the world. Since 2007, there have been so many wars and terror attacks created by mankind and different kinds of deadly virus diseases have been spreading all over the world. A lot of people from Mexico got the deadly swine flu sickness with high fever; over hundred thousand people died in Mexico because of swine flu sickness. The cause of this swine flu sickness was due to the drug war in the northern part of Mexico. Over thousands of drug smugglers got killed by the government in Mexico in 2007, but the Mexican government did not immediately clean up the dead bodies from the environment and left all the dead bodies above the ground in the hot weather; the heat from the hot weather caused all the dead bodies to rot and the bad chemical fluid from the dead bodies vaporized in the air in the form of moisture or gas state, spreading all over the nearby cities in Mexico. When the weather cooled down, the chemical moisture or gases from the dead bodies changed into the form of solid powder and dropped on all corners of the nearby cities in Mexico. When the people from nearby places or nearby cities breathed in or contacted these bad chemicals from the air or from the ground, they got the swine flu sickness. Then these sick people carried on the swine flu sickness to other people all over the world by traveling from one country to another in a short period of time.

A lot of people from Hong Kong got sick with the swine flu disease. The Chinese government was afraid that this sickness would spread all over China, so they tried to separate the sick people who got this swine flu sickness from the crowd, but the situation got worse and the swine flu sickness spread all over the world. The Hong Kong government kept all the travelers inside hotels and would not allow them to go out of the hotels until there was no sick person in the hotel, and then the government released the people from the hotel. The people who lived in Hong Kong had got SARS sickness and a lot of people had died many years ago. They had experienced SARS sickness; they were so afraid that the flu would spread all over Hong Kong and kill a lot of people again. We also had over hundred thousands of people getting the swine flu sickness and thousands of people including children were dying due to this swine flu sickness in our country. Research scientists have invented the swine flu shot and changed the name of swine flu sickness to H1N1 flu sickness, giving free shots to the people who most need them. Even though the people were getting the H1N1 flu shot, some of them were still dying after they got the flu shot. There were so many different kinds of flu sickness and HxNx, x=1, 2, 3 . . . level types of flu shot were created all over the world. Flu sickness is one of the biggest human disasters that has made a lot of people suffer from sickness and dying. The doctors can save the patients' lives that have some type of flu sickness, but the doctors can do nothing to save the patients' lives that have a different type of sickness. The only way we can do is to get rid of the bad materials or plants that cause the people to get sick and die.

We have been getting all kinds of big and small disasters in the past many decades due to climate change, for example, big fires in California and Colorado; heavy strong winds, tornados, hurricanes, heavy rains, and heavy flooding in America; volcano explosions in Hawaii and Iceland; tsunami flooding in the Indian Ocean and Pacific Ocean; big earthquakes in different countries like China, Taiwan, Haiti, and Chile; and strong cyclonic winds in Burma, Japan, Philippines, and Taiwan. These kinds of environmental disasters have destroyed a lot of buildings and houses, causing a lot of people to die. Because of all these disasters, the leaders from all over the world had gathered together for a meeting in Copenhagen, Denmark, during the first two weeks of December 2009 to discuss about the climate changes and the shortage of water that might occur all over the world.

On January 13, 2010, I heard on the television that Haiti got several earthquakes of 5, 5.6, and 7 magnitudes on different days, and most of the buildings in Port-au-Prince city in Haiti collapsed and were destroyed. A lot of people were trapped under the building rubble. People from all over the world went to Haiti to rescue the people that were trapped underneath the rubble to save their lives. I heard on the television that more than two hundred thousand people from Haiti were dead in this earthquake. On January 19, 2010, I heard on television there was another earthquake 6.1 in magnitude in Haiti. The aftermath of the Haiti earthquake really made me upset; all the people in Haiti did not aggressively go out and hunt for their own food. They just stayed underneath the trees, and they waited to get help from the people of other countries to come and rescue them. It seemed like the people in Haiti did not know how to organize to overcome the disaster problems and move forward to take care of their own lives. One of the television reporters in Haiti was blaming Mother Nature, saying that she had buried people buried underneath the rubble, and another media reported that the people of Haiti would die if they did not get any water or food in time after the earthquake. I did not understand how the people would die when there was a big ocean near Haiti; they could use the water in the nearby ocean temporarily as drinking water when they were dealing with this kind of disaster. Where did the people of Haiti get water to drink before the earthquakes? How did they survive before the earthquakes? The people of Haiti were acting just like people without knowledge who relied on the people of other countries to get water and food. The Haiti government did not even come forward to save their own people's lives when this disaster happened. The Haiti government should have organized the people of Haiti to take care of their own people. They could have got food and water from the nearby cities to feed the people from the disaster areas, or they could have asked all the people in the disaster areas to move to nearby towns or cities to get water and food. The countries from all over the world should have been prepared to guide their people to learn to take care of their own people when they had this kind of disasters in their own country. Anyway, we took the lead in asking the Americans to donate money to Red Cross to help all Haiti earthquake victims.

On February 27, 2010, I heard the news on television that Chile had got an 8.8 magnitude earthquake in the city and tsunami on the beach. Most of the buildings were damaged in the city. Luckily, only around hundred people died in this earthquake. On March 2, 2010, and March

5, 2010, Taiwan got 6.5 magnitude earthquakes on both days, but no building collapsed and no one was hurt. On April 18, 2014, Central and Southern Mexico got 7.2 magnitude earthquake. Chile got over 7 magnitude of earthquake in April 2014; luckily no one died. California was also getting many earthquakes of different magnitudes, but luckily we got very little damage. But we had bad flooding disasters caused by heavy storms and rains, which destroyed a lot of buildings and houses all over the United States.

Since we have been getting so many kinds of environmental disasters caused by Mother Nature in our country and all over the world, we need to know how the earth, the sun, the moon, and the stars were made in the space and how science is playing an important role in our daily lives along with the objects in the space. We can research and use the best techniques to prevent all kind of disasters that might happen to us in the future if we know the cause of disasters. All the objects created by Mother Nature are related to each other to protect the environment and to prevent sickness for mankind due to environmental disasters. I had been working and researching in my backyard for so many decades, by digging the ground so many feet deep; planting, removing, and researching the plants; and observing the environment; this made me understand the reason the earth become so violent and was causing so many disasters to destroy all the properties by Mother Nature in our country and in other countries all over the world.

Mother Nature created sun, moon, stars, Mars, the earth, and many other objects in round shape to turn slowly in space to create morning, noon, evening, and night on the earth and let the earth alternately in a day get heat from the sun at daytime and coolness from the moon, the stars, and many other icy cube balls from space in the nighttime. When the sun, the moon, the earth, and other objects turn, they create winds to circulate the hot and the cold air in the sky and in the space. The winds blow in the range of five to ten miles per hour every day when the earth spins regularly. If the heat from the sun creates great pressure of air in space, strong winds form; it depends on the pressure of the air. It produces strong winds with stronger ranges. The acceleration ranges of the wind depend on the pressures of the air. Sometimes the acceleration of the wind is 60 miles per hour; sometimes it is 80 miles per hour, depending on the pressure of the winds. The liquid or the water from the ground vaporizes when they get strong heat from the sun. The liquid shoots up from the ground if the ground is heated up by the sun; some of the liquids vaporize into moisture or gas state in the air. Because the pressure of the cool air above the ground is stronger than the pressure of the hot moisture air that shoots up from the hot ground, the winds and the pressure of the surrounding cool air push the hot moisture air, which shoots up from the ground and twists, forming small twister winds. The surrounding cool air or moisture air above the ground cools down the nearby extremely hot moisture air that shoots up from the ground, slowly forming clouds. The pressure of the cold air above the ground is stronger than the pressure of the moisture air that shoots up from the ground and pushes the clouds, twisting and forming small twister clouds; then repeatedly the cool air from the surroundings cools down the nearby shot-up hot moisture air, slowly forming clouds and becoming a larger twister cloud. The nearby cool air and their pressure of the air forces the twister cloud to turn and move rapidly with the top spinning concept; the moisture from the surrounding areas makes the twister clouds become larger and stronger, turning strongly and moving rapidly. When they move to a certain distance, where there is warmer air, the strong twister clouds slowly melt and disappear. The small or big twister storms are formed depending on the pressure and the moisture that shoots up from the ground and the outer pressure from the nearby surrounding cool air. It is described in the *Britannica Encyclopedia* that when funnel-shaped clouds with strong winds move with a velocity of over twenty miles per hour they become strong tornado storms, and if the strong clouds with strong winds move with a velocity over seventy miles an hour, they become a hurricane storm. Mostly the strong twister storms were found in the Midwest United States in winter and early spring. The strong twister storms has destroyed so many cities in the Midwest United States in the past decade and led to big environmental disasters for the people who lived there. A sandstorm is created when the surface of the desert is too dry and hot; the heat from the desert heats up the underground wet sand while the liquid or the water from the underground desert vaporizes and become gases and moisture, shooting up into the air from the ground with great pressure and forming strong winds and strong storms. Then they push up the dry sand from the surface of the deserts and blow the dry sand all over the places. We saw big sandstorms in Arizona.

Mother Nature created the earth with mankind, livestock, animals, ocean species, plants, trees, chemicals, underground hollows, tunnels, clays, sands, stones, metals, soils, and many other things. Mother Nature created the sun to give light and heat to warm up the earth. Mother Nature created the moon, Mars, stars, orbitals, and other objects with ice in space to cool down and protect the earth from the heat of the sun. Mother Nature created moisture, clouds, rains, air, and the winds in the sky in space to circulate in the environment, to recycle the water, and to protect human beings from the heat and the hot air caused by the sun. Otherwise the earth would be destroyed by the heat of the sun, the whole planets would get burned, and the people, livestock, animals, plants, and trees would get different kinds of diseases and sickness from the heat waves. Scientists are searching the cause of disasters to create and design different kinds of fans, electric fans, air-conditioners, refrigerators, and buildings with roofs to cool down the heat waves from the sun and protect the people from getting sick.

One of the bridges that was built centuries ago in Minnesota collapsed due the heat waves of the sun; luckily, no commuter died in this incident. The hot waves of the sun heated up the cement concrete and the metal bars holding the cement concrete due to it being the hottest temperature on the day the Minneapolis bridge collapsed; the metal that held the bridge became soft due to the heat; it slid and bent down slowly due to the weight of the cement concrete and a part of the bridge collapsed. The Twin Towers of the World Trade Center were solidly built. The collisions of the airplanes with the tall Twin Towers in New York caused big explosions and heated up the buildings, due to which the metals holding them reached the melting point and the Twin Towers bent and collapsed. Because the metals became soft and due to the weight of the cement concrete, the Twin Towers collapsed all the way to the ground floor. These terror attacks became the biggest horrible disaster in the history of the United States of America.

We have water and chemical substances underground. When the heat waves of the sun heats up the chemical substances to the boiling point under the ground day by day, then if the hot liquid substance is water, the water becomes extremely hot and boils up, and the extremely hot water starts flowing out from the underground streams through the soft wet clay to the above ground due to the pressure of the hot water. We find this kind of hot water streams in southern parts of California. If these liquid substances from underground the mountains are explosive kind of chemicals, then if these chemicals are heated up by the heat waves from the sun day by day, they become extremely hot, causing big explosions under the ground of the mountains, pushing up the clay, the rocks, the hot burning liquid chemical substances, and gases from underground the mountains and the hot burning liquid chemical substances flow out from the undergrounds. These hot burning liquid substances from underground the mountains form lime and carbonate stones due to the cold air, after they flow out from the underground. The scientists call these explosive mountains as volcanoes. There are many volcanic mountains in California, Hawaii, Japan, Iceland, and many other countries.

When the volcanic mountain causes strong explosion due to the heat waves of the sun, the clay, the rocks, the hot burning liquid chemical substances, and gases from underground the mountain flow out with enormous pressure due to the explosion and create strong winds. The pressure from the explosion of the volcanic mountain is so strong that they push the strong winds to further distance. When the volcanic mountain in Iceland was exploding, it created strong winds due to the pressure of the explosion and pushed the strong winds all the way to India; these strong winds destroyed a lot of old houses in the poor community, causing the biggest disaster in India. The explosion from the volcanic mountain would not stop until all of the chemical fluid from the underground burned out; the heat from the active volcanic mountain could cause the explosion in the nearby volcanic mountains to continuously carry on to another nearby volcanic mountain, then to another nearby volcanic mountain in another country. The volcanic mountains in the North Pole and Europe were inactive before, because heavy snow covered them up. When the snow and the cool air in the surrounding areas are cleared out by the climate change, the volcanic mountains get direct heat waves from the sun, making the volcanic mountain active again.

When the weather is extremely hot, the heat waves from the sun heat up the liquid chemical substances in the ground and vaporize as moisture and gases to the airs, causing the ground to dry out; sometimes the water from the rivers and the oceans dry out due to the heat waves of the sun and cause shortage of water. The moisture and gases from the liquid chemical substances in the air float as high as possible into the sky and into the space, depending on the atomic weights of the chemical substances and their densities. When they reach above the sky, because of the coolness of the space and the densities of the liquid chemical substances, they form clouds in the sky. These clouds become heavy and come back down to the sky and lead to rains by heat waves of the sun, and they come back down to the earth; otherwise they float in space as icy cube stones; since the icy cube stones are very sticky, sometimes they form big icy cube stones or icy balls in space. If they get heat waves from the sun, sometimes the big icy cube stones or icy balls get back to the moisture state and become clouds; these clouds slowly form big clouds. Sometimes these clouds melt and become rain and come back down to the earth. Sometimes there are some icy chemical stones in space that cause collisions by the reactions of the chemicals and form explosions in the sky accompanied by explosive noises, creating electric lights and thunderstorms in the sky.

The strong storms are created by the pressure and volume of the clouds in the sky; the pressure of the strong storms create strong winds, causing flood disasters in the cities that are located in the path of the strong storms that pass by. There are many underground hollows and underground tunnels created either by Mother Nature or mankind in the earth. The underground hollows and tunnels are held up above by hard clay and small and big stones. When it rains, depending on the volume of the rain that falls from the sky, depending on the times and the depth of the sopping in the grounds, which makes the soil and the clay in the underground become wet and soft, if the hard clay in the underground becomes wet and soft all the way to the top of the underground hollows and tunnels, then the soft wet clay sinks down and forms land and muck, which slide into the underground hollows and tunnels. It forms sinkholes in that areas; depending on the number of cars and houses in that areas, the cars and the houses are buried inside the sinkholes. These kinds of sinkholes are found in California and Florida. If there are small or big stones on top of these soft wet clay, when the land and the muck slide into the underground hollows and tunnels, the small or big stones fall on the surface; depending on the depth of the land and muck sliding areas and the accelerated speeds of the heavy weight of the stones that drop in the underground, they open up the grounds; then they expand the opening of the grounds to so many hundred miles and form small and big earthquakes on the earth. If this kind of land and muck sliding happens underneath the oceans, it forms earthquakes underneath the oceans. If there are heavy stones above the surfaces of the land and muck underneath the oceans, then land and muck slide underneath the oceans; if the heavy stones from the surface drop on the surface of the oceans, depending on the land and muck sliding accelerated speed and the weight of heavy stones that drop on the surface underneath the oceans, it causes the underwater to rise and form strong and enormous tsunami waves, causing big flooding on the shores and washing away all the objects including human beings from the shores and from the island. When tsunamis were formed in the Indian Ocean, causing big flooding on the shores, the strong waves washed away everything from the shores of Indonesia and Sri Lanka, killing over hundred thousands of people. The military of United States took the lead in rescuing the tsunami victims in Indonesia and Sri Lanka.

If there are cliffs near the rivers or oceans, the clay and the soil under the cliffs soak in excess of water and become soft. The soft clay and the soft soil at the edges of the cliffs cannot stay strong and form land and muck sliding on the cliffs, washing away all the objects from the cliffs. If there are heavy rains, the water from the heavy rains cause the land and the hard clay in the underground to become soft; if there are trees, the roots of the trees grow and push down into the underground. If there are underground hollows or underground tunnels, the roots grow all the way down to the top of the hollows and tunnels; then the hard clay becomes wet and soft if they get excess of water, causing underground land and muck sliding and forming earthquakes in the ground underneath. We can prevent this kind of disaster by not letting the trees grow so big and not letting the big trees' roots grow so deep all the way down to the underground hollows and tunnels. There was an underground landslide with a 7 magnitude earthquake in the Qinghai province in China in April 2010. When the miners were trapped inside the mines, they had to use the skin of the tree roots as food to survive inside the underground mines. If we let the trees grow so big, this will also cause big disasters.

We had so many forest fires in the United States, especially in California, in the past many decades. The forest fires were either created by Mother Nature or by human error. The forest fires heated up our environment, causing the air to become extremely hot; the hot air cleared out the clouds from the sky. Then we got the direct heat waves from the sun, which heated up our environment and made it extremely hot, and the water in the ground, the rivers, and the oceans vaporized and formed more hot air in the sky, and the hot air in the sky spread to the nearby cities, states, and countries by strong winds. For example, the strong winds from the southern part of Pacific Ocean in America blew in and pushed the cool air from the southern parts of America to the middle parts of America. The hot air from the middle parts of America was pushed to spread to the northern parts of the countries. Because the extreme hot air was spreading, it caused the snow from the mountains to melt in the northern part of the countries. All the snow from the mountains broke down piece by piece and fell into the oceans in Alaska and the northern part of the countries. The hot vaporizing air cleared out the clouds from the sky and formed drought in the areas that had no rains. These are the reasons we have water-shortage problems in the nearby areas, especially in California.

I was very upset at NASA scientists when I heard television reporters announcing that NASA scientists had arranged to bomb the moon in the month of November 2009, to find whether there was any water underneath the moon; they also announced that NASA scientists had already built a bomb to get ready to bomb the moon. After a few days, I heard television reporters announced that they would show live on televisions how they were going to bomb the moon. Then I saw on television how NASA was bombing the moon, and a lot of white materials shot out from the moon. NASA scientists announced that it would take a couple of weeks to review the white materials that shot out from the moon. I was getting very annoyed when I saw the situation on the section of the moon that they were bombing. I saw that the section of the moon that they had bombed was already very deep; some areas formed sharp and bumpy edges and the corners of that section's shapes looked just like an ice cube melting down, just like when an ice cube is chopped with a knife, leaving this kind of bumpy shape to it. If the readers are interested to find out why the moon had this kind of shape with bumpy edges, they can use a big ice cube to test them at home. I did not know how long NASA scientists had been bombing the moon; they had already damaged the moon to leave it with this kind of bad shapes with bumpy edges. If they kept bombing the moon, they would destroy the whole moon and make it disappear from the space.

NASA had sent out many space shuttles with many astronauts to land on the moon so many decades ago; most of the time, they brought back materials from the moon when they came back. If they have done the analysis of those materials that they brought back from the moon, they should know what kind of materials was inside there; they should find out whether the materials that they brought back from the moon have any disease or not. NASA scientists also sent up the scraper machine with a space shuttle to the moon to find out what was underneath the moon. The scraper machine scraped and cleaned the top black dirt layer of the moon and found a white layer of materials underneath the dirt layer on the moon. Then the scraper machine scraped the white layer of the materials, kept them in a container, and brought it back to the earth. If they sent the container with the materials that NASA brought back from the moon to the laboratory to analyze what kind of materials was inside the container, they would know what kind of substances was inside the container; if they know the kind of substances in the container, then they have already got the answer what is underneath the moon. We do not need to keep bombing and destroying the moon. Finally, I decided to stop NASA scientists from continuing their research on the moon.

On Monday, November 9, 2009, I called Sirena to suggest that NASA should stop bombing the moon again and suggested leaving the moon alone and let Mother Nature take care of the moon. After I stopped NASA scientists from continuing bombing the moon, they asked the White House whether they should continue their research on the moon. I did not say anything and waited for the White House to respond to them. After a week, they said they would continue their mission of research on the moon. In the third week of November, every night I could not sleep. I tried to figure out how to stop NASA scientists from continuing bombing the moon. I was thinking what the white materials were that shot out from the moon after NASA bombed the moon, which we saw on television. Then I figured out the white materials that shot out from the moon were melted by the heat that was produced by the bombing and disappeared; we can tell those white materials from the moon were nothing but white ice pieces. I called Sirena again to send out messages to NASA scientists to let them know that the white materials that came out from the moon were nothing but small pieces of ice that had melted after NASA scientists bombed the moon. Then I asked Sirena to suggest that NASA scientists should study the sun instead of interrupting the moon.

NASA scientists have been researching the space for so many decades; they had listed in detail all the objects that they brought back from the moon. If they studied that list of objects from the moon, they would get the answers how moon was made. NASA had sent out so many space shuttles and astronauts to space before to research the materials and objects that were floating in space. When those objects in space dropped onto the surfaces that were closer to the earth, the gravity of the earth pulled them down to the earth; then those objects would fall on to the ground of the earth. NASA did announce so many decades ago a big object had fallen from space onto the ground and a tremendous loud noise on the ground in Siberia was heard. They tried to find the place where the big object had fallen on the ground. They found the place was in Siberia, but they could not find any object on the ground except they found that the place was left with a deep, round, big football-field-sized shape on the ground when the big heavy object from space fell on that ground. They did not know what kind of object fell on the ground, as it had disappeared after it hit the ground. We all could use our human brains to predict what kind of big object would have disappeared after it hit the ground; this big object would be nothing but a big icy cube ball. Only an icy cube ball has the ability to melt and disappear. Now we all know that the fallen big object was a big icy cube ball, as it melted and disappeared after it hit the ground. I continuously heard NASA scientists announce and release the information on television that a lot of big and small black stones were falling from space on to the earth. They had to use missiles to shoot and destroy the big black stones that were falling on to the earth and crack them into small pieces. All these small pieces of black stones had fallen onto the earth and had disappeared. I did not understand why NASA scientists did not search and find out where all those small pieces of stones were after they used a missile to crack down the big stones that fell on the earth. If they did, they would find out the answer as to what kind of materials they were. According to the information released from NASA scientists about all the stones falling from the space, we can predict that they all were nothing but icy cube balls, covered with polluted black or brown dirt. We can make the assumption from the white materials that came out from the moon when NASA bombed it and all sizes of the stones falling from space that are described above that Mother Nature created the moon with the combination of water and chemical liquid in the shape of a big icy ball and all the big and small stars are small icy cubes, and any other objects in space are icy balls or icy cubes, coated with chemical substances or dirt soil in the cold space.

The gravity at the center of the earth is holding all the materials and the objects including mankind and the different kinds of species on the earth. We need to be aware of the gravity of the earth. If the earth has less gravity, then the earth cannot hold the objects on the earth; if the gravity of the earth is very strong, the possibility of pulling down the objects from the sky and space is higher. If the gravity of the earth has enough strength to pull down tremendous big objects like the moon and Mars from space and drop on to the earth, a big object like the sun would burn all the objects of the earth if the sun fell on to the earth and the coolness from the moon would freeze all the objects of the earth if the moon fell on to the earth. If the sun or the moon fell on to the earth with great force, it could break the earth into many pieces. The aftermath of these incidents would be that small broken pieces of the earth would be left; if the small broken pieces of the earth do not have gravity, they would not hold any mankind, any species, and any object. The mankind, the species, and the objects on the earth would be floating in space, and all the mankind and the species would not survive. If all the broken pieces of the earth have gravity, all the small earths would hold all the mankind, the species, and the objects on their surfaces of the smaller earths in space; they would become the mankind and the species of that smaller earth. If we assign the different smaller earths with different names, we could call the people of the smaller earths just like we name a country America and call the people of America Americans. We can use the same concept to name all the smaller earths and name all the mankind and the species on the smaller earths. But it is not a good idea to let the original earth break apart; we need and we should protect the earth either by not making the gravity of the earth get stronger or we need NASA scientists to keep an eye on the space to destroy with a missile all the falling big and small objects from space to protect and safeguard our earth.

On Thursday, February 11, 2010, I was very happy and relieved after I heard NASA scientists announce on television that they were going to study the sun instead of the moon and would stop interrupting the moon. Then NASA scientists moved their cameras to the sun to show the pictures of the sun on television. After I saw the huge red sun on television, I tried to figure out how the sun was made. I had heard before that General Electric Company was making diamonds from carbon material, using very high-temperature (over thousand degrees Fahrenheit) compressor oven to compress and heat up the carbon material to make diamonds. I predicted the sun must be a huge round-shaped diamond, because only diamonds could withstand tremendous high heat. Mother Nature created the sun as a huge diamond fire ball to produce light, heat up the space, and light up the whole universe. The sun produces clean air by burning down all the chemicals in the space. The mankind and plants on the earth are getting light and heat from the sun and the oxygen from the clean air. The mankind, the species, and all the plants are using oxygen from the air to survive. Mankind blows out carbon dioxide and carbon monoxide from their lungs into the air. Carbon dioxide, some carbon monoxide, and their relative chemical gases in the leaves and the trunks of the plants are sprayed out into the air at night. Sometimes you will find fluid or sticky oil in their leaves, branches, and trunks when the weather is very hot. Different kinds of plants have different kinds of chemicals that produce different kinds of colors and odors. The fluid, the moisture, and the gases that come out from their flowers, leaves, branches, and trunks must be their original color when they contact with light and heat. If all these different colored moisture and gases from the plants reside in one corner section outside in the yard, then this corner section is heated up by the sun. When I sprayed this heated-up corner section with water, I saw most of the time white smoking gases coming out from the ground. I saw a few times a rainbow of three to four different colors above the ground, which was related to the flowers' color of the plants when I sprayed water in this corner section. The relative chemical moisture and gases escape from the plants in the daytime when they are heated up by the sun; depending on the atomic weight of the chemical gases, they float up above the ground and go up to the sky or to the space as high as they can from the earth. Once the chemical gases are above the sky, they become icy chemical stones, floating in space. The sun is turning slowly in space and when it comes in contact with those icy chemical stones and nearby surrounding chemical gases and oils that moving in big fires flash out from the sun. The sun burns all the chemical gases and oils from the space and forms dirt soil, which floats in space. This dirt soil lands on the surface of the moon, the orbiters, and many objects in space. When the astronauts first landed on the moon many decades ago, we saw a lot of deep round shapes on the moon's surface from the pictures that the astronauts took; those deep round shapes on the moon were formed by the collision of other big and small icy chemical stones on the moon.

The sun, the moon, the earth, and other orbiters are spinning in space; the earth is rotating around the sun, and the moon is rotating around the earth to form day and night. When the earth is rotating around the sun, the sun burns all the surrounding chemicals and cleans up the space. The sun keeps burning and cleaning the chemicals in space in every corner that comes in contact with it, producing clean air. If the sun dies down, the whole space will become very dark and cold; the space will fill up with all these chemicals and sticky oil from the earth, which will get thicker and thicker; the chemical fluid in space will form bigger icy chemical stones and they will float in space. The dying sun does not have any heat to burn the chemicals and the icy chemical stones in space; the dying sun cannot produce any pressure to push away all the huge Mars, orbiters, and the icy chemical stones in space when they move closer to each other. It will cause a big collision and break them apart; all the big or small pieces of the sun, Mars, orbiters, and the icy chemical stones will floating up in space. Some of them will float down a distance so that the gravity of the earth can pull them down to the earth. The space will start getting cooler and cooler without the heat of the sun, and the cold air from the space will push down to the earth and make the earth very cool. All of the water on the surface of the lakes, rivers, and oceans will form hard ice. Because the cool air keeps pushing down from the space, making the earth become cooler and cooler, the coolness of the water in the lakes, the rivers, and the oceans will spread down to the deeper underground oceans and form hard ice and all different kinds of fishes and species in the lakes, the rivers, and the oceans will freeze to death. Even though the human beings can use their wisdom to produce light and heat to survive, in the long term, the liquid and fluid in the human bodies will be frozen by the coolness from the space. All the plants will be frozen and will die with no human beings producing heat and food in a very cold environment; all the different kinds of species from the planet cannot survive without any food. Finally, the whole earth will be filled with nothing but dead bodies of mankind, the different kind of species including animals, livestock, fishes, insects, the dead plants, and trees above the ground and underneath the frozen lakes, the frozen rivers, and the frozen oceans. This kind of worst-case scenario and environmental disaster will happen to us if we do not protect the sun, the moon, or any objects in the space. We need to protect them by not letting any objects get into collisions and protect them from breaking and disappearing. We need to protect the sun, the moon, the orbiters and many other objects in the space to balance the environment of the earth and the beauty of the space. Mother Nature has filled up the sky with neon or blue color as the base in the space; when the sun rises and the sun sets, we see the most beautiful colors like red, green, yellow, and purple up in the sky and sometimes we see a colored rainbow and sometimes we see double-colored rainbows up in the sky in daytime. Depending on the reflection of the sunlight from the sun, we can see from the earth the shining lights of the moon and the stars on a cool night create the beauty of the night, giving out encouragement and enjoyment to mankind on the earth.

I have spent time in studying the environments of different places and have used my scientific theoretical concepts to compare and make the above assumptions of the creation of the planet by Mother Nature and how they are protecting the mankind from space. I tried to give out the worst-case scenario to point out the kind of environmental disasters that could happen to the planet if NASA scientists keep interrupting to bomb and destroy the moon and the sun, making them disappear in space, and what kind of the worst disasters that could impact the people who live on the earth if the moon and the sun are destroyed. The people must be prepared not to let any kind of environmental disasters happen to the earth; we need to find the causes of the disasters and the techniques to protect the earth before the disasters happen. We can protect environmental disasters of human creation if we know their causes. We can use human wisdom to create and design technologies to take precaution in avoiding the disasters to protect our environments. For example, by manufacturing medicines to help the sick people get better, designing good machines to be used to build all good materials to protect mankind from the weather disasters, planting good trees to provide good shade so as to prevent sickness from heat, getting rid of bad plants that contain bad chemical substances, preventing the factories from producing bad chemicals in the neighborhoods, we can prevent allergies and sickness in the environment. All these factors can help save lives and save the earth by preventing environmental disasters.

Environmental chemical substances disasters are created not only by Mother Nature but also by the mankind with the worst violation, destroying the communities and the countries in the whole world. There are basic human disciplines that we learn when we are young to become a disciplined and good-hearted people to take part in serving or getting involved in the community. Every adult is a role model for the young generation; we should let all of this young generation learn from those adults to carry on their generations to be good-hearted and disciplined people just like the adults they have learned it from. We can prevent human disasters in our environment if all the human beings apply the human discipline with dignity, responsibility, fairness, respect, and mutual understanding. The three most important bad characteristics given below can lead to the worst human disasters. These are:

1: Anger/Temper
2: Greed/Possession
3: Jealousy

We can learn to control the above three bad characteristics by meditating and not letting the worst human disasters happen in our lives. If we do not learn to control the three bad characteristics that are described above, we will extend to have five bad action behaviors with or without any intention, which are described as follows:

1: Accusing or attacking others without any reason
2: Lying to others without any reason
3: Stealing or forcing and taking away other people's belongings or property
4: Destroying others or breaking apart others' family
5: Killing or murdering

There are three types of human environmental disasters that are created by mankind as described as follows:

1: Family disaster
2: Religious disaster
3: Community and territory disaster

1: Family disaster
The family will create the worst family disaster if the family members, including the husband and wife and the children, lack in love, trust, respect, mutual care, and understanding with each other. If

any of the family members including parents and the children have the three bad characteristics from the above, if the family members listen to outsiders who come in with bad intentions, and if the family members do not take good care of the family budget and welfare, it will lead the family into big arguments and ugly treatments with each other, and they will use force to attack each other, making the family members become very violent in their daily life.

The family members should push away all the bad behaviors and bad attitudes that could lead and destroy the family to the worst family disaster. If the family members know how to simplify their lives with understanding, they all can live together happily.

2: Religious disaster

There are many kinds of religions in this world. All the people of different religions and churches can live in peace and harmony in the community together if the religious leaders and their followers from different temples and churches give respect to each other and follow the good rules and regulations that are set for the people to follow, if the religious leaders and their followers from different temples and churches do not use their wrong ideas and concepts to manipulate and mislead the people in the wrong direction, and if the religious leaders and their followers from different temples and churches do not use politics to fight for the expansion of their territory in the community. The expansion of the religious territory fights of different temples and churches would lead to the worst religious disasters in the whole world.

3: Community and territory disaster

If the people in the community have the three bad characteristics described above, the people in the neighborhood can never have good relationship among the people in the community. They would create all kinds of arguments without any agreement, and they would never take any responsibility, having disrespectful manners and no fairness in solving any problem for the people in the community. The people from the community would be attacking, fighting, murdering, and making the community not peaceful and very unsafe. This kind of situation would lead to the worst community and territory disaster and would force the people in the community to become terrorists, terrifying the communities. These kinds of outrageous fights would never end if we do not stop the people by pointing out their unacceptable concepts and ideas to fight for their civil rights and their human rights.

We can protect our community from all kind of disasters if we can avoid family fights, religious fights, and community and territory fights, reasonably treating each other with understanding and respect. Unfortunately, there are so many kinds of violations happening all over the world. We have all kinds of criminals, murder cases, civil rights movement fights, and wars on terrorism being fought in our country and all over the world.

One of the most dangerous characteristics that ruin the people's lives in our country is their anger/temper. If the people do not have any anger or temper in their lives, they can live peacefully with harmony and fairness wherever they are; whoever the people they meet, they would give consideration to others with respect. But most of the people never learn to control their anger; they get so angry when they meet people who refuse to listen to them or people who do not want to cooperate with them or fight back at them, so they get into big arguments, and then they have the intention of using force or their guns to shoot and kill others. If one of the person dies from a gun wound, they both have to pay a high cost for their lives; one has to stay in jail for the rest of his life under the rules of law because he has killed someone, and the other, who died of the gun wounded, also pays a high cost for his life by arguing and fighting back with the other. The people in the real world are never aware of the kind of costs that they have to pay when they fight and argue with each other. No one takes the time to point out the conclusion of how the anger, the fights, and the killing would make people spend the rest of their lives in jail under the rules of law. If they know ahead what would happen in the aftermath of fighting and killing, they would learn to control their anger. They will also learn that it is not worth it for them to argue and fight for something which is not important. All the people should learn the use "give and take" concept, working and sharing in the community together with respect for each other. We should train to control ourselves not to use the five bad action behaviors that were described above; we can gain respect in our communities if we use our good manners and good behaviors to treat other people with sincerity and fairness. There have been a lot of murder trial cases in this country; all these can be prevented if they all learn to control their anger/temper, try to use "forgive and forget" attitude, and ignore all the unpleasant problems and walk away.

For example, see the NFL football player Aaron Hernandez murder trial case in Boston, Massachusetts, and Michael Dunn/Jordan Davis loud music murder trial case in Florida.

Greed/possession and jealousy are bad characteristics that can ruin people's lives. We can simplify our lives and live happily with our family in this world if we are satisfied with the amount of money that we earn. We do not need to be greedy and be possessive type of people to live in this world. We do not need to be jealous of others if other people can live better than us. We can use our own ability to try our best to work hard to improve our lives to live better in this world. We do not need to get upset and angry at ourselves if we cannot make the kind of money like any other rich people. If we have satisfaction in our lives, we will live happily forever with our own family and friends. We should always wish the best for others whether they are rich or poor. But unfortunately, a lot of people are greedy and possessive; they want to get rich, and they use all kind of techniques to make money to get rich. Some people use illegal techniques to cheat on other people to make big money, some people get into illegal drug businesses and fight for their territory, some of them get killed, and some of them get arrested under the rule of law and have to spend the rest of their lives in jail. Some of the people borrow money from the banks or from their friends to buy stocks in the stock market, and when they lose all their money in the stock market, they cannot afford to pay back to the banks or to the person from whom they took the money to play stocks. Whatever the techniques all these people used to cheat on other people's money, when they get caught and arrested, they have to spend the rest of their lives in jail. So many decades ago, a group of people from Hong Kong wanted to get rich; they liked to gamble. They hoped they could make big money in the stock market, and they put their lives in jeopardy by borrowing money from the banks to buy stocks in stock markets. Unfortunately, they lost all their money from the stocks; even after they sold all their stocks and their properties, there was not enough money to pay back their debts. When the banks started pushing them very hard to pay back their debts, they had nowhere to borrow the money to pay back the debts and they had to end their lives by jumping down from tall buildings. This was one of the biggest human disasters in the history of Hong Kong.

The civil rights movement fight is also one of the human disaster fights that are happening in our country. The black people are using the civil rights movement to fight for their rights, for their equality, attacking the white people without giving any consideration of the white people's civil rights. They force other people to accept them; if other people do not want to accept them or if they do not get their way, they gather on the street to strike, and they use outrageous action in destroying business buildings, breaking all buildings' glasses, and going inside the stores to loot and destroy the stores. They created a lot of criminals and murder cases when they were around in the neighborhoods. They looted, they robbed, and they killed the people on the streets and in the stores, terrifying the community and making the people scared of them. The Burmese lady Daw Khin Win Min got killed by the black guy Barry White in San Francisco for San Francisco jewelry slayings was tied to price dispute. The Burmese people wanted The National Association for the Advancement of Colored People (NAACP) and President Obama to take accountability for Daw Khin Win Min murder case in San Francisco just like they took accountability for Trayvon Martin murder case in Florida. There were so many other similar criminals and murder cases in this country. The killers were using criminal acts to destroy the family in the neighborhood, making the victim's family and the children living in a very difficult situation grow up.

The black leaders from NAACP and other civil rights black organizations should get up and stop their black people from looting, from robbing, from killing, and from murdering people. They should realize it is not an appropriate action for them to keep striking and using the "racist" word to attack and take the advantage of other people if they don't get their way. They should take the lead in guiding their own black people and not creating all kinds of criminals and murdering conflicts in the neighborhoods; they should teach and guide their own people to give out consideration and respect to other people's civil rights and human rights. They should guide their own people for taking their own responsibility to work hard for themselves and live peacefully in the community. If we all treat each other with dignity and fairness with no criminals and murderous conflicts, we can avoid all kinds of human environmental disasters in our neighborhoods and in our communities.

There were conflicts among black and white teenagers in this country. The black teenagers, jealous of the white teenagers, complained and kept attacking them for no reason; they thought all the white teenagers got everything from their parents and the society. They wanted to get all the things that all the white teenagers got, and they got upset when they saw all the white teenagers were earning their own money, buying their own things, and helping their family and friends in the community. They never realized the parents of those white teenagers never spoiled their children and they helped them out at home to stay out of trouble and trained them to go out and work; they trained them to earn money with their own labor and to save money for their college. They should find out the truth about the life of the white teenagers instead of hating them. This kind of jealousy fights among black and white teenagers should not be happening in this country. If we all train our children to be polite, respectful persons, having good manners in treating other young and old people, and give respect to others, they would be out of trouble and gain respect from other people. I would like to see all the children of all races to be trained properly to grow up to be very useful men and women and serve their communities with great pride by guiding their own people and their next generations to continue the circle of human lives in their own neighborhood and communities.

We have had so many terror attacks in our country since September 11, 2001, when Al-Qaeda terrorists brought down the Twin Towers of the World Trade Center in New York, attacked the Pentagon military building in Washington DC, and blew up the American Airlines in Pennsylvania. Over three thousand people were killed on September 11, 2001, by terror attacks; this unexpected terror attack made all American people very upset. President George W. Bush had to declare war on Afghanistan in 2001 after September 11, 2001, terror attacks and war on Iraq in 2003. We managed to win these two wars, but many thousands of soldiers got killed and many hundred thousands of soldiers were wounded after these two wars. We kept getting terror attacks in this country without solving any conflict between the Middle East and America. We had Boston marathon bombing in Massachusetts in 2013, which left so many people hurt, who had to go through the terrible tragedies for the rest of their lives. We also have had terror attacks in the American embassy compound in Benghazi, Libya, by the terrorists who killed Ambassador Chris Stevens and three other Navy SEALs on September 11, 2012, and destroyed the American embassy compound in Benghazi, Libya; these terror attacks would never have happened and Ambassador Chris Stevens and three other Navy SEALs would not have died, if they had given full protection to the American embassy compound in Benghazi, Libya. These were the biggest terrible disasters when the terrorists came in to attack and destroy our people and our country.

The aftermath of the wars made all the people exhausted and restless. The people from the war-zone countries became homeless; they had nowhere to go but had to live in refugee camps to avoid further disasters. The sight in the aftermath of wars was terrible; there were a lot of damaged houses and buildings with a lot of rubble, bricks, and broken pieces of concrete all over the neighborhood. There were also burned-down wrecked cars and military tanks on the streets of the cities and in suburban areas from war-zone countries. It was really heartbreaking to see all of mankind was left with bad human and environmental disasters in the war-zone countries.

We can stop all these human and environmental disasters by setting unifying rules and regulations to make all the countries agree and follow the rules and regulations that we set for all the countries to follow. We can find the best solutions and technologies to protect our environment to save our lives and our planets. We can create and design new things to decorate and brush the earth to be the most shining, colorful planet just like the rainbows. We should show our appreciation and respect for the creator of the world and let our generations to carry on our most beautiful and shining earth and the space. We should live and die with dignity in this world with no guilt.

I have taken the lead in advising, making decisions, rescuing, and saving lives in government and public affairs in United States since 1987 till date. I took the lead in fundraising to help the disaster victims from the countries all over the world, which are briefly described as follows:

- I advised using aircrafts to attack Iraq in the 1991 Iraq War, and we managed to capture all Iraqi soldiers and won the war, but we did not remove Iraq President Saddam Hussein and his administration.
- I advised using the profit from US Postal Service's fund to offset the Medicare shortage fund in 1993.
- I advised US military to use war-fighting airplanes to attack the mountains, underground tunnels, and caves and captured all Al-Qaeda and Taliban terrorist ground compact troops in Afghanistan and won the Afghanistan War in 2001.

- In the aftermath of the Afghanistan war, I funded billions of dollar worth of foods and medicines to help the people of Afghanistan.
- I gave advice that resulted in winning the second Iraq War again and successfully removed Iraq President Saddam Hussein and his administration from power in Iraq in March 2003. Then we got involved in many other countries in Europe, Middle East, Asia, and South America.
- In the aftermath of Afghanistan War and Iraq War, most of the big banks, auto industries, and many other big companies in our country collapsed and became bankrupt. I worked with US treasurer Henry Paulson to bail out the banks, auto industries, and some other big companies. I had all the banks and big companies, including auto industries, pay back all the bailed-out money with interest to the federal government.
- I advised buying back the companies of the United States that were sold to other countries and the bankrupt companies to keep jobs back in the United States.
- I bought out Afghanistan, Sudan, and all African countries with the agreement of the people of these countries.
- I funded millions of dollars to Palestinian people in Gaza when they had shortage of medicines in Palestine country.
- I advised saving all the sick babies from dying in the Somalia crisis.
- I advised saving all the women in Africa, Congo, Sudan, and Somalia, who were the victims that were attacked and raped by the rebels in their own countries, cleaning up of the territories and environments that were occupied by the rebels, and rebuilding the countries for them.
- I advised and helped in getting rid of diseases and sickness in Africa to improve their healthy living standard.
- I advised US military and US National Guards for rescuing and saving all the Katrina tornado disaster victims that were tracking in flooding zones inside New Orleans city and nearby cities when Katrina tornado touched down in Louisiana in 2005.
- I fundraised to help Haiti earthquake disaster victims and the Haiti people for taking care of over ten thousand of their own babies.

- I advised to look for the terrorist leader Osama Bin Laden and managed to find him and captured him in Pakistan.
- I advised and fundraised to help the disaster victims in Indonesia, India, Sri Lanka, Pakistan, Tibet, Philippines, and Burma when tsunami, earthquakes, and typhoons touched down in these countries.
- I suggested searching and creating new technology to save all the coal miners after only one out of thirteen coal miners survived in the deadly mine explosion disaster inside the Sago coal mine in West Virginia on January 5, 2006.
- I advised rebuilding all the old bridges after I explained the cause for the Minneapolis bridge collapse in Minnesota in August 2007.
- I guided Louisiana state governor Bobby Jindal and the people from New Orleans to clean up BP oil rig explosion in Gulf of Mexico in April 2010 and guided US Army Corp Engineers to seal the BP underground broken oil rig pipeline in Gulf of Mexico in Louisiana.
- I advised US Army Corp Engineers to fix and dig the Mississippi river deeper and reconstruct the Mississippi river during its flooding in 2011.
- I advised protecting and saving the most populated areas of Mississippi and Louisiana during flooding disasters in 2011.
- I advised fundraising to help New Jersey and New York Hurricane Sandy disaster's victims in 2012 and guiding to organize the electricians from different states to reinstall the electricity for the cities in New Jersey and New York after Hurricane Sandy touched down and destroyed the New Jersey and New York power grids. Governor Robert McConnell from West Virginia State also sent out the electricians from his state to help reinstall the electricity in New Jersey and New York.
- I informed Caltrans engineers to fix the Bay Bridge commuting problem after forty accidents happened on the new Bay Bridge.
- I informed UC Berkeley to open the fishing game research term to raise small salmons and other fishes from fish eggs, and raise them in the lakes and rivers to be used as human food.
- I advised setting a policy to use marijuana as a medical prescription drug to help the people who are in need and to

reduce the marijuana users in California and in any other states of America.

- I helped science research team to research diseases in Bay Area.
- I advised using Western dances to exercise and fix human bodies.
- I changed the healthcare insurance law to allow children up to twenty-three years old cover their health care under their parents' healthcare insurances.
- And many more…

After we went through so many terrible environmental disasters that happened in our country and all over the world, we are fortunate we can still stabilize our economy by managing all the disasters to fix and get things done in a short period of time. Throughout the year, I helped manage this country from home, and at the same time I searched to find the proof that the birch trees are the allergic trees, causing people to get allergies and sickness in our neighborhood and our communities in this country. The people were mistakenly planting the "Betulaceae" biological family type of birch family trees in the residential neighborhoods all over the United States. This type of plants contain betulinic acid that causes substantial burning on human bodies and form bad redness, pimples, blisters, rashes, and hives on people's skins and bodies, causing people's lips, ears, and bodies to get a bad itch and leading to pale spots being formed on human faces and bodies and causing people to get diabetes, ear infections, eye diseases, and bad allergies and sickness. I urge the people to get rid of all the "Betulaceae" biological family type of birch trees from the neighborhoods to clean up the environment in the community. I also urge people to get rid of the worst poisonous plants such as poison ivy, poison oak, and poison sumac from the communities if there are any. Only when we get rid of all these bad poisonous plants can we live healthily with no allergies and sickness in our neighborhoods and communities.

There are still many plants all over the world ingredients and chemicals of which we do not know. Some plants are touchable and eatable plants, some plants are touchable but are not eatable plants, and some plants are untouchable and uneatable plants. Only when we know the ingredients and the type of chemicals in the plants can we make an assumption which plants are good plants so that we can keep them in our environment and which plants are bad plants so that we can get rid of them from our environment. Only when we know the ingredients and the chemicals in the plants can we protect our environments, and we can also use the good chemicals in the good plants to produce good medicines to save human lives. I would like to open an analytical laboratory to get more research scientists to search and analyze the ingredients and chemicals in the plants about which we do not know yet. I would like to make this project possible in the near future with the help of all the readers and friends.

Abbreviations

ACS: American Cancer Society
AECH: Animal Eye Care Hospital
ASTCC: Advanced Sports Therapy Chiropractic Center
BMC: Beth Medical Center
EKG: Electro Kinetic Cardiogram
HAH: Hopyard Animal Hospital
KPMC: Kaiser Permanente Medical Center
NAACP: National Association for the Advancement of Colored People
NASA: National Aeronautics and Space Administration
NYCPRC: New York C. P. Radiology Center
NYEAEINCMC: New York Eye and Ear Infirmary National Care Medical Center
PG&E: Pacific Gas and Electric
VCMC: Valley Care Medical Center
WTC: World Trade Center

Index

Hernandez, Aaron, 351
Hilton, Lois, 42
Hoey, Beverly, 40
Hoffman, Linsi and Tim, 49
Holly, 34, 38, 49, 98, 144, 146, 148, 181, 199, 220, 283
Houck, Cara, ix, 165–66, 169–72, 174–75, 180, 182, 185, 189, 191–92, 329
Hughes, Howard, 1

J

Jennifer, B. C., 193, 195–96, 198, 204–8, 211–12, 218–21, 224, 254–57, 260–61, 279–84, 288–89, 291–92, 296, 298, 300
Jindal, Bobby, 356
Joan (nurse), 59, 224, 255–58, 264
Jodi R., 208

K

Kedziora, Joan. A., 59
Kevin S. W., 169, 177
Khaw, Daisy, 2, 232
Kim (office secretary), 89, 93

L

Lakshmi M., 296
Landsittel, Jody, 81
Larry S., 85–86, 304
Lee, Mr. Judge, 82, 84, 87
Lins, C. J., 8–9, 11–13, 81
Liskin, Howard, 22, 24–25, 33–34, 45
Lundgren, Ada, ix, 4–7, 11, 21, 72
Lydia, 202

M

Ma Aye Myint, ix, 8, 135–36, 145–47, 149, 151–55, 157, 161–62, 164–66, 168–69, 192–93, 199, 292, 298–99, 329
Makjcour, Kurt, 66
Makjcour, Linda, 65
Martin, Trayvon, 352
Martin (gardener), 267, 329, 352
McConnell, Robert, 356
McQueeney, Robert, 120
Michael C., 72, 75–77
Muniza M., 145

N

NASA, 341–44, 347
Noel E. T., 9, 11, 13
Nonette (medical assistant), 91
Novel, Bob, 22, 50
Nugent, Catherine, 4–5, 7, 40–41, 50, 72, 79–80, 83, 85–86, 90, 92, 242

P

Patty S., 105
Paulson, Henry, 355
Perko, Renee, ix, 35, 54–55, 67, 88–89, 92–93, 113, 130–31, 133, 151–52, 166, 171, 182, 191, 284
Peterson, Marlene, ix, 80–81, 114, 130, 132, 152, 156, 159, 162–66, 175, 180–81, 185, 189–92, 284, 302
Pono V. A., 30–32, 34–38